Infant, Child and Adolescent Nutrition

Infant, Child and Adolescent Nutrition

A Practical Handbook

Second Edition

Judy More BSc. RD, RNutr

Paediatric Dietitian
Child-nutrition.co.uk Ltd
Honorary Lecturer,
School of Health Professions,
University of Plymouth, Plymouth, UK

CRC Press
Taylor & Francis Group
Boca Raton London New York

CRC Press is an imprint of the
Taylor & Francis Group, an **informa** business

First edition published 2013
by CRC Press
6000 Broken Sound Parkway NW, Suite 300, Boca Raton, FL 33487-2742

and by CRC Press
2 Park Square, Milton Park, Abingdon, Oxon, OX14 4RN

CRC Press is an imprint of Taylor & Francis Group, LLC

Library of Congress Cataloging-in-Publication Data

ISBN: 978-0-367-55455-2 (pbk)
ISBN: 978-0-367-55456-9 (hbk)
ISBN: 978-1-003-09365-7 (ebk)

Typeset in Minion Pro
by MPS Limited, Dehradun

Contents

Preface vii
Author Bio viii

Section 1 Nutritional requirements and healthy eating

1 **Nutritional requirements** 3
2 **Principles of a balanced nutritious diet for children over 1 year** 17
3 **Social and cultural influences on food choices** 33

Section 2 Assessment of growth and nutritional intake

4 **Measuring and assessing growth** 49
5 **Assessing nutritional intake** 61

Section 3 Prenatal nutrition

6 **Preconception and fertility** 75
7 **Pregnancy** 81

Section 4 Infants: 0-12 months

8 **Milk feeding** 99
9 **Complementary feeding** 121
10 **Common feeding problems in infancy** 137
11 **Preterm infants** 147

Section 5 Preschool children: 1-4 years

12 **Preschool children 1–4 years** 161
13 **Common nutritional problems in preschool children** 177
14 **Feeding preschool children in childcare settings** 187

Section 6 School-age children

15 **Primary school-age children 5–11 years** 195
16 **Nutrition for adolescents** 205

Section 7 Nutrition for chronic conditions

17 **Food hypersensitivity – food allergies and intolerances** 219

18 **Childhood obesity** 233

19 **Nutrition for children with chronic diseases and syndromes** 245

Appendix 1: Function and Food Sources of Nutrients 267

Appendix 2: Growth Charts 273

Appendix 3: BMI and Waist Circumference Charts 283

Glossary 289

Index 293

Preface

From conception through to adolescence, nutritional intake and status affect the health and wellbeing of children during their childhood and on into their adult years. Myths and confusion surrounding the topic of nutrition for children can compromise the health of some children. To combat this, evidence-based information has been compiled in this book to provide a comprehensive guide to the theory behind nutrition from preconception to adolescence.

In this second edition, I have reviewed and updated the evidence where science and practice have recently advanced – examples of some such areas covered are the importance of iodine in preganancy and for children's brain development, changes in food allergy prevention and treatment, recommendations on complementary feeding in infancy and revised recommendations on UK vitamin D supplements. The discussion on understanding and managing fussy faddy eating in toddlers has been expanded.

Putting the theory into practice is a challenge that requires an understanding of how children's feeding skills develop, how children learn to like foods, how their attitudes to eating food change with age and why families and children choose the foods and drinks that they purchase and consume. These topics are explored in this text to help parents, careers, caterers, health advisors and educators manage mealtime behaviour and provide suitable nutritious meals and snacks for children.

Health professionals working with children – be they paediatricians, general practitioners, nurses, health visitors, social workers, nursery nurses, school nurses, practice nurses, breast feeding counsellors, allied health professionals or dietitians – can use this text to find reliable nutritional information to pass on to parents and children. It is an essential reference for them and for students in all medical and social care courses.

Judy More

Author Bio

Judy More is a Registered Dietitian and a Registered Nutritionist specialising in children's nutrition. She is a past chairman of the Paediatric Group of the British Dietetic Association. Her current interests are in public health and after setting up her company Child-nutrition.co.uk Ltd., she is a consultant to government departments and several infant formula and children's food companies. She teaches at several UK universities, writes books and nutrition articles for professional and consumer publications, develops resources, gives media interviews and advises nurseries, schools and private patients. She has developed and published evidence-based portion sizes for children of different ages. As an expert member on the Infant and Toddler Forum, www.infantandtoddlerforum.org, she was lead author for their resources and publications. She edited the nutrition section of the e-learning Child Health Programme for the Royal College of Paediatrics and Child Health, which is a government sponsored programme to support professionals working with under-fives.

Section 1

Nutritional requirements and healthy eating

1 **Nutritional Requirements**

2 **Principles of a Balanced Nutritious Diet for Children Over 1 Year**

3 **Social and Cultural Influences on Food Choices**

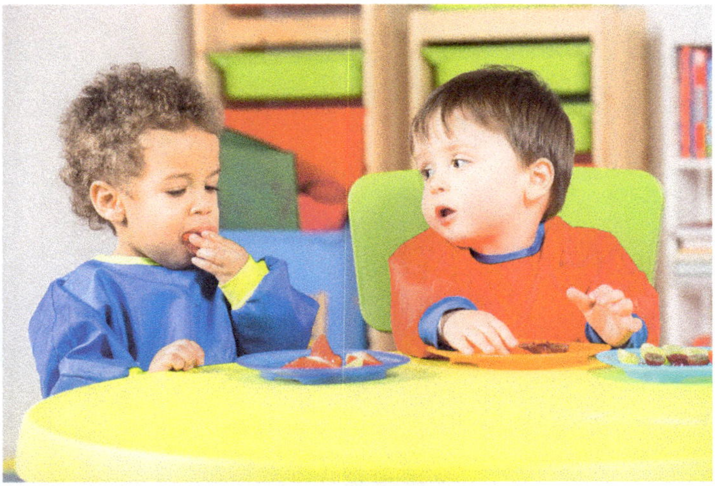

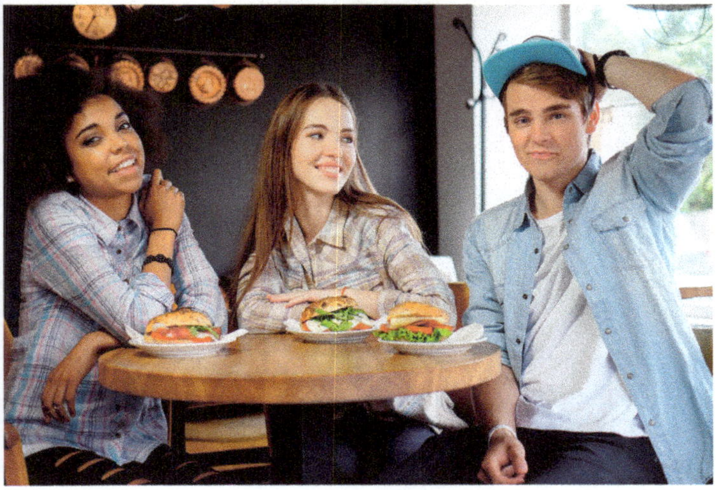

1

Nutritional requirements

Summary

- Nutritional requirements increase as children grow and are theoretically defined for different age groups of children.
- Reference Nutrient Intakes (RNIs) are used to define the average daily amount of protein and each essential micronutrient that different age groups of children need.
- Energy requirements depend on weight and activity and are theoretically defined by Estimated Average Requirements (EARs) for each age group.
- There are no set fluid requirements for children over 1 year of age as the kidney functions well and can cope with varying amounts of fluid intake; however, dehydration should be avoided by offering 6–8 drinks per day.
- Different nutrients have different functions in the body and a combination of all the nutrients is required to maintain health and sustain growth and development.

Food and drinks provide water, energy and nutrients that are required for growth, development, health and a strong immune system to fight infection. When a diet is balanced and nutritious, it provides adequate amounts of water, energy and all the nutrients.

In general, energy and nutrient requirements increase with age as children grow, but to support rapid rates of growth in infancy, there are some exceptions: daily calcium, iron and phosphorus requirements are higher in infancy than in the following 3 years.

Water

Water makes up about 75 per cent of a newborn infant's body weight and about 70 per cent of that of a toddler. Throughout childhood, this percentage slowly decreases to about 60 per cent of an adolescent. Infants and young children have a larger skin area in relation to their size than older children and can dehydrate very quickly, and, so, need regular fluid intakes throughout the day.

Infant milk feeds are about 90 per cent water and a young infant's water intake can come entirely from milk feeds. Once solid food is introduced, some water will be obtained from food as well as drinks. Older children obtain about 60 per cent of their water intake from food and the remaining 40 per cent is from drinks. The kidneys can cope well with small or large intakes of fluid from around 4–6 months of age so there are no set fluid intakes but as a guide:

Daily average fluid requirements for infants and children advised by Dietetic Department Great Ormond Street Hospital for Children NHS Trust 2018 are:

- 0–6 months: 150 mls/kg body weight;
- 7–12 months: 120 mls/kg body weight;

Table 1.1 Estimated Average Requirement (EAR) for energy for children in the United Kingdom (Scientific Advisory Committee on Nutrition 2011)

Age	Estimated Average Requirement for energy				
		Kilocalories/day		Megajoules/day	
	Kilocalories/kg/day	Males	Females	Males	Females
1–2 months*	96 (120)	526 (598)	478 (550)	2.2 (2.5)	2.0 (2.3)
3–4 months*	96	574 (622)	526 (598)	2.4 (2.6)	2.2 (2.5)
5–6 months*	72 (96)	598 (646)	550 (622)	2.5 (2.7)	2.3 (2.6)
7–12 months*	72	694 (742)	646 (670)	2.9 (3.1)	2.7 (2.8)
1 year		765	717	3.2	3.0
2 years		1004	932	4.2	3.9
3 years		1171	1076	4.9	4.5
4 years		1386	1291	5.8	5.4
5 years		1482	1362	6.2	5.7
6 years		1577	1482	6.6	6.2
7 years		1649	1530	6.9	6.4
8 years		1745	1625	7.3	6.8
9 years		1840	1721	7.7	7.2
10 years		2032	1936	8.5	8.1
11 years		2127	2032	8.9	8.5
12 years		2247	2103	9.4	8.8
13 years		2414	2223	10.1	9.3
14 years		2629	2342	11.0	9.8
15 years		2820	2390	11.8	10.0
16 years		2964	2414	12.4	10.1
17 years		3083	2462	12.9	10.3
18 years		3155	2462	13.2	10.3

* Figures are for breastfed infants 1–12 months. Where figures vary for formula-fed infants, they are given in brackets.

1 megajoule = 1000 kilojoules (kJ)

- Children over 10 kg: 100 mls/kg for first 10 kg, +50 mls/kg for next 10 kg, + 20 mls/kg thereafter – up to about 2.5 L/day maximum.

Energy

Energy requirements in children must provide for (Wiskin et al. 2011):

- basal metabolic rate, which is around 60–70 per cent of energy expenditure;
- physical activity, which varies considerably and can be up to 30–40 per cent of energy expenditure;
- growth – the energy required varies throughout childhood as the rate of growth changes, as described in Chapter 4.

Throughout childhood, energy requirements increase as weight increases and individual requirements vary specifically with activity levels and growth rate. Estimated average energy requirements for children devised by the UK Scientific Advisory Committee on Nutrition (SACN) are listed in Table 1.1. Inadequate energy intakes will reduce weight gain and if intakes are very low, growth and development can slow down. An excess energy intake will be stored on the child's body as excess fat, causing overweight or obesity.

Energy intake is from foods and drinks, and is measured in either kilojoules (kJ) or kilocalories (kcal); 1 kcal = 4.18 kJ. Energy is derived from the protein, fat, carbohydrate and alcohol in the foods. Differing amounts of energy are provided by each gram of these substances, as shown in the following text:

Protein	4 kcal/g (17 kJ/g)
Fat	9 kcal/g (37 kJ/g)
Carbohydrate (excluding fibre)	3.75 kcal/g (16 kJ/g)
Fibre	2 kcal/g (8.4 kJ/g)
Alcohol	7 kcal/g (29 kJ/g)

In a balanced diet for children over 5 years of age, the energy from each component is around (Scientific Advisory Committee on Nutrition 2015, Scientific Advisory Committee on Nutrition 2019):

Protein	15 per cent
Fat	35 per cent
Carbohydrate	50 per cent

For infants, these percentages change as the diet changes from milk only, providing 8 per cent of energy from protein, 47 per cent from fat and 45 per cent from carbohydrate towards the figures above as their milk intake decreases as food intake increases.

Nutrients

Nutrients can be classified into two groups:

- macronutrients: protein, fat and carbohydrate;
- micronutrients: vitamins and minerals.

Protein

Proteins are needed for building and maintaining all the cells in the body. During growth, vast numbers of new cells are created and extra protein is needed for this. Protein is made up of long chains of amino acids linked together. Some amino acids can be made by the human body (non-essential amino acids) but others cannot; these are called 'essential amino acids' and must be provided by food. All the essential amino acids needed are found in the protein in animal foods, such as milk, eggs, meat and fish. Proteins in plant-based foods contain some but not all of the essential amino acids. However, the combination of a starchy food, such as cereals and their flours, bread, pasta, potatoes or rice, together with pulses or nuts will provide all the essential amino acids together. Examples of this combination are baked beans on toast, rice and peas or a hummus or peanut butter sandwich.

Carbohydrate

Carbohydrates provide energy and fibre. The energy from the starches and sugars are metabolised into glucose, which is used by the cells. The brain almost exclusively uses glucose for energy. Other cells can use glucose or fat.

Starch

Starches are long chains of sugar molecules that do not have a sweet taste.

Sugars

Sugars in food are either *monosaccharides,* for example,

- glucose;
- fructose – the main sugar in fruit.

or *disaccharides*, for example,

- lactose – the sugar in milk – composed of glucose and galactose;
- sucrose – white table sugar made from sugar cane or root vegetables – composed of glucose and fructose;
- maltose – the main sugar formed when starch breaks down – composed of two glucose units.

Free sugars are:

- all monosaccharides and disaccharides added to foods by the manufacturer, cook or consumer;
- sugars naturally present in honey, syrups, fruit and vegetable juices;
- sugars naturally present in fruit and vegetable purees and pastes and similar products in which the cellular structure has been broken down;
- lactose and galactose added as ingredients.

Free sugars are the most harmful to teeth.

Sugars not classed as free sugars are:

- those present in non-processed fruits and vegetables (fresh, frozen or dried) where the sugars remain within the intact cells of the fruit and vegetables;
- naturally occurring lactose in milk and products such as plain yogurt and cheese.

Fibre

Fibre is a term used for the particular types of carbohydrates that are not digested by the enzymes in the small intestine for absorption into the blood. They pass intact through to the large intestine ensuring the digestive system functions appropriately, preventing constipation and diarrhoea.

Soluble fibre (pectin, gums, mucilage extracted from psyllium husk, β-glucan, fructans and some hemicellulose) is resistant to digestion in the small intestine but is partially or totally fermented by colonic bacteria to short-chain fatty acids in the large intestine. These short chain fatty acids provide small amounts of energy and maintain or alter the intestinal microbiota.

Insoluble fiber (lignin, cellulose and some hemicellulose) passes through the digestive tract intact and is excreted in the faeces.

Prebiotics

Prebiotics are the types of fibre that encourage the growth of beneficial bacteria in the intestine. Prebiotic fibre is found in fruits and vegetables, such as onions, leeks, garlic and bananas.

Fat

There are different types of fat, all of which provide energy. Triglyceride fats are the most common in foods and can be:

- saturated – no double bonds within the fatty acid chains;
- monounsaturated – 1 double bond within the fatty acid chains;
- polyunsaturated – 2 or more double bonds within the fatty acid chains.

The fat in foods is a mixture of all the types of fat but certain foods have more of 1 type than the others. Complex fats, such as cholesterol, account for a very small proportion of the fat in foods.

Saturated fat

About 60–70 per cent of the fat in meat, butter, cream, milk and cheese is saturated fat. About 90 per cent of the fat in coconut oil and 50 per cent in palm oil is saturated. A lot of the saturated fat in processed commercial foods such as biscuits, cakes, pastries and ready meals is hydrogenated fat. This is because hydrogenating unsaturated fats to change them into saturated fat extends the shelf-life of the foods; unsaturated fat is more likely to oxidise and become rancid than saturated fats.

Trans fats

Trans fats are found naturally in milk and milk products and are not harmful, whereas the trans

Table 1.2 Names and food sources of the various essential omega 3 and omega 6 fats

	Omega 3 fats	Omega 6 fats
Short-chain form – from plants		
Names	ALA (alpha-linolenic acid)	LA (linoleic acid)
Main food sources	Walnuts, linseeds and their oils	All nuts, seeds and vegetable oils
	Rapeseed oil	
	Olive oil and soya oil have smaller amounts	
Long-chain form – from animal foods		
Names	EPA (eicosapentaenoic acid)	GLA (gamma linolenic acid)
	DHA (docosahexaenoic acid)	AA (arachidonic acid)
Main food sources	Best source are oily fishes.[a]	Fish, meat and egg yolks
	Other sources are red meat and egg yolks depending on how the animals and chickens are fed.[b]	

[a] Oily fishes are: salmon, mackerel, trout, fresh tuna, sardines, pilchards and eel.

[b] Animals that have grazed on grass rather than been fed cereals have higher amounts of omega 3 in their meat. Egg yolks from chickens fed a special feed high in omega 3 fat will be a good source of omega 3 fats.

fats produced during processing food are now known to raise cholesterol in the same way that an excess of saturated fat does.

Unsaturated fats – monounsaturated and polyunsaturated

Most vegetable oils, nuts and seeds contain more monounsaturated and polyunsaturated fat than saturated fat.

Essential fats: omega 3 and omega 6 fats

These two groups of polyunsaturated fats are essential because the body cannot make them (Table 1.2). Plant foods provide these in a shorter chain form and some are converted to the long-chain form within our cells. Food from animal sources provides these essential fats directly in the long-chain form. The long-chain form of omega 3 fat is particularly needed for the growing brain, the nervous system and for good vision. Infants can only make limited amounts of the long-chain form and rely on getting plenty of long-chain omega 3 in breast milk or infant formula as well as some oily fish during complementary feeding. Children over 1 year of age should be able to make adequate amounts of the long-chain forms even if they eat a vegetarian diet without fish. Research shows, however, that children who regularly eat oily fish a couple of times per week and have a good intake of omega 3 fat in the long-chain form are less likely to get asthma.

Balancing omega 3 and omega 6 fats in diets

The balance of these 2 groups of essential fats affects health. Up until about 50 years ago diets had about equal quantities of omega 3 and omega 6 fats, but nowadays we eat a much higher proportion of omega 6 fats and very little omega 3 fat. This change is thought to be one of the factors causing increased rates of inflammatory responses such as allergy, asthma and hay fever in children.

Vitamins

Vitamins are chemicals that are needed for the proper functioning of the human body but cannot be made within the body. They are made by certain plants, animals or bacteria and thus the vitamins are acquired by eating those plant and animal foods. Certain bacteria in the gastrointestinal tract provide two of the vitamins – vitamin K and vitamin B12.

Vitamins A, D, E and K are fat-soluble vitamins and are found within the oils and fats in some foods. When an excess of these vitamins are eaten, reasonable amounts of them can be stored in the body. Vitamin C and the B vitamins are water-soluble and any excess amounts of them consumed are excreted in urine. The stores of water soluble vitamins that are built up are much smaller and it is thus crucial to have a regular supply in the diet.

Vitamin A

Vitamin A comes in two forms: retinol in some animal foods (full-fat milk, butter, margarine, egg yolks and liver) and carotene in fruits and vegetables. Carotene is the orange coloured pigments in fruits and vegetables, and is also present in dark green vegetables such as spinach and broccoli.

Vitamin A is important for growth and development as well as vision. As an antioxidant, it is part of the immune system helping to prevent infections and illness. In the developing world, many children have impaired vision due to a deficiency of vitamin A. Fortunately, this extreme deficiency is not seen in the United Kingdom.

Excess vitamin A taken in the form of too many supplements could be a problem for children as excess amounts are stored in the body. Liver is very high in vitamin A now that animal feed is enriched with it. The Food Standards Agency recommends that children and adults should only consume liver once per week (Scientific Advisory Committee on Nutrition 2005).

B vitamins

The B vitamins are thiamin, folic acid, niacin (nicotinamide), riboflavin, pyridoxine, biotin, pantothenic acid and vitamin B12. They play roles in growth and development of a healthy nervous system, and are needed to convert food into energy. Vitamin B12 and folate are important for preventing types of anaemia. Good sources of B vitamins include meat, milk products, fish, eggs, cereals, seeds and vegetables. Dark green vegetables, liver and pulses are high in folate.

Vitamin C

Vitamin C, also known as ascorbic acid, is essential for increasing the iron absorption from plant foods, protecting cells from damage and for maintaining blood vessels, cartilage, muscle and bone. Vitamin C is also involved in wound healing. A severe deficiency causes scurvy.

Vitamin D

Vitamin D is key for bone health and the immune system. It is sometimes called the 'sunshine vitamin' as most is made in exposed skin when we are outside in daylight. The action of ultraviolet (UV) radiation of wavelength 290–310 nm converts 7-dehydrocholesterol to vitamin D3 (via its precursor). Skin synthesis is affected by many factors, including the following:

- Skin type: Synthesis is higher in white populations than in darker pigmented skins of children of Asian, African and Middle Eastern origin.
- Individual genetic variations in the skin, which affect the cutaneous synthesis of vitamin D.
- Latitude: The intensity of the sunlight decreases with increasing distance from the equator. In the United Kingdom, vitamin D is only made in the skin during the summer months from April to September. Hence, in summer, a store of vitamin D must be built up to last through the winter. This is now considered unlikely with modern lifestyles in the United Kingdom.
- Climate: Cloud cover decreases the intensity of the sunlight.
- Air pollution: This reduces the critical UV light waves available for skin synthesis.

- Lifestyle habits with regard to time spent outside or clothing. People who cover most of their skin when outside have limited synthesis and are more likely to be deficient in vitamin D.
- Sunscreen use, as sunscreens prevent skin synthesis. Although it is important not to let children's skin burn in the sunshine, it is also important for them to spend time outside everyday in summer in order to make plenty of vitamin D and build up a good store. Sunscreens should be used to prevent sunburn when children are outside for extended periods in the middle of the day. If sunburn is unlikely, then children should be encouraged to play outside without sunscreen.

The liver enzyme 25–hydroxylase converts endogenously synthesised vitamin D3 and diet-derived D2 and D3 to 25 hydroxyvitamin D. In the kidney, 25 hydroxyvitamin D can be converted to 1,25-dihydroxyvitamin D, the active hormone, which has several roles in the body, which are:

- the absorption of calcium from food and for depositing calcium and other minerals into bone to give it strength;
- maintaining calcium levels in the blood – low levels of calcium can cause tetany and fitting, which is seen in young infants who are deficient in vitamin D;
- as a component of the immune system.

Very few foods contain vitamin D – oily fish is the best source. Meat and egg yolks contain small amounts. In the United Kingdom, margarines, formula milks and some breakfast cereals are fortified with vitamin D. Other countries, such as USA, Canada and Finland, fortify milk and milk products with vitamin D. Because this vitamin is necessary to support the rapid rate of bone growth in children, in the United Kingdom, daily vitamin D supplements are recommended to meet the Reference Nutrient Intake (RNI):

- from birth for all children up to 4 years of age;
- in autumn and winter for older children;
- all year round for older children who do not spend time outside each day in spring and summer months with bare skin exposed to the sunlight.

However it is prudent for all children to take a daily suppement of 10 μg vitamin D3 as exceeding the upper tolerable intake levels is very unlikely. Historically, vitamin D was taken in a cod liver oil supplement but vitamin drops or tablets are now recommended.

Vitamin D deficiency is seen in about one third of UK children during the winter (Food standards Agency and Public Health England 2018). Over 60 UK children each year have clinical consequences of deficiency, which include rickets, cardiomyopathy, hypocalcaemic seizures, delayed gross motor development and bone fractures. Cardiomyopathy can cause death (Julies et al. 2020). Under-fives and adolescents are at higher risk of rickets due to their rapid growth rates. Children with dark skins are particularly at risk as they need longer in the sun to make enough vitamin D.

Debate continues around the ideal daily supplement recommendations for the United Kingdom due to individual genetic variations (Cashman et al. 2020).

Vitamin E

Vitamin E is an important antioxidant that protects cell structures in the body. It is found in many foods such as vegetable oils, butter and margarines, meat, fish and eggs. Children usually have plenty of vitamin E in their food.

Vitamin K

Vitamin K is needed for bone health and to ensure normal blood clotting. It is provided mostly by the bacteria in the intestine. Green leafy vegetables are the best food source of vitamin K.

Minerals

Calcium has many key functions in the body and is needed for the structure of healthy bones and teeth. The calcium in bone acts as a store so that there is always a ready supply enabling the muscles, including the heart, to contract and the nerves and cells to function as necessary. Milk, cheese and yogurt are the best sources. Soya beans are a reasonable source of calcium but soya milk needs to be fortified with extra calcium to provide the same amount as cow's milk. White bread has been fortified with calcium since the 1940s and tinned fish with bones such as sardines is another good source. Calcium carbonate is usually used in calcium supplements and food fortification and calcium in this form is less bioavailable than that in milk and milk products.

Copper is involved in energy and protein production. Tiny amounts are present in all foods. Children usually get enough from their food.

Fluoride strengthens tooth enamel making it more resistant to attack by the acid produced by plaque bacteria. Frequent acid attack overtime causes in tooth decay. The two main sources of fluoride are toothpaste and tap water. Teeth should be cleaned twice a day using a fluoride-containing toothpaste:

- up to the age of 3 years – a smear of toothpaste containing 1000 ppm of fluoride;
- 3–7 years – a pea-sized amount of toothpaste containing 1000 or 1350–1500 ppm of fluoride;
- from the age of 7 years – use toothpaste containing 1350–1500 ppm of fluoride.

There are areas of the United Kingdom where tap water is fluoridated or the water naturally contains adequate levels of fluoride. However, there are large areas of the United Kingdom where water does not contain adequate fluoride. Dentists may recommend fluoride tablets or drops for children who are at high risk of dental disease. That is those who have:

- a family history of a high caries level;
- medical conditions where treatment for dental caries should be avoided (e.g. bleeding disorders, cardiac problems);
- a mental or physical disability, which can make treatment for dental disease particularly difficult.

Advice from a dentist on giving supplements is crucial as too much fluoride can cause dental fluorosis – permanent brown spots on the teeth.

Iodine forms part of the hormone thyroxine, which has several key roles in the body – converting food into energy and enabling growth and physical and mental development. Iodine deficiency is common in some areas of Europe and is increasingly of concern in the United Kingdom. The United Kingdom is now classified as mildly iodine deficient by the World Health Organization, based on a 2011 national study of 14–15-year-old schoolgirls. Fish, milk, yogurt and eggs are good sources.

Iron is part of the structure of haemoglobin, the chemical that carries oxygen to all the cells in the body via the blood. Oxygen is needed by cells to produce energy. Many under-fives and adolescents do not eat enough iron in their diet, and anaemia due to iron deficiency is fairly common among these 2 age groups in the United Kingdom. It causes tiredness, delayed growth and development and more illness as iron is also part of the immune system. Poor appetite is another consequence; this can create a vicious circle as less iron will be eaten by a child with a poor appetite. See page 178 for more information on iron-deficiency anaemia.

The 2 forms of iron in food are:

- haem iron, which is readily absorbed – good sources are red meat such as beef, lamb, pork, dark poultry meat such as chicken legs and thighs and oily fish;
- non-haem iron, which is poorly absorbed unless vitamin C is present – good sources are eggs, pulses, nuts, fortified breakfast cereals, dried fruit and some vegetables.

Magnesium is also involved in the process of converting food into energy as well as building

Table 1.3 Salt/sodium intake recommendations

Age	Daily recommended maximum intake (Scientific Advisory Committee on Nutrition 2003)		Reference Nutrient Intake (Department of Health 1991)
	Salt (g/day)	Sodium (g/day)	Sodium (g/day)
0–3 months	1	0.4	0.21
4–6 months	1	0.4	0.28
7–9 months	1	0.4	0.32
10–12 months	1	0.4	0.35
1–3 years	2	0.8	0.5
4–6 years	3	1.2	0.7
7–10 years	5	2	1.3
11 + years	6	2.4	1.6

bone and protein production. The best sources are wholegrain bread, breakfast cereals, milk and yogurt. Other good sources are meat, eggs, pulses and some vegetables.

Phosphorus forms the main structure of bones along with calcium. It is found in milk but unlike calcium, it is also found in most other foods, so children usually have plenty in their food.

Potassium plays a key role in fluid balance, muscle contractions and proper nerve function. The best sources are potatoes, nuts, fruit and vegetables.

Selenium is an antioxidant and plays a role in the production of the thyroid hormone as well as energy production. The best sources for children are bread, meat, fish, eggs and other foods made from flour. Brazil nuts and cashew nuts are particularly rich.

The amount of selenium in the soil determines how much is in the food grown on that soil. Selenium levels in UK soil are on the low side compared to those in the United States where levels are higher.

Sodium plays a key role in fluid balance and maintaining blood pressure and is necessary to maintain growth in children. Sodium is found in several foods but the main source is in salt, which is used to preserve some foods and added to enhance flavour in most processed food. Too much salt can raise blood pressure in older children and adults, creating a higher risk of heart disease, but there is no evidence of harm in younger children. Children eating a lot of processed snack foods and ready meals, which all have added salt, may exceed the recommendations on salt/sodium intake published by the Scientific Advisory Committee on Nutrition (SACN) in 2003, as listed in Table 1.3.

However, the SACN recommendations are not evidence based for children, are very difficult to achieve and are only slightly above the recommended intake expressed as the RNI. Average intakes in the United Kingdom are above those set by SACN.

Zinc helps wounds to heal and is part of the immune system. In children, it is important for growth as it is part of two hormones – growth hormone and insulin. The best food sources are meat, fish, milk and eggs. Bread and breakfast cereals are also good sources.

Other beneficial components in food

Phytochemicals

Phytochemicals are compounds that occur naturally in plants (phyto means 'plant' in Greek) and have biological significance but are not established as essential nutrients. They include antioxidants, which are the brightly coloured pigments in plant foods – that is in fruits, vegetables, spices, herbs, nuts, cocoa beans and foods made from cereals. Tea and coffee also contain them. They are subdivided into various groups such as phytoestrogens, phytosterols and flavonoids, flavanols and

Table 1.4 UK Reference Nutrient Intakes for protein for children

Age	Protein RNI (g/day)		Protein (g/kg body weight/day)
	Males	Females	
0–3 months	12.5	12.5	2.1
4–6 months	12.7	12.7	1.6
7–9 months	13.7	13.7	1.5
10–12 months	14.9	14.9	1.5
1–3 years	14.5	14.5	1.1
4–6 years	19.7	19.7	–
7–10 years	28.3	28.3	–
11–14 years	42.1	41.2	–
15–18 years	55.2	45	–

isoflavones. Some of the commonly known phytochemicals are:

- lycopene in tomatoes;
- quercetin in apples, onions, grapes and berries;
- anthocyanins in berries.

There are thousands of these chemicals in plant foods, and research indicating that they may be protective against various cancers and cardiovascular disease has only been published in the last 30 or so years. Their mode of action in cancer prevention is by:

- increasing the body's ability to break down carcinogens;
- acting as an antioxidant to mop up free radicals before they damage cells in the body;
- enhancing the immune system;
- altering hormones, which are associated with the onset of cancer.

They help prevent cardiovascular disease by:

- decreasing blood cholesterol;
- altering the profile of fats in the blood;
- reducing the oxidation of fat present in arterial walls.

They have not been shown to be of critical importance for the day-to-day health of children, but during childhood, it is important for children to learn to like the foods that contain them and to learn that eating fruit and vegetables at all meals is normal because of their likely disease prevention later in life.

Table 1.5 UK recommended intakes for fibre for children

Age group (years)	Recommended intakes (g/day)
2–5	15
5–11	20
11–16	25
16–18	30

Probiotics

Probiotics are bacteria in food that colonise the intestine and provide health benefits. Beneficial bacteria in the intestine help the intestine to function optimally and may help to prevent diarrhoea in children. Examples of beneficial bacteria are bifidobacteria and lactobacilli that are found in live yogurt. Fermented foods

Table 1.6 UK Reference Nutrient Intakes for vitamins for children

Age	Vitamin A (µg/day)	B vitamins						Vitamin C (mg/day)	Vitamin D (mg/day)
		Thiamin (mg/day)	Riboflavin (mg/day)	Niacin (mg/day)	Vitamin B6 (mg/day)	Vitamin B12 (µg/day)	Folate (µg/day)		
0–3 months	350	0.2	0.4	3	0.2	0.3	50	25	8.5–10
4–6 months	350	0.2	0.4	3	0.2	0.3	50	25	8.5–10
7–9 months	350	0.2	0.4	4	0.3	0.4	50	25	8.5–10
10–12 months	350	0.3	0.4	5	0.4	0.4	50	25	8.5–10
1–3 years	400	0.5	0.6	8	0.7	0.5	70	30	10
4–6 years	400	0.7	0.8	11	0.9	0.8	100	30	10
7–10 years	500	0.7	1.0	12	1.0	1.0	150	30	10
Males									
11–14 years	600	0.9	1.2	15	1.2	1.2	200	35	10
15–18 years	700	1.1	1.3	15	1.2	1.2	200	40	10
Females									
11–14 years	600	0.7	1.1	12	1.0	1.2	200	35	10
15–18 years	600	0.8	1.1	14	1.2	1.5	200	40	10

provide a wider variety of probiotic strains than supplements which only provide a few different strains.

Dietary requirements

In general, the amount of energy and each nutrient that children need to stay healthy increases as they grow. In the United Kingdom, energy and nutrient requirements have been set for different age groups of children in 1991 by the Committee on Medical Aspects of Food Policy (COMA) (Department of Health 1991). COMA was the forerunner of the current SACN (www.sacn.gov.uk).

The relevant units used for dietary requirements are as follows:

- Reference Nutrient Intake (RNI) – the average daily amount of a nutrient that is considered to be enough to meet the requirements of 97 per cent of the population of each age group of children. This means only 3 in 100 children would require an amount higher than this. It is used as the daily recommendation for protein, vitamins and minerals.
- Lower Reference Nutrient Intake (LRNI) provides the daily amount of a nutrient to meet the dietary requirements of the lowest 3 per cent of a population.
- Estimated Average Requirement (EAR) is the daily mean/average requirement for each age group and would only be enough for 50 per cent of a population. It is used for energy requirements.

These recommended values vary somewhat from country to country.

Macronutrients

RNIs for protein have been set for different age groups of children but an individual protein requirement can be calculated more specifically for individual infants and young children depending on their body weight (Table 1.4).

Table 1.7 UK Reference Nutrient Intakes for minerals for children

Age	Calcium (mg/day)	Chloride (mg/day)	Copper (mg/day)	Iodine (µg/day)	Iron (mg/day)	Magnesium (mg/day)	Phosphorus (mg/day)	Potassium (mg/day)	Sodium (mg/day)	Selenium (µg/day)	Zinc (mg/day)
0–3 months	525	320	0.2	50	1.7	55	400	800	210	10	4
4–6 months	525	400	0.3	60	4.3	60	400	850	280	13	4
7–9 months	525	500	0.3	60	7.8	75	400	700	320	10	5
10–12 months	525	500	0.3	60	7.8	80	400	700	350	10	5
1–3 years	350	800	0.4	70	6.9	85	270	800	500	15	5
4–6 years	450	1100	0.6	100	6.1	120	350	1100	700	20	6.5
7–10 years	550	1800	0.7	110	8.7	200	450	2000	1200	30	7
Males											
11–14 years	1000	2500	0.8	130	11.3	280	775	3100	1600	45	9
15–18 years	1000	2500	1.0	140	11.3	300	775	3500	1600	70	9.5
Females											
11–14 years	800	2500	0.8	130	14.8	280	625	3100	1600	45	9
15–18 years	800	2500	1.0	140	14.8	300	625	3500	1600	60	7

Table 1.8 Safe intakes for certain micronutrients

Nutrient		Safe intake
B vitamins	Pantothenic acid	Infants: 1.7 mg/day; Chidlren: 3–7 mg/day
	Biotin	10–200 μg/day
Trace minerals	Chromium	0.104–1.976 μg/kg body weight/day
	Fluoride	0.12 mg/kg body weight/day
	Manganese	16.5 μg/kg body weight/day
	Molybdenum	0.480–1.534 μg/kg body weight/day

RNIs are not set for the other macronutrients but the SACN in their various recent reports have made the following recommendations:

- **Carbohydrate**: at least 50 per cent of total energy from total carbohydrates
    - Free sugars: 5 per cent of total energy – but this is very difficult to achieve and other countries recommend about 10 per cent of total energy;
    - Fibre: Average approximate daily intakes for different age groups are shown in Table 1.5
- **Fat**: a maximum of 35 per cent of total energy;
- **Saturated Fat**: a maximum of 10 per cent of total energy for children 5 years and over. A flexible approach for children under 5 years (Scientific Advisory Committee on Nutrition 2019).

Micronutrient requirements

UK RNIs for vitamins and minerals for children are listed in Tables 1.6 and 1.7.

For some of the micronutrients that are only required in very small amounts, 'safe intakes' are set (Table 1.8).

Ensuring adequate energy and nutrient intakes

Children can store a certain amount of nutrients within their body and hence eating to meet the RNI for each nutrient each day is not necessary. An average daily intake over a few weeks is adequate.

In general, it is not necessary to calculate the nutrient intakes of children and compare them to the RNIs because foods can be grouped into food groups with all the foods in each food group providing a similar range of certain nutrients. By combining foods from each of the food groups in average portion sizes each day, all the nutrients needed will be automatically provided.

How to meet energy and nutrient requirements through food and drinks in a balanced nutritious diet is discussed in Chapter 2.

References and further reading

Cashman KD, Kiely ME, Andersen R et al. (June 2020) Individual participant data (IPD)-level meta-analysis of randomised controlled trials with vitamin D-fortified foods to estimate Dietary Reference Values for vitamin D. *European Journal of Nutrition*. doi: 10.1007/s00394-020-02298-x

Department of Health (1991) *Report on Health and Social Subjects No. 41. Dietary Reference Values for Food Energy and Nutrients for the United Kingdom*. London: The Stationery Office.

Dietetic Department Great Ormond Street Hospital for Children NHS Trust (2018) *Nutritional Requirements for Children in Health and Disease*, 7th edn. London: Great Ormond Street Hospital Trust.

Food Standards Agency and Public Health England (2018) Results of the National Diet and Nutrition Survey (NDNS) rolling programme for 2014 to 2015 and 2015 to 2016. www.gov.uk/government/statistics/ndns-results-from-years-7-and-8-combined (Accessed 01 November 2019.

Julies P, Lynn RM, Pall K *et al.* (16 January 2020) Nutritional rickets under 16 years: UK surveillance results. *Archives of Disease in Childhood* Published Online First. doi: 10.1136/archdischild-2019-317934

Scientific Advisory Committee on Nutrition (2003) *Salt and Health*. London: The Stationery Office.

Scientific Advisory Committee on Nutrition (2011) *Dietary Reference Values for Energy*. London: The Stationery Office.

Scientific Advisory Committee on Nutrition (2015) *Carbohydrates and Health*. London: The Stationery Office.

Scientific Advisory Committee on Nutrition (2019) *Saturated Fats and Health*. London: The Stationary Office.

Scientific Advisory Committee on Nutrition (2016) *Vitamin D and Health*. London: The Stationery Office.

Scientific Advisory Committee on Nutrition (2005) *Review of Dietary Advice on Vitamin A*. London: The Stationery Office.

Shaw NJ (November 2016) Prevention and treatment of nutritional rickets. *The Journal of Steroid Biochemistry and Molecular Biology* **164**: 145–147. doi: 10.1016/j.jsbmb.2015.10.014. Epub 19 October 2015.

Revez JA, Lin T, Qiao Z et al. (2020) Genome-wide association study identifies 143 loci associated with 25 hydroxyvitamin D concentration. *Nature Communications* **11**(1). doi: 10.1038/s41467-020-15421-7

Wiskin AE, Davies JH, Wootton SA and Beatties RM (2011) Energy expenditure, nutrition and growth. *Archives of Disease in Childhood* **96**: 567–572.

2

Principles of a balanced nutritious diet for children over 1 year

Summary

- Nutritious foods can be divided into 5 food groups based on the nutrients they contain.
- An average daily combination of a number of portions from 8 food groups along with adequate fluid and a vitamin D supplement provides nutritional adequacy.
- The food groups and number of portions children require are:
  1. bread, rice, potatoes, pasta and other starchy foods – include at each meal and some snacks: 4–5 portions;
  2. fruit and vegetables – include at each meal and some snacks: about 5 portions;
  3. milk, cheese and yogurt – 3 portions per day;
  4. meat, fish, eggs, nuts and pulses – 2 portions per day or 3 for vegetarians;
  5. oils, butter and fat spread - small amounts in food preparation.

Extra food groups add enjoyment and palatability along with additional nutrients:

6. Cakes, biscuits & puddings: 1 portion per day;
7. Sauces, and sweet/savoury spreads: 2 portions per day;
8. Sweet drinks, confectionery and high fat packet snacks: 1 portion per week of either sweet drinks, confectionery or savoury snacks.

- Between six and eight drinks should be offered each day.
- Sweet foods should be limited to 4 times per day.
- The number of average daily portions of each food group is the same throughout childhood from 12 months of age but portion sizes of food and drinks increase as children grow and their energy and nutrient requirements increase.
- Assessing the average number of daily portions from each food group can be used to help parents and children make changes to improve the nutritional adequacy of their diets.

Balanced nutritious diet

It is not necessary for children to eat the exact Reference Nutrient Intakes (RNI) of each of the nutrients each day as outlined in Chapter 1. Most nutrients are stored in the body and these stores last some time. Children may eat more of some nutrients on certain days and less on other days, depending on the foods offered and the quantities consumed.

Foods are grouped together according to the nutrients they contain and so all the foods within each food group provide a similar range of nutrients. Over a period of 2 weeks or so, on a balanced diet with a reasonable variety of foods from each of the first five food groups, along with adequate fluid and a vitamin D supplement, children will be getting on average what they need.

The food groups and the nutrients they contain along with the recommended number of average daily portions from each food group are set out in Table 2.1. The first five food groups in Table 2.1 provide most of the nutrients. Foods within the Extra Food Groups provide fewer nutrients and/or are high in energy. However they are eaten to add flavour, palatability and enjoyment to meals and they provide some nutrients. When devising the portion sizes for different age groups More, Lanigan and Emmett were able to include these extra food groups within a theoretical meal plan that met all nutrient requirements within the estimated average energy requirements for children on the 50th percentile for weight (More et al. 2021).

Most foods are based on more than 1 food group. For example, pizza provides a serving from 3 or 4 food groups depending on the ingredients used:

- Pizza base contains flour – providing a portion from food group 1.
- Cheese on top provides a portion from food group 3.
- If a meat is included it provides a portion from food group 4.
- If diced vegetables are included in the topping they provide a ½ or whole portion from food group 2.

Drinks

Fluid requirements vary depending on the weather and each child's physical activity. The kidneys can cope with a wide range in fluid intake and pale yellow urine indicates a child is well hydrated. Between six and eight drinks per day provide adequate fluid, although children may need more in very hot weather or after extra physical activity. Water and milk are the safest drinks to offer between meals as they do not cause tooth erosion or increase the risk of dental decay. Milk and yogurt drinks are included in food group 3. Up to 3 drinks per day can be milk but more than this can decrease the appetite for foods from the other food groups that contain iron.

Sweetened drinks and fruit juices and smoothies are high-sugar drinks that also contain acid which can cause dental decay if given frequently. They should be limited to once per week as in Table 2.1.

Pictorial guides for food groups

The UK Eatwell Guide is the visual representation developed by Public Health England describing how to combine the food groups on a daily basis (Figure 2.1). It has been devised for children over 5 years and adults. There is no UK visual representation of a combination of the five food groups for children under 5 years old.

This five food group combination can be applied to whichever cultural diet families eat. The wider the variety of foods eaten within each food group the better the balance of nutrients provided.

***Limitations of the Eatwell guide*:**

1. The inclusion of substitute drinks for milk in food group 3 may lead to nutrient deficiencies in children if the substitutes used are not fortified with calcium, riboflavin, iodine and vitamin A. Excluding all dairy protein in a child's diet may limit growth.
2. The emphasis on low dairy fat in the UK Eatwell Guide is not appropriate for growing children as it could limit vitamin A intakes for children who refuse most fruit and vegetables.

Most countries have developed their own visual representation of combining food groups to provide a balanced nutritious diet according to their food cultures. The principles are the same and the food groups vary very little from the UK Eatwell Guide.

For example, in the United States and Singapore plate models are also used (Figures 2.2 and 2.3), Thailand has the 'Nutrition Flag' (Figure 2.4) and in St. Lucia in the Caribbean the food groups are displayed as a cooking pot (Figure 2.5).

Table 2.1 Food groups and recommended number of daily portions

Food groups	Foods included	Main nutrients supplied	Recommendations: Infants 6–12 months	Recommendations: Preschool children 1–4 years	Recommendations: School children 5–18 years
1. Bread, rice potatoes, pasta and other starchy foods	Bread, chapatti, breakfast cereals, rice, couscous, pasta, millet, potatoes, yam and foods made with flour such as pizza bases, buns and pancakes	Carbohydrate B vitamins Fibre Protein Some iron, zinc and calcium	3 portions a day	Serve at each meal and some snacks 3–5 portions per day	Serve at each meal and some snacks 3–5 portions per day
2. Fruit and vegetables	Fresh, frozen, tinned and dried fruits and vegetables	Vitamin C Phytochemicals Fibre Carotenes	3–4 portions a day	Offer at each meal and some snacks – about 3 small portions fruit per day and 3 small portions of vegetables	Serve at each meal and some snacks – aim for 3 portions per day of fruit and 3 portions per day of vegetables
3. Milk, cheese and yogurt	Breast milk, infant formulas, follow-on and growing up milk formulas, cow's milk, goat's milk, yogurts, cheese, milk puddings, and tofu	Calcium Protein Iodine Riboflavin	Demand feeds of breast milk or infant formula as main milk drink	3 portions per day	3 portions per day
4. Meat, fish, eggs, nuts and pulses	Meat, fish, eggs, nuts and pulses (lentils, dahl, chickpeas, hummus, kidney beans and other similar starchy beans)	Iron Protein Zinc Magnesium B vitamins Vitamin A Iodine Omega 3 long-chain fatty acids: EPA and DHA from oily fish	1–2 portions a day; 2–3 for vegetarians	2 portions perday or 3 for vegetarians Fish should be offered twice per week and oily fish at least once per week[a]	2 portions per day or 3 for vegetarians Fish should be offered twice per week and oily fish at least once per week[a]

(*Continued*)

Table 2.1 (Continued)

Food groups	Foods included	Main nutrients supplied	Recommendations		
			Infants 6–12 months	Preschool children 1–4 years	School children 5–18 years
5. Oils, butter and fat spreads	Cream, butter, margarines, cooking and salad oils, and mayonnaise	Vitamin E Omega 3 and omega 6 fatty acids		Small amounts in food preparation	Small amounts in food preparation
Fluids	Drinks	Water Fluoride in areas with fluoridated tap water	Milk feeds and drinks of water offered with meals	6–8 drinks per day More in hot weather or after extra physical activity	6–8 drinks per day More in hot weather or after extra physical activity
Vitamin supplements			Vitamin D from birth	Vitamin D	Vitamin D Folic acid for adolescent girls who could become pregnant and during pregnancy
Extra food groups					
6. Cakes, biscuits and puddings	Biscuits Cake/muffins/croissant Fruit-based puddings Ice cream	Carbohydrate including free sugars Fat Small amounts of protein, B vitamins and other nutrients	–	From 2 years: 1 portion per day	1 portion per day
7. Sauces, and sweet/savoury spreads	Jam/honey/syrups Gravy Tomato or vegetable or curry sauce Ketchup/savoury sauce Fruit juices	Free sugars Fat Salt	–	From 2 years: 2 portions per day	2 portions per day

(Continued)

Table 2.1 (Continued)

Food groups	Foods included	Main nutrients supplied	Recommendations		
			Infants 6–12 months	Preschool children 1–4 years	School children 5–18 years
8. Sweet drinks, confectionery and high fat packet snacks	Fruit juices Sweetened drinks Chocolate/Indian Sweets Crisps/other packet snacks	Free sugars Fat Salt	–	From 2 years: 1 portion per week if at all	1 portion per week if at all

[a] Oily fish should be limited to 2 portions per week for girls and 4 portions per week for boys.

DHA, docosahexaenoic acid; EPA, eicosapentaenoic acid

Brazil has taken a completely different approach and emphasises the use of fresh food cooked from scratch and avoiding processed foods in their ten dietary guidelines shown in Table 2.2:

Portion sizes

Portion sizes of foods increase as children grow and have higher energy and nutrient requirements. However, the recommended number of

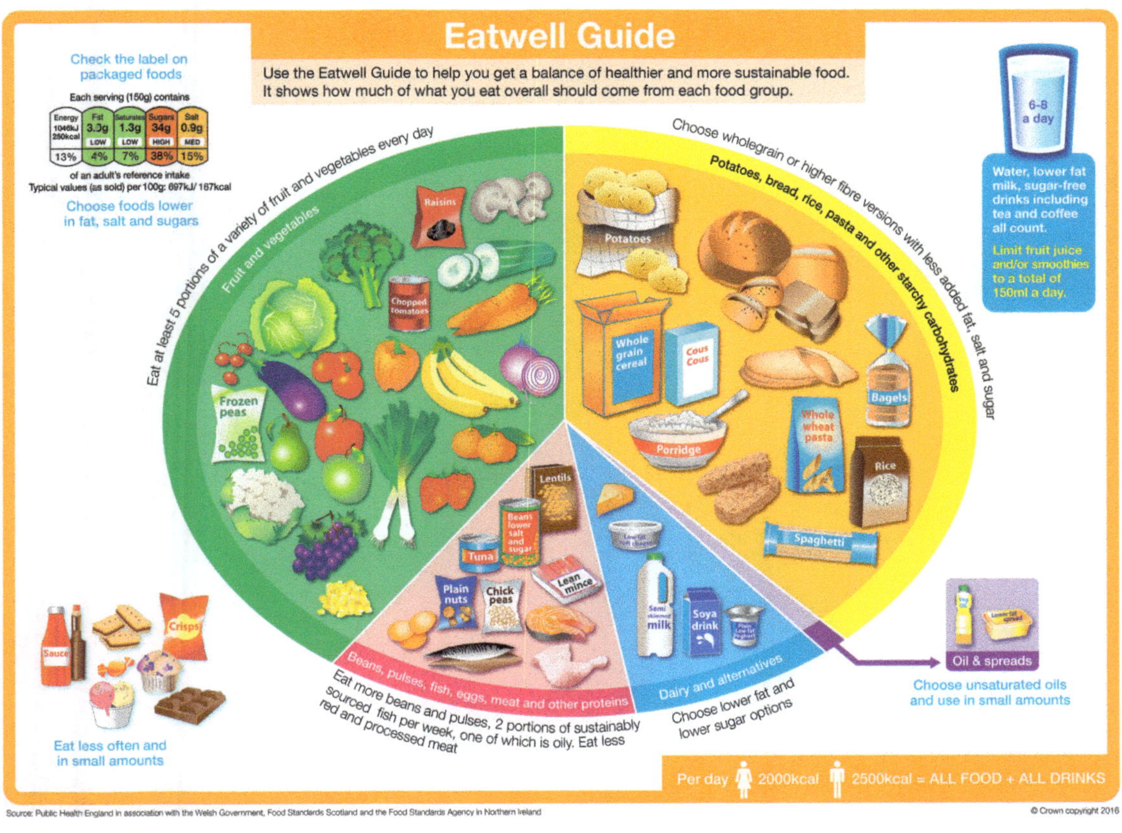

Figure 2.1 The 'Eatwell Guide'. Copyright: Food Standards Agency

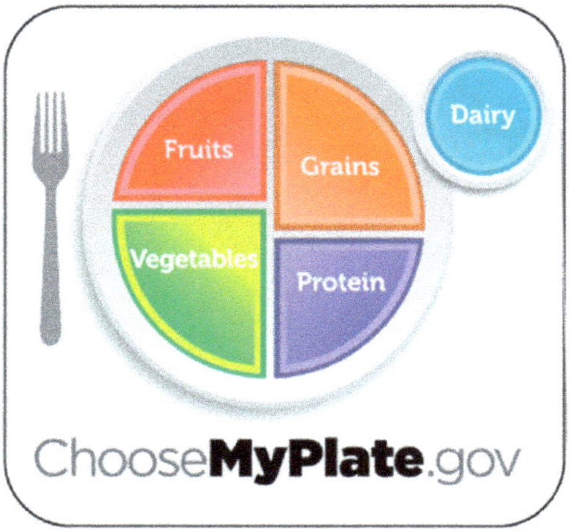

Figure 2.2 The US 'MyPlate'

daily portions from each of the food groups is applicable for all children from 1 year of age. Portion sizes for different age groups are included in Chapters 12, 15 and 16.

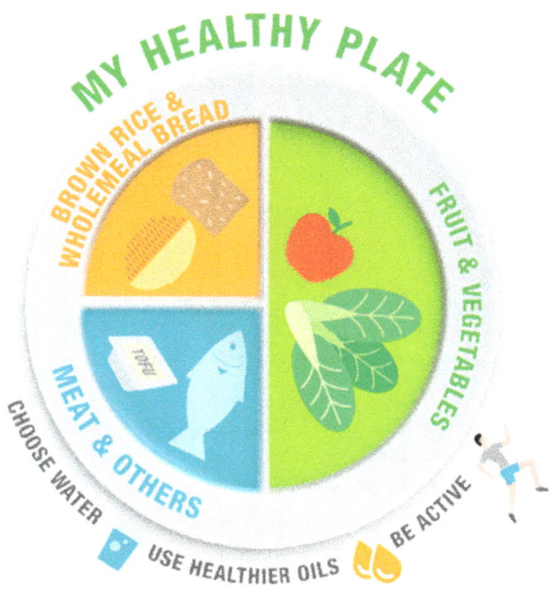
MY HEALTHY PLATE
BROWN RICE & WHOLEMEAL BREAD
FRUIT & VEGETABLES
MEAT & OTHERS
TOFU
CHOOSE WATER
USE HEALTHIER OILS
BE ACTIVE

Figure 2.3 Singapore My Healthy Plate

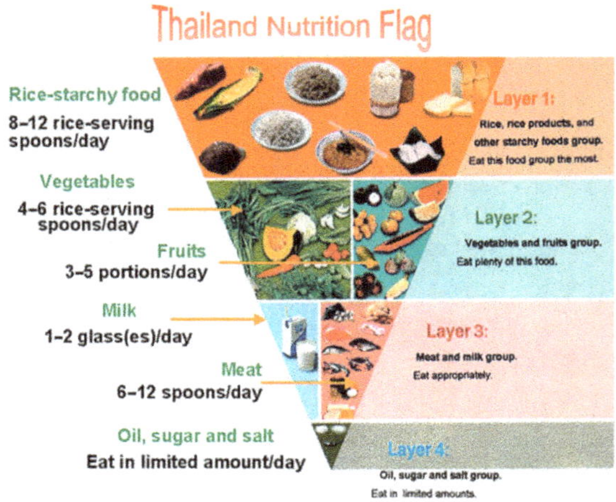
Thailand Nutrition Flag
Rice-starchy food
8–12 rice-serving spoons/day
Vegetables
4–6 rice-serving spoons/day
Fruits
3–5 portions/day
Milk
1–2 glass(es)/day
Meat
6–12 spoons/day
Oil, sugar and salt
Eat in limited amount/day
Layer 1:
Rice, rice products, and other starchy foods group.
Eat this food group the most.
Layer 2:
Vegetables and fruits group.
Eat plenty of this food.
Layer 3:
Meat and milk group.
Eat appropriately.
Layer 4:
Oil, sugar and salt group.
Eat in limited amounts.

Figure 2.4 Thailand Nutrition Flag: 'Healthy Eating for Thais'

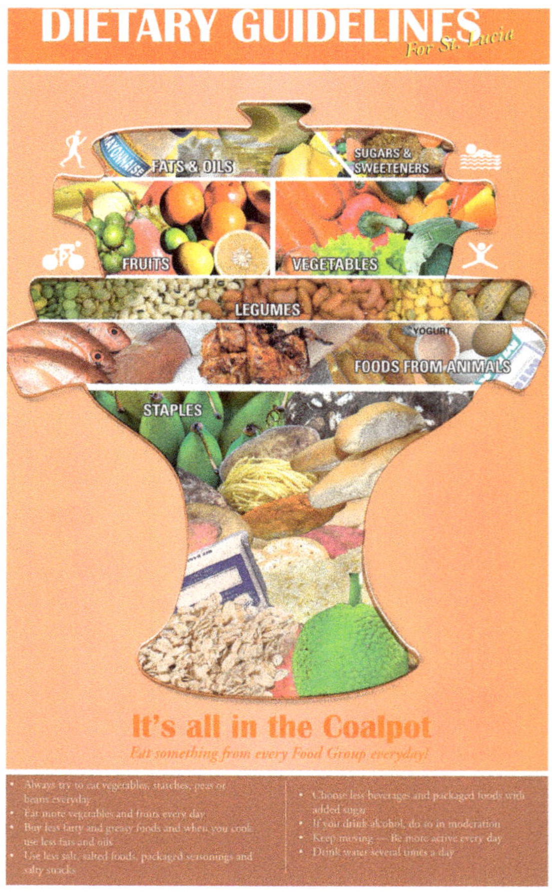
DIETARY GUIDELINES
For St. Lucia
FATS & OILS
SUGARS & SWEETENERS
FRUITS
VEGETABLES
LEGUMES
YOGURT
FOODS FROM ANIMALS
STAPLES
It's all in the Coalpot
Eat something from every Food Group everyday!

Figure 2.5 Dietary guidelines for St. Lucia

Table 2.2 Brazilian 10 steps to healthy diets

1. Make natural or minimally processed foods the basis of your diet	Natural or minimally processed foods, in great variety, and mainly of plant origin, are the basis for diets that are nutritionally balanced, delicious, culturally appropriate and supportive of socially and environmentally sustainable food systems. Variety means foods of all types – cereals, legumes, roots, tubers, vegetables, fruits, nuts, milk, eggs, meat – and diversity within each type – such as beans and lentils, rice and corn, potato and cassava, tomatoes and squash, orange and banana, chicken and fish.
2. Use oils, fats, salt and sugar in small amounts when seasoning and cooking natural or minimally processed foods and to create culinary preparations	As long as they are used in moderation in dishes and meals based on natural or minimally processed foods, oils, fats, salt and sugar contribute to diverse and delicious diets without making them nutritionally unbalanced.
3. Limit consumption of processed foods	The ingredients and methods used in the manufacture of processed foods – such as vegetables in brine, fruits in syrup, cheeses and breads – unfavourably alter the nutritional composition of the foods from which they are derived. In small amounts, processed foods can be used as ingredients in dishes and meals based on natural or minimally processed foods.
4. Avoid consumption of ultra-processed foods	Because of their ingredients, ultra-processed foods such as salty fatty packaged snacks, soft drinks, sweetened breakfast cereals and instant noodles, are nutritionally unbalanced. As a result of their formulation and presentation, they tend to be consumed in excess and displace natural or minimally processed foods. Their means of production, distribution, marketing and consumption damage culture, social life and the environment.
5. Eat regularly and carefully in appropriate environments and, whenever possible, in company	Make your daily meals at regular times. Avoid snacking between meals. Eat slowly and enjoy what you are eating, without engaging in another activity. Eat in clean, comfortable and quiet places, where there is no pressure to consume unlimited amounts of food. Whenever possible, eat in company, with family, friends or colleagues: this increases the enjoyment of food and encourages eating regularly, attentively and in appropriate environments. Share household activities that precede or succeed the consumption of meals.
6. Shop in places that offer a variety of natural or minimally processed foods	Shop in supermarkets and municipal and farmers markets, or buy directly from producers or other places, that sell varieties of natural or minimally processed foods. Prefer vegetables and fruits that are locally grown in season. Whenever possible, buy organic and agro-ecological based foods, preferably directly from the producers.
7. Develop, exercise and share cooking skills	If you have cooking skills, develop them and share them, especially with boys and girls. If you do not have these skills – men as well as women – acquire

(*Continued*)

Table 2.2 (Continued)

	them. Learn from and talk with people who know how to cook. Ask family, friends and colleagues for recipes, read books, check the internet and eventually take courses. Start cooking!
8. Plan your time to make food and eating important in your life	Plan the food shopping, organise your domestic stores and decide on meals in advance. Share with family members the responsibility for all activities related to meals. Make the preparation and eating of meals privileged times of conviviality and pleasure. Assess how you live so as to give proper time for food and eating.
9. Out of home, prefer places that serve freshly made meals	Eat in places that serve fresh meals at good prices. Self-service restaurants and canteens that serve food buffet-style charged by weight are good choices. Avoid fast food chains.
10. Be wary of food advertising and marketing	The purpose of advertising is to increase product sales and not to inform or educate people. Be critical and teach children to be critical of all forms of food advertising and marketing.

Vegetarian diets

Vegetarianism can be divided into five main groups:

- partial vegetarian– red meat and offal are excluded but poultry and fish are eaten;
- pescatarian – all meat and offal are excluded but fish is eaten;
- lacto-ovo vegetarian – red meat, offal, poultry and fish are excluded but milk and eggs are eaten;
- lacto-vegetarian – red meat, offal, poultry and fish and eggs are excluded but milk is included;
- vegans – all animal products including eggs and milks are excluded.

Vegetarian diets, but not vegan diets, can provide a balanced, nutritious diet for optimal growth and development as long as they are well planned. Iron is the main nutrient at risk for children who do not eat meat as it is less well absorbed from plant-based foods than from meat and oily fish. Omega 3 fats may be low in diets that exclude all fish.

Nutritional requirements for growth and development can be achieved in the vegetarian diet by:

- offering 3 portions/day of the vegetarian foods in food group 4 (i.e. eggs, nuts and pulses) and offering a food high in vitamin C at each meal to increase the iron absorbed from the plant-based foods;
- including starchy foods from food group 1 in combination with nuts and pulses from food group 4 (e.g. as baked beans on toast, rice and dahl, rice and peas or peanut butter sandwich) as the amino acids in the protein of starchy foods complement the amino acids in the protein in nuts and pulses to provide together all the essential amino acids needed for growth and development;
- offering breakfast cereals which are fortified with added iron rather than those that are not;
- including dried fruit at meal times, often, as it is a good source of iron
- increasing omega 3 fats from plant sources for those not eating fish, by using rapeseed oil for cooking, walnut or olive oil for dressings and walnuts in place of other nuts or giving a supplement of omega 3 fatty acids.

Vegan diets

Epidemiological research shows that children brought up on vegan diets grow to be shorter adults than children who eat meat and milk

(Grasgruber et al. 2014, Gat-Yablonski et al. 2017, Millward 2017, Morency et al. 2017). Meat and milk proteins are thought to promote optimal growth by exerting a positive influence on the growth plate of growing children.

Vegan diets are unlikely to provide adequate calcium, vitamin B12, iron, iodine, vitamin A and omega 3 fats unless they are extremely well planned with appropriate supplements given. Substitute drinks for milk and milk products are not all fortified with the calcium, iodine, riboflavin and vitamin A to the same level as that found in milk. A vegan diet is not recommended for the under-fives (see Chapter 12).

More restricted diets

Diets more restricted than a vegan diet, such as Zen macrobiotic, fruitarian or raw food diets, are not recommended for children as they cannot provide all the energy and nutrients for growth and development. A referral to social services and for a dietetic assessment are essential if parents reject this advice.

Free sugars and dental health

Dental decay is caused by constant exposure to acid that is either contained in food and drink or produced by bacteria in the plaque on teeth as the bacteria break down the sugar present in food and drink. Acid is present in all drinks and fruit juices except water and milk.

When there is sufficient time between these acid attacks, saliva neutralises any acid and the tooth enamel recovers its structure. Research has shown that by limiting sugar and sugar-containing foods to 4 times per day or less the risk of dental caries is reduced (Moynihan and Petersen 2004).

Free sugars have a place in balanced nutritious diets, enhancing flavour and enjoyment. As outlined in Chapter 1 the UK Scientific Committee on Nutrition have recommended that free sugars should be restricted to about 5 per cent of total energy intake but this is very difficult to achieve without decreasing palatability and enjoyment of food. Other countries recommend limiting free sugars to 10 per cent of total energy intake. In practice a diet with 5–10 per cent of total energy as free sugars allows the inclusion of foods with small amounts of free sugars up to 4 times per day as discussed above in Table 2.1. An example of including foods with small amounts of free sugars at 3 meals and 1 snack is:

- breakfast – a breakfast cereal with added sugar, honey or syrup OR jam or honey on toast
- midday – a second course of a flavoured yogurt;
- evening meal – a second course of a pudding containing free sugars OR biscuit, cake or muffin alongside fruit;
- 1 snack per day containing free sugars, such as tea bread, scone or hot cross bun.

Free sugars added to food come in a variety of forms and include: honey, all syrups (corn, maize, agave, golden, glucose, fructose etc), sucrose, glucose, maltose, dextrose, fructose, hydrolysed starch, molasses, treacle, raw/brown sugar, demerara and fruit juice.

Foods high in free sugars such as confectionery, chocolate and sweet drinks should be limited to once per week and are best eaten in small quantities at the end of a meal rather than in between meals.

Brushing teeth

Tooth caries (decay) and gum disease can be avoided by twice daily brushing with a fluoride toothpaste as brushing reduces the plaque coating teeth that contains the bacteria that convert sugar into acid.

A regime of brushing teeth last thing at night and one other time in the day should be encouraged, assisted and supervised by an adult until a child is at least 7 years old. Children should be guided not to swallow the toothpaste but to spit it out and not rinse the teeth with water after brushing as this rinses away the fluoride before it is absorbed into the tooth enamel.

Regular Dental Checkups are essential and are offered when children are registered with a dentist.

Sugar-containing medicines

Children who require frequent and multiple medications are particularly at risk of dental decay if sweetened medicines are used. If a sugar-free alternative is not available, the medicine should be given at mealtimes if possible.

Salt

Salt is added to preserve some foods and to enhance flavour in others. Unfortunately, it is a very cheap flavour enhancer and has been used to excess in the food industry. The recommendations for restricting salt and sodium intake are listed in Table 1.3 but these recommendations are not evidence based and are very difficult to achieve. Furthermore, it is very difficult for families to estimate the intake of salt as some fresh foods naturally contain some sodium. Children will certainly not get ill or be harmed if they exceed these recommendations, but if they learn to prefer only salt-flavoured foods they may continue to eat mostly salt-flavoured foods as adults and then would be at risk of raised blood pressure.

In practice, limiting salt intake to a reasonable intake in children means:

- including nutritious foods preserved with salt, such as bread, cheese, Marmite, ham, bacon and salamis as they also contain important nutrients;
- not adding salt to food at the table;
- using herbs and spices rather than extra salt to flavour food in cooking;
- choosing tinned foods without added salt over those tinned with salt;
- limiting the amount of processed foods offered as these usually have a higher salt content than home-cooked foods;
- limiting salty snack foods such as crisps and other packet snacks to once per week at the most.

Saturated fat

Milk, cheese, yogurt, meat and eggs contain a mixture of fats, including saturated fat, but these foods should not be cut out of a children's diets as they are nutritious foods. By limiting the foods high in fat to small quantities as outlined on Table 2.1, the saturated fat content of children's food will be around 10 per cent total energy as recommended in Chapter 1. The foods to reduce are:

- crisps and similar high fat packet snacks;
- fried foods and pastry;
- commercially prepared cakes, biscuits and pastries with a long shelf life.

Caffeine

Excess caffeine can cause interrupted sleep, anxiety and behavioural changes and increased blood pressure. In 2015, The European Food Safety Authority concluded that for children single doses of caffeine up to 3 mg/kg body weight and daily intakes of caffeine up to 3 mg/kg body weight do not raise safety concerns. For a 10-year-old child weighing 30 kg, this would work out to around 90 mg of caffeine, which is just over one 250 ml can of energy drink.

Colours and preservatives in food and drinks

The UK Food Standards Agency currently advises that the following colours should be avoided as research indicates they may affect children's behaviour:

- Tartrazine (E102);
- Ponceau 4 R (E124);
- Sunset yellow FCF (E110);
- Carmosine (E122);
- Quinoline yellow (E104);
- Allura red AC (E129).

Most manufacturers are working towards removing these substances from foods and replacing artificial colourings with natural food dyes.

Meals and snack routines

A planned routine of 3 meals and 1–2 nutritious planned snacks ensures children are not going for long periods of time without an energy boost from food, thus ensuring fairly even blood sugar levels throughout the day. When meals contain 2 courses of different foods they provide a wider range of foods and nutrients. The second course can be something simple like yogurt and fruit or it may be a nutritious pudding. Including a sweet second course after the savoury course makes the meal more of an occasion and more enjoyable for children. As discussed above, it can be included within the recommendations on limiting free sugar intake.

Examples of nutritious puddings are those that contain 1 of more of the following ingredients: milk, flour, eggs, fruit, dried fruit, ground or chopped nuts. For example:

- yogurt with fruit;
- fruit crumble with custard;
- fruit pie with custard;
- other fruit-based puddings such as apple Charlotte or summer pudding;
- bread and butter pudding with dried fruit;
- rice pudding served with fruit;
- quick mixed milk puddings, such as Angel Delight, served with some fruit slices;
- Bakewell tart served with fruit slices;
- sponge cake with custard;
- unsweetened tinned fruit with evaporated milk or ice cream;
- jelly with fruit pieces;
- fruit sponge cakes, such as apple sponge cake;
- egg custard with fruit slices;
- fruit salad with cream;
- fresh fruit, such as strawberries, with cream;
- fresh fruit with a biscuit or piece of cake.

Snacks

Children, particularly young children, may not be able to eat enough in just 3 meals to satisfy their energy and nutrient requirements, so including nutritious foods from food groups 1–4 in their snacks ensures adequate nutrient intakes.

Examples of nutritious snacks are:

- fresh fruit (dried fruit can be cariogenic (decay-causing) when eaten as a snack so it is not advised);
- vegetable sticks, such as carrot, cucumber, pepper, baby corn with dips based on yogurt, cream cheese or pulses such as hummus;
- wholegrain breakfast cereals with milk;
- cheese cubes and crackers/breadsticks or chapatti;
- unsalted nuts (not whole nuts for children under 5 years);
- sandwiches, filled rolls and pitta breads;
- French toast or toast with a range of spreads;
- slices of pizza with a plain dough base that has not been fried;
- yogurt and fromage frais;
- crumpets, scones, pitta bread with a spread;
- currant buns, scones and teacakes;
- pancakes, fruit muffins and plain biscuits;
- home-made plain popcorn;
- cakes containing dried fruit or vegetables or nuts (e.g. fruit cake and carrot cake).

Suitable drinks for meal times include:

- still water;
- milk (plain or flavoured);
- vegetable juices.

The best drinks to offer between meals and with snacks are water and plain milk which do not have the same damaging effect on teeth as acidic and sugary drinks. Water has become a more popular drink in the United Kingdom in recent years but some parents may never offer children water to drink as they do not drink water themselves and some think it is cruel to offer water in place of flavoured drinks.

Daily meal plans combining the food groups

A variety of different eating plans, depending on a family routine, can provide a healthy eating regime with the desired combination of the food groups. There are 2 examples below. They both meet the principles of a balanced nutritious diet having:

- 3 meals;
- 2 snacks;
- 6 drinks;
- 2 courses at each main meal;
- bread, rice, potatoes, pasta and other starchy foods (group 1) at each meal and some snacks;
- fruit and vegetables (group 2) at each meal and some snacks;
- 3 portions of milk, cheese and yogurt (group 3);
- 2–3 portions of meat, fish, eggs, nuts or pulses (group 4);
- oils, butter and fat spreads (group 5) used in food preparation;
- 1 portion of cake, biscuit or pudding to add enjoyment to 1 meal per day (group 6);
- free sugars offered only a maximum of 4 times per day.

Example eating plan 1

In this example, breakfast is a quick meal based on cereal with fruit and milk – a quickly prepared breakfast that would suit a family that has little time in the morning. The midday meal might be served at nursery or school and the evening meal is a cooked meal that the family might eat together.

The 3 milk portions are taken at breakfast, mid-morning snack at nursery or school and for the evening meal pudding.

Figure 2.6 Example eating plan 1

		Food groups included	Sample menu
Breakfast		Bread/rice/potatoes/pasta/starchy food	Breakfast cereal
		Milk/cheese/yogurt	½ portion milk on cereal + ½ glass milk to drink
		Drink	
		Fruit	Banana slices
Snack		Fruit	Pear
		Drink	Milk
Midday meal	1st course	Meat/fish/eggs/nuts/pulses	Meatballs in a tomato and herb sauce topped with grated cheese
		Milk/cheese/yogurt	
		Bread/rice/potatoes/pasta/starchy food	Pasta
		Vegetables	Broccoli florets
	2nd course	Fruit pudding	Apple crumble
	Drink	Drink	Water
Snack		Bread/rice/potatoes/pasta/starchy food + oils/butter/fat spreads	Crackers with butter and Marmite
		Drink	Water to drink
Evening meal	1st course	Meat/fish/eggs/nuts/pulses + Bread/rice/potatoes/pasta/starchy food	Fish and potato piesticks
		Vegetables	Carrot and cucumber
	2nd course	Milk/cheese/yogurt	Yogurt and strawberries
		Fruit	
	Drink	Drink	Water

Example eating plan 2

In this example there is a more substantial breakfast that might suit a family that is not rushed in the morning, for example on a weekend day. The evening meal is a lighter meal with no food from the meat/fish/eggs/nuts/pulses group as there are already 2 portions from this group – 1 at breakfast and 1 at lunch.

Figure 2.7 Example eating plan 2

		Food groups included	Sample menu
Breakfast		Meat/fish/eggs/nuts/pulses + butter + vegetable	Scrambled egg with grilled tomatoes
		Bread/rice/potatoes/pasta/starchy food	Toast
		Drink	Water
Snack		Milk/cheese/yogurt	Glass milk
Midday meal	1st course	Meat/fish/eggs/nuts/pulses	Chicken curry
		Bread/rice/potatoes/pasta/starchy food	Rice
		Vegetable	Green beans
	2nd course	Fruit Pudding + Milk/cheese/yogurt	Fruit sponge with custard
		Drink	Water
Snack		Fruit	Grapes
		Bread/rice/potatoes/pasta/starchy food	Bread sticks/Pretzels
		Drink	Water
Evening meal	1st course	Bread/rice/potatoes/pasta/starchy food + Milk/cheese/yogurt + Vegetable	Cheese and tomato sandwiches
	2nd course	Fruit	Peach slices and cream
		Drink	Water

> **Activity**
>
> Plan a 1-day menu using the appropriate number of portions from each food group for a family. For each meal, itemise the food and how it should be prepared.

Meal planner for a vegetarian diet

Figure 2.8 shows a meal plan for a balanced vegetarian diet including the extra criteria:

- 3 portions of foods from food group 4: 1 at each meal;
- a high-vitamin C food with each meal;
- 2 courses at each main meal;
- extra dried fruit and nuts to provide more iron.

Assessing nutritional adequacy using the food groups

A child's diet can be assessed for adequate nutritional intake by comparing a record of what they have eaten with the principles of healthy eating listed below in Figure 2.9.

How to assess the diet and help parents and children to improve a diet are discussed further in Chapter 5.

Figure 2.8 Vegetarian meal plan

	Day 1	Day 2	Day 3
Breakfast	Scrambled egg with toast and grilled tomatoes	Baked beans on toast	Muesli with added ground almonds and dried fruit
	Milk to drink	Fruit with yogurt	Milk on cereal and to drink
Midday meal	Chickpea curry with spinach and cauliflower	Lentil and parsnip soup with wheatgerm bread	Pasta with red kidney beans in bolognaise sauce
	Rice		Green beans
	Bread and butter pudding with dried fruit	Yogurt and strawberries	Custard and sliced banana
Evening meal	Vegetable soup and peanut butter sandwiches	Tofu and vegetable stir fry with noodles	Pitta bread with hummus
			Red pepper and cucumber sticks
	Raspberries and cream	Pear slices and a muffin	Kiwi fruit with a mini Bakewell tart

Figure 2.9 Prinicples of healthy eating

Food groups	Recommended number of daily age appropriate portions
1. Bread, rice, potatoes, pasta and other starchy foods	Included at each meal – and some snacks
2. Fruit and vegetables	Included at each meal and some snacks
3. Milk, cheese and yogurt	3 portions per day
4. Meat, fish, eggs, nuts and beans	2–3 portions per day
5. Oils, butter and fat spreads	Small amounts in food preparation
6. Cakes, biscuits & puddings	Maximum 1 portion per day
7. Sauces, and sweet/savoury spreads	Up to 2 portions per day
8. Sweet drinks, confectionery and high fat packet snacks	Maximum 1 portion per week
Sugar intake	Foods with free sugars limited to 4 times per day for dental health. No more than 1 portion of cake/ biscuits/pudding/ice cream per day
Drinks	6–8 per day or 1 with each meal and snack
Vitamin supplements	10 micrograms (400IU) Vitamin D3 daily

Energy intake assessment for children over 2 years is based on their Body Mass Index measurements.

References and further reading

Moynihan P and Petersen PE (2004) Diet, nutrition and the prevention of dental diseases. *Public Health Nutrition* 7(1A): 201–226.

More JA, Lanigan J, and Emmett PA (2021) The development of food portion sizes suitable for 4-18-year-old children used in a theoretical meal plan meeting energy and nutrient requirements. *Journal of Human Nutrition and Dietetics*. 00: 1–16. doi: 10.1111/jhn.12852.

Scientific Advisory Committee on Nutrition (SACN)/ Committee on Toxicity (COT) (2004) *Advice on*

Fish Consumption: Benefits and Risks. London: The Stationery Office.

Ministry of Health Brazil (2014) *Brazilian Dietary Guidelines for the Brazilian Population* http://bvsms.saude.gov.br/bvs/publicacoes/dietary_guidelines_brazilian_population.pdf (Accessed April 2020).

Reduced growth in vegan children

Grasgruber P, Cacek J, Kalina T, et al. (Dec 2014) The role of nutrition and genetics as key determinants of the positive height trend. *Economics & Human Biology* **15**: 81–100. doi: 10.1016/j.ehb.2014.07.002. Epub 7 August 2014.

Gat-Yablonski G and De Luca F (2017) Effect of nutrition on statural growth. *Hormone Research in Paediatrics* **88**(1): 46–62. doi: 10.1159/000456547. Epub 31 March 2017.

Millward DJ (2017) Nutrition, infection and stunting: the roles of deficiencies of individual nutrients and foods, and of inflammation, as determinants of reduced linear growth of children. *Nutrition Research Reviews* **30**(1): 50–72. doi: 10.1017/S0954422416000238.

Morency ME, Birken CS, Lebovic G, et al. (August 2017) Association between non-cow milk beverage consumption and childhood height. *American Journal of Clinical Nutrition* **106**(2): 597–602. doi: 10.3945/ajcn.117.156877. Epub 7 June 2017.

3

Social and cultural influences on food choices

Summary

- Cultural and religious food traditions vary widely within the United Kingdom.
- Food traditions vary from family to family so health professionals should not make assumptions about eating habits based on ethnic grouping or religion alone.
- Poverty and low income limits food choices and the ability to provide a healthy diet for children.
- Marketing and advertising influences children's food habits and requests for food.
- Parenting style affects the eating habits and foods consumed by children.

Throughout childhood, children tend to prefer to eat familiar foods. When given a choice of foods they will generally choose foods they have eaten before and enjoyed. They may need to be motivated to try new foods. From the beginning of complementary feeding children learn to like the foods their families choose to offer to them. Although adolescents may reject family foods, as young adults and parents, they are likely to revert to the eating habits they learned during their early childhood.

The very wide range of foods available within the United Kingdom today presents families with a huge choice of foods. Choices are based on:

- availability;
- cost and affordability, depending on socio-economic circumstances;
- cultural and religious traditions;
- family experience and choice of food fashions.

Poor food choices are key factors in the high rates of obesity, dental caries and iron-deficiency anaemia currently prevalent within the United Kingdom. Obesity in children is strongly associated with parental obesity and therefore family food habits.

Feeding practices are routed deeply in cultural and religious traditions. When health professionals understand why and how families make their food choices and engage in particular feeding practices they can give sensitive advice to help families improve their eating habits.

Cultural food traditions

Many different races have migrated to the United Kingdom, each bringing different cultural and religious traditions relating to food. Sharing food traditions and food restrictions can bind groups of people together and set groups apart from each other. This is seen in both religious and geographical food traditions.

Being fully aware of different food customs and practices is important but it is equally important that assumptions about a family's food habits are not made solely on the basis of their ethnic origin or religious grouping. There is enormous diversity in culture, traditions and food habits between and within different ethnic and religious groups and even within a family.

Migrant groups in the United Kingdom come from many different geographical areas. In the 2011 UK census 87 per cent of the population in England and Wales (48.6 million people) were born in the United Kingdom and 13 per cent of the population (7.5 million people) were born outside of the United Kingdom (Table 3.1).

86 per cent are white

8 per cent Asian/Asian British

3 per cent Black/African/Caribbean/Black British

London and the West Midlands are the most ethnically diverse (Figure 3.1).

On migrating to the United Kingdom, geographical groups tend to preserve their eating traditions (Table 3.2). This is seen particularly where larger groups have settled together and have a good source of traditional food through local markets and retailers. However, not all new migrants have access to their culturally acceptable foods – for example asylum seekers may be

Table 3.1 UK population census statistics 2011: ethnic groups

Ethnic Group	Number (thousands) and percentage			
	UK born		Non-UK born	
White	44,774	92.2	3,435	45.8
British	44,186	91.0	949	12.6
Irish	178	0.4	354	4.7
Gypsy or Irish Traveller	51	0.1	7	0.1
Other White	360	0.7	2,126	28.3
Mixed/Multiple ethnic group	985	2.0	239	3.2
White and Black Caribbean	401	0.8	26	0.3
White and Black African	113	0.2	53	0.7
White and Asian	271	0.6	71	0.9
Other Mixed	200	0.4	90	1.2
Asian/Asian British	1,770	3.6	2,443	32.6
Indian	606	1.2	807	10.7
Pakistani	631	1.3	493	6.6
Bangladeshi	232	0.5	215	2.9
Chinese	93	0.2	300	4.0
Other Asian	207	0.4	628	8.4
Black/African/Caribbean/Black British	873	1.8	992	13.2
African	323	0.7	666	8.9
Caribbean	358	0.7	237	3.2
Other Black	192	0.4	89	1.2
Other ethnic group	168	0.3	395	5.3
Arab	64	0.1	167	2.2
Any other ethnic group	105	0.2	228	3.0
		100		100
All	48,571	86.6	7,505	13.4

Source: 2011 Census.

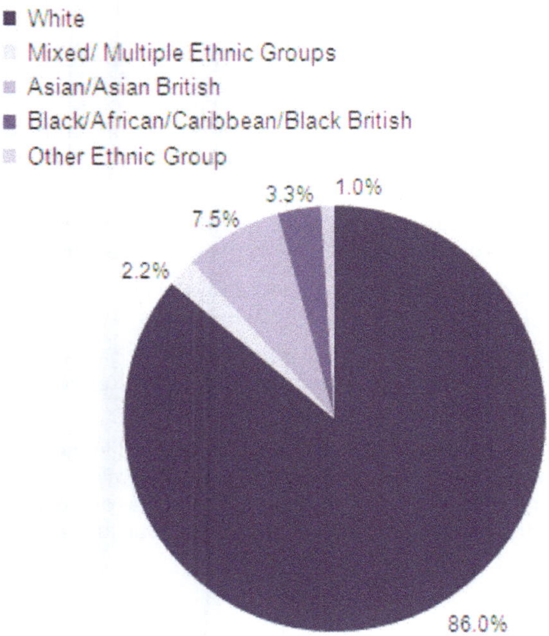

Figure 3.1 Distribution of total minority ethnic population by ethnic group in England and Wales in 2011. Data from Office of National Statistics: (www.ons.gov.uk)

housed in areas where their traditional foods are unobtainable.

Western influences also affect traditional eating patterns of migrant groups to a considerable extent. Younger generations born in the United Kingdom generally move away from traditional dietary practices of their migrant parents and adopt the traditions of their friends and peers.

Activity 1

Visit a shop specialising in foods of 1 of the geographical regions above and make a list of 20 unfamiliar foods and then find out how they are used in the preparation of dishes for that ethnic group.

When ethnic groups do not have access to their traditional foods, they may need advice on how to choose a balanced, nutritious diet from the vast array of foods available in the United Kingdom. However, motivation to seek professional advice is low in many ethnic groups. Factors that influence the uptake of nutritional advice are complex. Those in the lower socio-economic groups are less likely to follow advice if they have a lower educational attainment or are affected by poverty.

A community worker, health professional or facilitator who is trusted and recognised and who speaks the language can improve the outcome of nutritional interventions (*Stockley et al.* 2009).

Activity 2

Make a list of the main barriers to healthy eating for the ethnic groups in your area.

Activity 3

Make a list of factors that reduce motivation of ethnic families to seek professional advice on healthy eating.

Religious food traditions

Within each religious grouping, families decide which food traditions to adopt. In some families 1 parent may observe certain food traditions while the other parent may not. Some common traditions are listed in Table 3.3.

Fasting

Most religions have a tradition of fasting (i.e. not eating any food or excluding certain foods) for particular periods of time (Table 3.3). Pregnant women and young children are usually exempt from fasting, however, some pregnant women may choose to observe these practices.

Religious festivals

Celebratory meals and specific foods are often eaten at festival times, as shown in Table 3.4. Dates of festivals are approximate as they are often based on lunar calendars. (Table 3.5)

Table 3.2 Common traditional foods eaten by groups from different geographical regions that have migrated to the United Kingdom

Migration to the UK from	Traditional foods eaten
Caribbean Islands	Rice, sweet potatoes, yams, green bananas, plantain, dasheen, okra, cornmeal and coconut cream; Beverages based on condensed milk with added sugar or honey; Milk-based energy or malt drinks such as Nutriment, Nourishment, Supermalt, Mighty Malt
South Asia	Chapattis, parathas, puris, bhatura and naan are all types of bread made from wheat flour; Spices; Yogurt; Fried snacks – samosas and pakoras
East Africa	Maize, millet, sorghum, matoke/cooking banana, cassava, sweet potato, yam
West Africa mainly Nigeria and Ghana	Cassava, green bananas, yam, plantain, ground rice, cornmeal, gari and kenkey; Akra or black-eyed beans; Ground nuts and seeds are often part of the meal; Spices; Tropical fruits
China	Balance of yin (coldness) and yang (hotness) is usually observed in meals; Black beans; Soy products such as tofu and soya milk; Green leafy vegetables. Cereals vary: in the north: wheat-based foods such as dumplings and noodles; in the south: rice and foods made from rice flour such as noodles, cakes, vinegar

Socio-economic factors influencing food choice

Nutritional content of diets and ill-health show a marked socio-economic gradient. National nutritional surveys and research have shown that:

- poorer households have a less diverse diet and are less likely to experiment with new foods;
- socio-demographic status of mothers influences the type of diet eaten during pregnancy and the foods fed to her children;
- poverty and poor housing often have an effect on a mother's physical and emotional wellbeing and these in turn affect the choice of foods she makes for her children;
- although there is no significant difference in energy intake between different socio-economic groups, the intakes of most vitamins and minerals in children is lower in lower socioeconomic groups;
- dental caries and iron-deficiency anaemia are both more common in under-fives in low-income households.

Costs that a low-income family might prioritise over buying food include:

- rent/housing;
- heating and lighting;
- gas and electricity bills;
- clothes and shoes for children.

Food choices are limited in low-income families because:

- there may be no public transport links to large supermarkets where foods are cheaper than in smaller local shops;
- families cannot take advantage of better value bulk buys as their fridge and cupboard storage is extremely limited or non-existent;
- families are more likely to spend limited resources on cheap and filling foods that are less nutritious;
- relatively inexpensive sweet foods are given as treats in place of more expensive treats such as toys and branded clothes and shoes;
- the variety of fruit and vegetables available for purchase in small local shops may be limited and of poorer quality;
- families are unlikely to purchase fruit and vegetables again if the children did not like them.

Table 3.3 Common food traditions within religions

Religion	Food tradition
Buddhist and Jains	No meat or fish because of the belief of non-violence to all forms of life
Christian	Meat not eaten on Fridays
Jewish	No pork; Only fish with fins or scales; Milk and milk products are not served with meat
Orthodox Jewish	Kosher meat and milk products
Hindu	No beef or beef products because the cow is sacred; Pork often avoided also as considered unclean; Only fish with fins and scales; Some are vegetarians
Muslim	No pork. Other meats are halal[a]; No alcohol; Hand and feet washing before meals
Rastafarian	Sometimes vegan or no pork or shellfish
Sikh	No pork and sometimes no beef; Vegetarianism is common; No alcohol

[a] Halal meat is from an animal that has been ritually slaughtered by being blessed and allowing the blood to drain – usually after the animal is stunned.

Table 3.4 Common fasting traditions within religions

Religion	Fasting tradition
Christian	Individual choices of certain foods not to be eaten during Lent – 40 days prior to Easter
Hindu and Sikh	Fasting between dawn and dusk on 3 festival days each year – the birthdays of Lord Shiva, Rama and Krishna. Degrees of further fasting are individual choice (e.g. fasting may be 1 or 2 days per week when only milk, yogurt, fruit, potatoes and nuts are eaten). More common in women than men
Jewish	24-hour fast over Yom Kippur
	Certain foods not eaten during Passover
Muslim	Fasting between dawn and dusk during the lunar month of Ramadan. Pregnant women, the elderly and children under 12 years are exempt

Government-funded schemes to support the nutritional intake of children in low-income families include:

- Healthy Start scheme;
- free school milk for young children and subsidised milk for others;
- free school meals.

Entitlement varies and is changed from time to time by governmental policy.

Healthy Start Scheme

This scheme is the latest version of a UK Government-funded scheme to give nutritional support to low-income families with pregnant women and children under 4 years (www.healthystart.nhs.uk). Eligibility to join the scheme depends on family income except for pregnant teenagers under 18 years who are all entitled to join irrespective of their financial circumstances.

Under the scheme low-income families and pregnant teenagers are entitled to:

- weekly vouchers to buy fruit, vegetables, milk and infant formula;
- free vitamin supplements for pregnant and breastfeeding women and children under 4 years of age.

Table 3.5 Religious festivals observed by different religions

Religion	Festival
Buddhist	Veska – birth enlightenment and death of Buddha – usually during May full moon
Christian	Easter – March/April
	Christmas – December/early January
Hindu	Mahashrivatri – birthday of Lord Shiva – March
	Ram Navmi – birthday of Lord Rama – April
	Janmastami – birthday of Lord Krishna – late August
	Navaratri – nine nights October
	Holi – March
	Raksha Bandhan – August
	Diwali – Festival of Lights and New Year – October/November
Jewish	Rosh Hashana New Year – September/October
	Yom Kippur Day of Atonement – ten days later
	Passover – eight days in April
Muslim	Eid al-Fitr ('little Eid') – at the end of the Ramadan
	Eid al-Adah ('big Eid')
Sikh	Baissakha – New Year's day – April
	Diwali – Festival of Light – October/November
	Birth of Guru Nanak – November

Activity 4

Make a list of factors that need to be addressed around food and nutrition in low-income families.

Cultural variations in feeding practices

Cutlery

Some families use cutlery or chopsticks while others only use their hands; some only eat food with their right hand.

Eating environment

This may be a table, food on laps in front of the television, or eating while sitting on the floor. Some families always eat with the television on, others never with the television or distractions.

Self-feeding by infants and toddlers

Some families encourage self-feeding from the beginning of complementary feeding, other parents prefer to take control of all the infant and toddler feeding and these children do not get the opportunity to learn to self-feed until older.

Mealtime routines

Some families do not eat around a planned daily routine of 3 meals and 2–3 snacks and allow grazing on food throughout the day.

Marketing and media influences on food choices

Eating behaviours and food choices can be strongly influenced by advertising, food packaging and presentation of food content.

Children are increasingly targeted with advertising and marketing. Large sums of money are spent targeting them with food advertising to build brand loyalty and persuade them to want particular food products, starting from when they are toddlers. Children younger than eight years are especially vulnerable because they lack the cognitive skills to understand the persuasive intent of television and online advertisements (Calvert 2008).

Marketing experts know that toddlers and children have considerable purchase influence and successfully negotiate purchases through 'nag factor' or 'pester power'. Requests are often for brand name products and food accounts for over half of total requests, with parents honouring these requests 50 per cent of the time (Story and French 2004). The most requested item is breakfast cereal, followed by snacks, drinks and toys.

Media messages about food are targeted at children through:

- television, radio, internet and social media advertisements;
- in-store displays;
- child-friendly packaging, including familiar cartoon characters on the packaging;
- stealth marketing techniques such as embedding products in the programme content in films, online and in video games.

High-fat, high-sugar and low-fibre foods are regularly advertised and often feature messages implying that low-nutrient foods are beneficial. These implications, although not technically false, may nonetheless confuse children and their parents about what makes a particular food a healthy choice. Older children exposed to advertising chose advertised food products significantly more often than those who were not exposed (Story and French 2004).

Several studies point towards the contribution of food marketing to the rising levels of childhood obesity (Boyland et al. 2016). In Australia and Canada industry self-regulation initiatives to restrict low nutrient food advertising to children have not shown any success (Smithers et al. 2014, Potvin Kent and Wanless 2014).

Activity 5

- Make a note of the foods advertised to children on television during several periods of children's television viewing time (e.g. 16:00–19:00) and calculate the percentages of nutritious and non-nutritious foods advertised.

Activity 6

- List the negative effects that television viewing has on children's eating habits and health.

Food fashions

Food choices change over time and food fashions can influence the nutritional quality of food consumption and health. Environmental factors such as plastic packaging on food and cleaning chemicals in the home have now been shown to influence the gut microbiome and consequently health (Mei et al. 2020). Following some food fashions may be nutritionally adequate for adults but may compromise the nutritional quality of children's diets which need to be more nutrient dense than adults' diets to support their optimal growth and development.

Recent positive food fashions

- Sustainable food choices may be based on 1 or more philosophies e.g.:
  - locally grown and seasonal foods;
  - less processed foods and foods cooked from basic ingredients means less chemical additives in food (Gultekin et al. 2019);
  - avoiding plastic packaging reduces plastic pollution and also lowers intake of food contaminated with chemicals from plastic.

Recent food fashions with a negative effect for children

- Meat and dairy are excluded because of perceived carbon footprint – these are both nutritious foods and limited quantities in children's diets ensure a more nutritious diet – both meat and dairy protein ensure optimal growth in height by exerting positive influences on the growth plate in the long bones of children.

- Only plant based or vegan diet to reduce cost and carbon footprint – without meat and milk protein in the diet children will grow to be shorter than their genetic potential (see page 24). Additionally vegan substitute foods can be highly processed with chemicals and additives to provide a required texture.
- Dairy free – chosen for perceived health benefits without the medical need to investigate or manage a milk protein allergy. Without supplements to compensate for the key nutrients in milk – calcium, riboflavin, iodine and vitamin A, long term effects can be poor bone health and hypothyroidism with limited growth and brain development.
- Gluten free – chosen for perceived health benefits without the medical need to treat coeliac disease or gluten sensitivity. Wheat is a nutritious cereal and using less nutritious cereals such as rice and maize in place of wheat reduces a child's iron and B vitamin intake.
- Low carbohydrate – this may help with weight loss for some but may cause very low blood sugar levels in some children. The effects of low blood sugar levels can be irritability, poor behaviour, poor concentration and lethargy.

Influence of family feeding practices and parenting skills

The mother is often the key decision-maker in feeding children, however, this is not so in all cultures and families. Other household members who may purchase the foods for the children and prepare and cook meals and snacks are:

- father;
- maternal grandmother or grandfather;
- paternal grandmother or grandfather;
- most elderly member or other members of the household;
- older sibling who can speak English while other members of the household do not;
- staff at the nursery the infant or young child attends;
- babysitters;
- child minders;
- other carers.

Family meals

Eating together as a family in a relaxed and enjoyable way is an important social time in family life as well as a learning opportunity for children: they learn to eat different foods and improve their feeding skills.

Parents are very strong role models for young children who learn by copying. When parents eat nutritious foods themselves and offer the same foods to their children, the children have the opportunity to learn to like those nutritious foods. Young children are less likely to try new foods that they have not seen other people eating.

However, eating together as a family has become less common due to:

- parents' long working hours and long commuting times;
- shift work;
- preference of parents not to eat at the same time as their children.

With many young children eating separately from their parents, the concept of 'children's food' has developed. When young children are given control over what is served they tend to choose familiar foods, thereby narrowing down the range of foods they eat and forgoing the experience of a wider range of foods and the opportunity to learn to like the foods adults are eating.

Older children who consume more meals with their families have:

- better nutritional intakes (Gillman et al. 2000, Sweeting and West 2005);
- a lower risk of obesity (Taveras et al. 2005).

Videon and Manning (2003) found parental presence at the evening meal was associated with a higher consumption of fruits, vegetables, milk, yogurt and cheese, as well as less skipping of breakfast in adolescents.

Parenting styles

A parent or carer's role is to offer nutritious meals and snacks to young children in pleasant social environments but to allow each child to decide when they have had enough to eat, so that they develop an understanding of feeling hungry and eating to satisfy that feeling.

Parenting styles influence the range and type of foods that children are prepared to eat. A positive parenting style makes mealtimes enjoyable and improves nutritional intakes through a wider range of nutritious foods being eaten.

Rudolf (2009) has described four parenting styles that relate to responsiveness and control (Figure 3.2). Positive parenting is being responsive to children's emotional and physical needs while being in charge and setting appropriate and clear boundaries. This is the *authoritative* style and parents using this style will buy a range of nutritious foods and encourage and prompt children to eat them while making allowances for their individual tastes and preferences. Children will be allowed to decide when they have had enough to eat.

The *authoritarian* parenting style takes control beyond any consideration of a child's needs, feelings or preferences. Parents may insist children eat certain foods and may resort to coercing and forcefeeding. Children may be forced to finish all the food on their plates even when they have indicated they have had enough. Certain foods that the parent deems unsuitable may be denied altogether, making them very desirable in the child's mind.

The *indulgent* parenting style is responsive to the child's wishes and demands even when they are not in the child's best interests. This will include giving children full control over what food is to be served, thereby narrowing the range of foods they eat. In addition giving in to demands for frequent portions of sweet or high-fat foods which will provide less nutrients and excess energy, these children will also be at risk of dental caries.

A *neglectful* parenting style is where the parent is neither in charge nor responsive to the child. There may be no routine of meals and planned snacks and nutritious foods, that maintain health and growth, may not be offered.

Positive and negative feeding practices are described in Table 3.6.

Using food and drinks as rewards, treats or for comfort

The most desirable reward for young children is their parents' attention. However, sweet, energy-dense, low-nutrient foods are often used as a substitute for this and given outside of meal and planned snack times to:

- show love and affection;
- receive affection from the child;
- comfort them;
- reward for good behaviour;
- bribe young children to modify their behaviour;
- bribe young children to eat a food or meal they are refusing.

Encouraging such foods to be regarded as desirable is not compliant with teaching healthy eating.

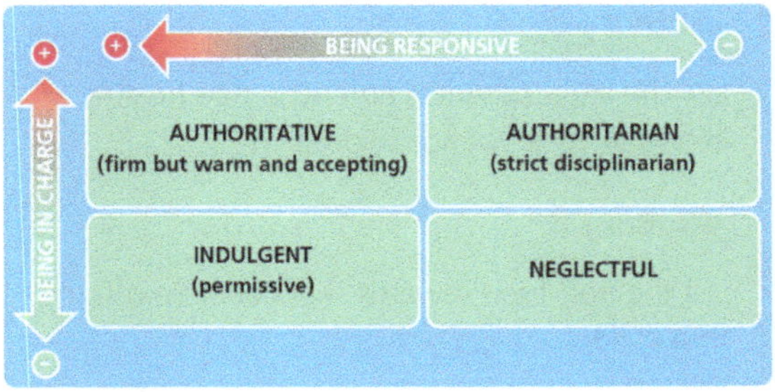

Figure 3.2 The model of parenting proposed by Mary Rudolf has four styles relating to responsiveness and control

Table 3.6 Positive and negative feeding practices by parents and carers

Positive feeding practices	Negative feeding practices
Praising when food is eaten	Coercion or coaxing children to eat healthy foods
Taking away uneaten food without comment	Coercion or coaxing children to eat more when they indicate they have had enough
Parents eating with children and eating the foods they want the young children to eat	Offering alternatives or rewards to encourage more food to be eaten
Pleasant interaction with young children during the mealtime	Encouraging children to finish up everything on their plate
Offering appropriate portion sizes	

Advantages of a meal and snack routine

Routines help young children to feel secure. A feeding routine of 3 meals and 2–3 planned nutritious snacks throughout the day:

- prevents grazing on less nutritious food throughout the day;
- prevents young children becoming over hungry or thirsty by going too long between eating occasions;
- avoids attempts to feed young children when they are ready to sleep and too tired to eat;
- prevents toddlers not being hungry at meal times because they have eaten snacks or had large sweet drinks just before the meal.

Activity 7

List the factors to consider before giving advice to families.

Activity 8

List the ways parents can encourage healthy eating in their young children.

Activity 9

List the non-food rewards that could be offered to a child.

Activity 10

List the disadvantages of not eating together as a family.

Social and cultural influences on infant feeding choices

Factors affecting infant feeding practices adopted by families and how they follow the infant feeding recommendations include:

- socio-economic status;
- parental age;
- personality;
- educational attainment of the mother;
- infant's birth order;
- consistency of advice from health professionals.

Breastfeeding vs. formula feeding

Although the health benefits of exclusive breastfeeding from birth until beginning complementary feeding for both infants and mothers are well documented, about 1 in 5 mothers in the United Kingdom do not initiate breastfeeding at birth and by 1 week of age less than half of infants are being exclusively breastfed. Breastfeeding rates are slowly increasing but for the past 80 years or so, infant formula milks (breast milk substitutes) have been widely available and have become accepted by many people as equivalent to breastfeeding. Formula feeding is often portrayed in the media as the socio-cultural norm and female breasts are associated with sexuality. As a result:

- many women are surrounded by family and friends who have not breastfed and have never seen a baby breastfeeding;

- many mothers feel embarrassed breastfeeding in front of others both outside and within the home;
- breastfeeding in public may be met with disapproval despite laws in both Scotland and England making it illegal not to allow breastfeeding in public places.

In addition:

- lack of appropriate staff training within health services leads to lack of knowledge, skills and confidence in health professionals and inappropriate practices and routines persist;
- breastfeeding is not a priority in all maternity units and promotion is often left to advocates;
- women may lack support to continue exclusive breastfeeding from health services and their social networks;
- breastfeeding support services are frequently short-term initiatives rather than embedded in mainstream services.

Many women find breastfeeding challenging and give up earlier than they wish to. As shown in Figure 3.3, breastfeeding rates are higher among mothers:

- from higher occupational groups;
- with highest educational levels;
- aged 30 or over;
- of first babies.

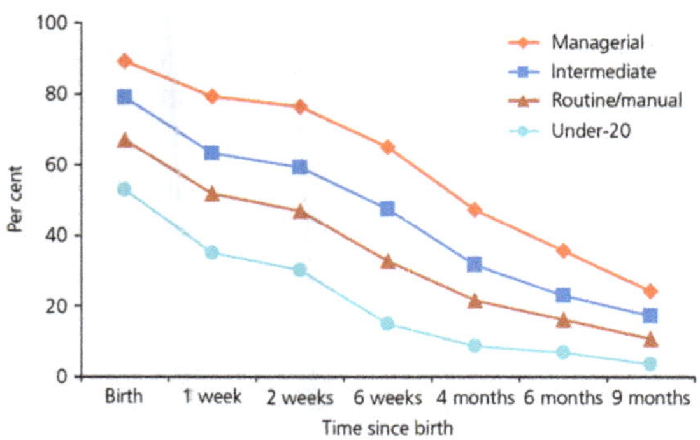

Figure 3.3 Duration of breastfeeding by mother's socio-economic group and age under 20 years. 2005

Some families are reluctant to change infant feeding practices from those handed down by previous generations, and certain cultural practices are at variance with the Department of Health infant feeding guidelines and can compromise the nutritional intake of infants. Such practices include:

- women not taking vitamin D supplements during pregnancy and breastfeeding – particularly those at higher risk of low vitamin D levels (see page 83);
- giving water rather than colostrum to newborn babies as colostrum is seen as having a poor nutritional value or being unhealthy;
- preference for formula feeding rather than breastfeeding because formula feeding is seen as a Western ideal and therefore assumed to be better for the baby;
- herbal teas given during infancy as they are deemed to have health benefits;
- boiled water and barley water given to infants as 'cooling' drinks to balance breast milk which is seen as a 'hot' food;
- cow's milk introduced in place of formula milk before 12 months of age because it is cheaper than formula milks;
- beginning complementary feeding very early, before 4 months, or late, after 6 months
- inappropriate complementary foods;
- convenience and sweet foods that are low in iron given due to limited availability of halal or nutritious vegetarian savoury complementary foods;
- little variety of complementary foods given (e.g. low-nutrient porridge given at all meals in the day);
- coercing infants to eat/drink to excess as a rapid weight gain or a 'bonny baby' is seen as an indicator of health and wellbeing.

References and further reading

Birch LL and Davison KK (2001) Family environmental factors influencing the developing behavioural controls of food intake and childhood overweight. *Pediatrics Clinics of North America* **48**(4): 893–907.

Boyland EJ, Harrold JA, Kirkham TC *et al.* (2011) Food commercials increase preference for energy-dense foods, particularly in children who watch more television. *Pediatrics* **128**(1): e93–e100.

Boyland EJ, Nolan S, Kelly B et al. (February 2016) Advertising as a cue to consume: a systematic review and meta-analysis of the effects of acute exposure to unhealthy food and nonalcoholic beverage advertising on intake in children and adults. *The American Journal of Clinical Nutrition* **103**(2): 519–533. Epub 20 January 2016.

Burgess-Champoux TL, Larson N, Neumark-Sztainer D, Hannan PJ and Story M (2009) Are family meal patterns associated with overall diet quality during the transition from early to middle adolescence. *Journal of Nutrition Education and Behavior* **41**(2): 79–86.

Calvert SL (2008) Children as consumers: advertising and marketing. *Future Child* **18**: 205–234.

Chiu K, Warner G, Nowak RA, Flaws JA and Mei W (2020) The Impact of environmental chemicals on the gut microbiome, toxicological sciences, kfaa065, https://doi.org/10.1093/toxsci/kfaa065.

Food Standards Agency and Public Health England (2018) *Results of the National Diet and Nutrition Survey (NDNS) Rolling Programme for 2014 to 2015 and 2015 to 2016.* www.gov.uk/government/statistics/ndns-results-from-years-7-and-8-combined (Accessed 1 November 2018).

Gillman MW, Rifas-Shiman SL, Frazier AL *et al.* (2000) Family dinner and diet quality among older children and adolescents. *Archives of Family Medicine* **93**(3): 235–240.

Gultekin F, Oner ME, Savas HB and Dogan B (2019) Food additives and microbiota. *Northern Clinics of Istanbul* **7**(2): 192–200. Published 17 July 2019. doi: 10.14744/nci.2019.92499.

Netto G, Bhopal R, Lederle N, Khatoon J and Jackson A (2010) How can health promotion interventions be adapted for minority ethnic communities? Five principles for guiding the development of behavioural interventions. *Health Promotion International* **25**(2): 248–257.

North K, Emmett P, Noble S and the ALSPAC Study Team (2000) Types of drinks consumed by infants at 4 and 8 months of age: socio-demographic variations. *Journal of Human Nutrition and Dietetics* **13**: 71–82.

Potvin Kent M and Wanless A (2014) The influence of the Children's Food and Beverage Advertising Initiative: change in children's exposure to food advertising on television in Canada between 2006–2009. *International Journal of Obesity* **38**: 558–562. doi:10.1038/ijo.2014.4.

Powell LM, Schermbeck RM, Chaloupka FJ (December 2013) Nutritional content of food and beverage products in television advertisements seen on children's programming. *Childhood Obesity* **9**(6): 524–531. Epub 8 November 2013.

Rudolf M (2009) *Tackling Obesity through the Healthy Child Programme. A Framework for Action.* Leeds: University of Leeds.

Smithers LG, Lynch JW and Merlin TJ (May 2014) Industry self-regulation and TV advertising of foods to Australian children. *Paediatrics and Child Health* **50**(5): 386–392. Epub 27 December 2013.

Stockley L and Associates (2009) *Review of Dietary Intervention Models for Black and Minority Ethnic Groups.* Cardiff: The Food Standards Agency Wales.

Story M, French S (2004) Food advertising and marketing directed at children and adolescents in the US. *International Journal of Behavioral Nutrition and Physical Activity* **1**: 3.

Sweeting H and West P (2005) Dietary habits and children's family lives. *Journal of Human Nutrition and Dietetics* **18**: 93–97.

Taveras EM, Rifas-Shiman SL, Berkey CS *et al.* (2005) Family dinner and adolescent overweight. *Obesity Research* **13**(5): 900–906.

Videon TM and Manning CK (2003) Influences on adolescent eating patterns: the importance of family meals. *Journal of Adolescent Health* **32**(5): 365–373.

Resources

The Ishmali Nutrition Centre – a guide to traditional foods of African, Central and South Asian, and Middle Eastern origin www.theismaili.org/nutrition (Accessed July 2020).

Healthy Start Scheme www.healthystart.nhs.uk (Accessed July 2020).

Working with homeless people https://www.qni.org.uk/nursing-in-the-community/homeless-health-programme/ (Accessed July 2020).

World Health Organization (2010) Recommendations on marketing foods and beverages to children. www.who.int/dietphysicalactivity/marketing-food-to-children/en/Index.html (Accessed July 2020).

World Health Organisation (2016) Tackling food marketing to children in a digital world: trans-disciplinary perspectives. https://www.euro.who.int/__data/assets/pdf_file/0017/322226/Tackling-food-marketing-children-digital-world-trans-disciplinary-perspectives-en.pdf (Accessed July 2020).

Section 2

Assessment of growth and nutritional intake

4 **Measuring and Assessing Growth**

5 **Assessing Nutritional Intake**

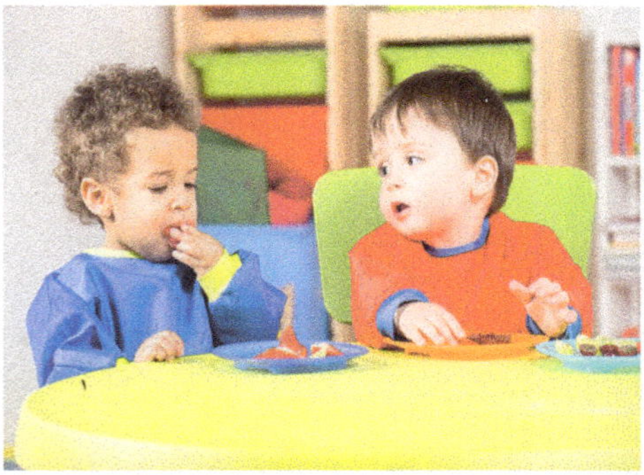

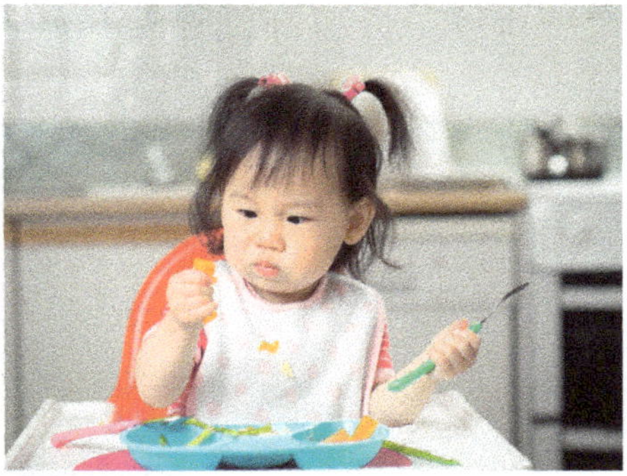

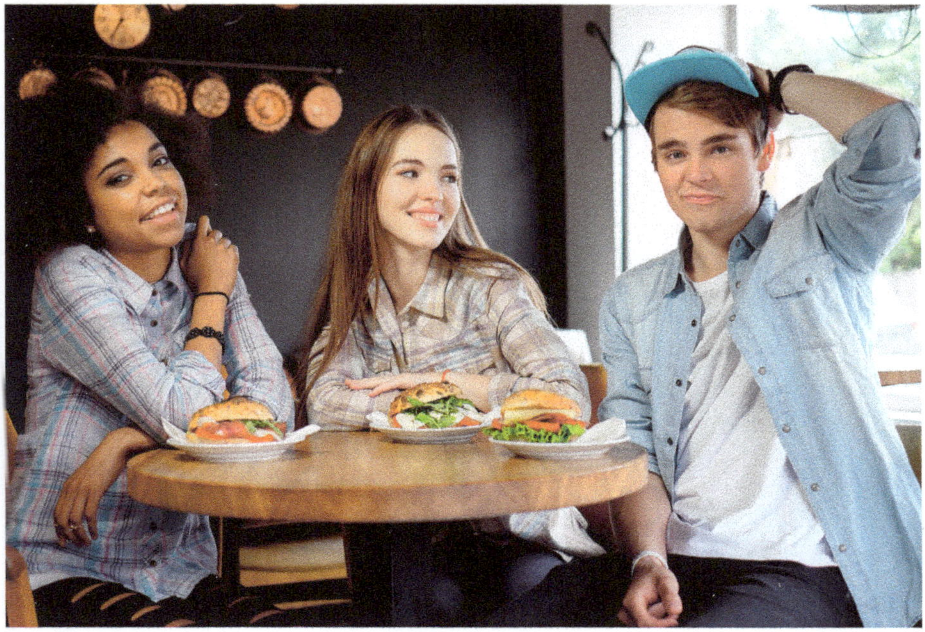

4

Measuring and assessing growth

Summary

- Growth is influenced by genetic inheritance and biological and environmental factors.
- Measuring growth is key to monitoring the nutritional, endocrine, emotional and physical health of children.
- Growth assessment requires training to take accurate measurements using calibrated equipment and to plot and interpret growth and body mass index (BMI) charts.
- Growth charts describe the normal range of weight and length/height children are expected to be at any age.
- Infants and children normally grow parallel to centile lines on growth charts although some variation is normal due to illness, cyclical growth and varying ages of the pubertal growth spurt.
- Frequent measurements are not necessary in normal healthy infants and children and can cause unnecessary stress and concern.

Measuring growth is a key tool in monitoring normal development and is used as part of a nutritional assessment. When energy intake from food and drinks is adequate, weight gain will be within normal parameters. Normal growth measurements can reassure health professionals and parents while variations from expected growth can be an important indicator in diagnosing obesity, growth faltering, endocrine disorders, emotional neglect and other medical conditions. Growth rates vary throughout childhood and knowledge of how and why they vary is important for interpreting growth measurements.

Biological drivers of growth

Growth is the product of many biological and environmental interactions spanning numerous cell and tissue types acting during pre- and postnatal development. Chondrogenesis, which is the biological process that drives height gain, occurs in the growth plates which are found near the ends of the bones. More than 100 genes are involved, hence the tendency for children's growth patterns to relate to their parent's stature. The on and off switches for the 88 growth genes acting on the chondrocytes in the growth plates are unknown. Bone growth drives muscle growth.

Growth is regulated by both positive and negative influences and the key drivers change as age increases.

Negative influences include: stress and anxiety, pathogens and infections.

The main positive influences (Table 4.1) include:

- nutrition including energy, micronutrients, protein and protein type – milk and meat

Table 4.1 Main drivers of growth at different ages

Age	Main drivers of growth in length or height
Prenatal	Maternal nutrition, IGF-1, IGF-2, EGF, FGF, TGF, insulin
Infancy 0–12 months	Nutrition, growth hormone, IGF-1
Childhood	Growth hormone, IGF-1, thyroxine
Puberty	Growth hormone, IGF-1, sex steroids: testosterone in boys and oestrogen in girls

proteins are believed to have positive influences and their absence in vegan diets results in a lower adult height;

- hormones;
- growth factors such as insulin-like growth factor 1 (IGF-I), insulin-like growth factor 2 (IGF-II), epidermal growth factor (EGF), fibroblast growth factor (FGF) and transforming growth factor (TGF);
- extracellular matrix molecules and intracellular proteins.

Growth rates throughout childhood

Prenatal growth is the most rapid phase of growth in children. Growth rate slowly declines during infancy and early childhood until during the primary school years when children grow at a fairly steady rate of about 5–6 cm/year. This declines to about 4–5 cm/ year just prior to the pubertal growth spurt, during which the growth rate increases rapidly for a period of about 3 years (Tables 4.2 and 4.3). The stages and physiological characteristics of puberty are shown in Table 4.4.

The age at which the pubertal growth spurt begins varies enormously as it is influenced by genetics, gender, ethnicity, physical activity and body weight. It occurs over about 3 years and is a period of rapid growth in height which occurs as a result of the synergistic effects of sex hormones and growth hormone. Adipose tissue stores also increase, with girls depositing adipose tissue at a greater rate than boys, laying down stores in the breast and hip regions. Fat deposition in boys tends to be more central.

In girls, the pubertal growth spurt begins at the commencement of puberty, at the time breast development begins, with the greatest height increase in the year preceding menarche. On average, girls grow a further 6 cm in height after menarche which occurs around 13 years of age. The age range for menarche is 10–16.5 years, with tall, heavy girls tending to begin menstruation earlier than their smaller, leaner classmates. Vigorous exercise, such as athletics, can delay menarche because of both the physiological effects of training and the depletion of body fat.

Boys start their growth spurt on average 2 years later than girls and will be the shorter of the 2 sexes for a period of time. Growth may not cease completely at the end of adolescence and a height increase of up to 2 cm can still occur between the ages of 17 and 28 years. Boys will eventually be on average 14.5 cm taller than girls.

Table 4.2 Average growth rates at different ages

Age/developmental stage	Weight gain (kg/ year)	Length/ Height gain (cm/year)
Infant	6.6	25
1–2 years	2.5	12
3 years-puberty	2	5–6
Female adolescent growth spurt	3.9	8 (6–10)
Male adolescent growth spurt	3.7	9 (6–13)

Table 4.3 Pubertal growth spurt statistics

	Girls	Boys
Average age of peak growth rate	11–11.5 years	13–13.5 years
Mean total gain in height over the 3-year growth spurt	20–25 cm	25–30 cm
Average final height	1.63 m	1.78 m

Table 4.4 Stages of Puberty showing physiological changes

	Pre-puberty	In Puberty	Completing Puberty
Girls	No signs of pubertal development	Any breast enlargement with nipples also enlarged	All of the following: Starting periods (menarche); Breast, pubic hair and auxillary hair development
Boys	No signs of pubertal development	Any of the following present: Slight deepening of the voice; Early pubic or armpit hair growth; Enlargement of the testes or penis	Any of the following present: Voice fully broken; Moustache and early facial hair growth; Adult size penis with pubic and auxillary hair

Anthropometric measurement

The most common measurements taken to assess growth are:

- weight using digital scales that are maintained and calibrated annually in line with medical devices standards;
- length for children under 2 years and height for children over 2 years (Figure 4.1a and 4.1c);
- head circumference measured around the widest part of the head (Figure 4.1b).

Additional measures can be used:

- waist circumference – a measure of the amount of fat stored centrally;
- mid upper arm circumference (MUAC) – used to screen for malnutrition in under-fives in the developing world. A MUAC<11 cm in infants 2–6 months and MUAC<11.5 cm in children 6 months to 5 years is used as 1 indicator of severe malnutrition;
- skinfold thicknesses – not regularly used but can be a useful measure when weight is inaccurate because of fluid retention such as oedema or ascites.

Assessing growth and body mass index on centile charts

Children's growth is assessed by plotting successive accurate measurements of weight and length/height on centile charts that describe weight for age and length/height for age, respectively. Accurate measurements must be taken on calibrated scales. Staff taking measurements, and plotting and interpreting growth charts should undertake training for this purpose. Practical training is usually done on the job with more experienced staff but online resources are available and are listed at the end of this chapter.

Body mass index (BMI) is a measure of thinness and fatness and is calculated by dividing the weight in kilograms by the square of the height in metres:

$$\mathbf{BMI} = \frac{\textbf{weight in kg}}{(\textbf{height in m})^2}$$

For example a young child weighing 13.2 kg and measuring 91 cm or 0.91 m will have a BMI of $13.2/(0.91)^2 = 15.9$. This figure can then be plotted on the BMI-for-age centile chart.

Recommendations for measuring children

Frequency of measuring infants and children

As a minimum, infants should be weighed at (National Institute for Health and Care Excellence 2014):

- birth;
- in the first week, as part of an overall assessment of feeding;
- times of routine immunisations at 8,12 and 16 weeks and at 1 year.

If there is concern, children should be weighed and measured as part of monitoring; however, weights measured too closely together are often misleading and can cause stress and concern. A full or empty

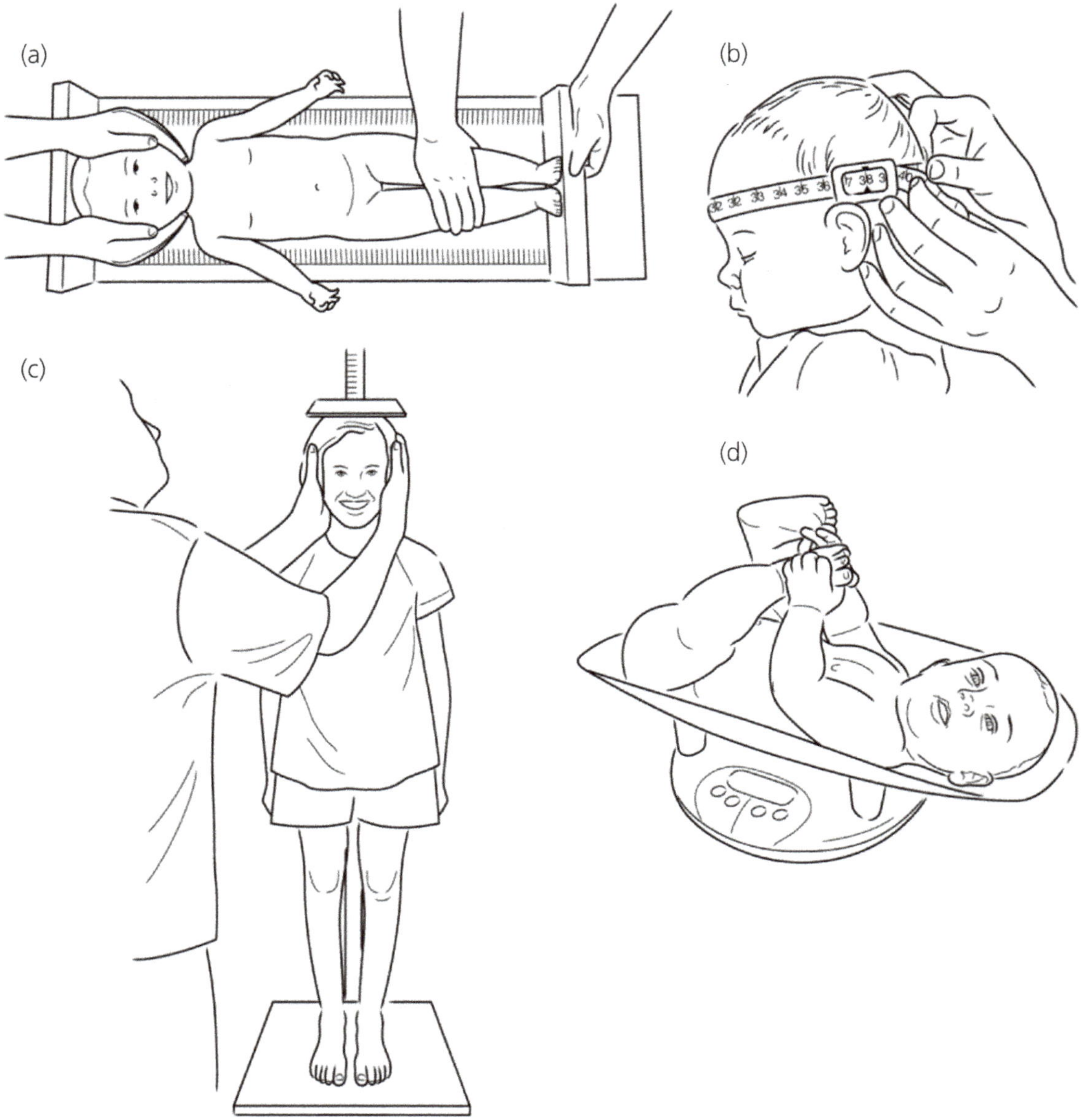

Figure 4.1 (a) Measuring length (b) Measuring head circumference (c) Measuring height (d) Measuring weight of an infant

bladder can make a significant difference to the weight of an infant. Weighing more frequently than:

- once a month up to 6 months of age;
- once every 2 months from 6 to 12 months of age;
- once every 3 months over the age of 1 year.

is not necessary in healthy children.

Length is not normally measured during infancy as it is hard to measure accurately and weight is an adequate indication of growth during the first year.

Head circumference is usually measured within 24 hours of birth and at 8 weeks; thereafter only if there are neurodevelopmental concerns.

Clothing

Infants and children up to 2 years should be weighed naked, without a nappy. Thereafter they can be weighed in underwear or very light clothing without shoes or socks.

Supine (lying on the back) length is measured up until 2 years and without clothing or a nappy as they can distort the hips and make the measurement inaccurate. Standing height is measured after 2 years of age and children can wear clothing but should remove shoes and socks. Any head wear such as topknots must also be removed.

Measuring equipment

Only class III clinical electronic scales in metric setting should be used to weigh children. These should be maintained and calibrated annually, in line with medical devices standards EC Directive 90/384 EEC.

Most equipment for measuring length and height is self-calibrating or should be adjusted with a standard measure.

Tapes for measuring head, waist, hip or limb circumferences should be made of a narrow, non-stretchable material such as paper or plastic.

Growth charts

Growth charts have been constructed by measuring a large number of healthy children at varying ages. Centile lines are then constructed showing the normal distribution of weight/height/head circumference measurements at each age. The 50th centile line is the median of the measurements for that age. Fifty per cent of children will have measurements below that line and the other 50 per cent will be above that line. The other centile lines are constructed using standard deviations from the median. The 25th and 75th centile lines are 2/3 of a standard deviation from the median. Twenty-five per cent of children's measurements will be below the 25th centile line and 75 per cent of children's measurements will be above that centile line.

The 2nd and 98th centiles are 2 standard deviations (or 2 *z* scores) above and below the median.

In the UK, 2 sources of data are used for the construction of the recommended reference charts (Table 4.5):

- The UK 90 reference data is from a large number of measurements of children living in the UK during the 1980s and up to 1990. These charts describe the average growth of children at this time before the epidemic of childhood obesity began. They are considered a reference for normal growth in the UK.
- The World Health Organization (WHO) Child Growth Standards were developed using data collected in the WHO Multicentre Growth Reference Study, which was a community-based, multi-country project conducted in Brazil, Ghana, India, Norway, Oman and the United States. In each of the six countries a sample of breastfed term infants from non-smoking, non-deprived mothers were measured longitudinally. Growth was found to be similar in all six countries and growth charts using the data describe the optimal growth 0–4 years for all children from different ethnic groups.

Table 4.5 Data sources for different age groups

Age group	Source of data
Preterm infants	UK 90 reference data
Term infants at birth	UK 90 reference data
2 weeks to 4 years of age	WHO data collected in the WHO Multicentre Growth Reference Study
5–18 years	UK 90 reference data

Growth charts recommended for use in the UK

The different growth charts in the UK (Table 4.6) all have 9 centile lines: 0.4th, 2nd, 9th, 25th, 50th, 75th, 91st, 98th and 99.6th. Each type comes in 1 version for boys and 1 for girls as boys and girls have slightly different growth patterns. The

Table 4.6 Growth charts recommended in the UK

Charts	Use for
Neonatal and Infant Close Monitoring Chart (NICM) – boys and girls	1. births before 32 weeks gestation 2. unwell neonates born after 32 weeks 3. term infants with significant growth and weight faltering
UK-WHO Growth Chart 0–4 years – boys and girls	Healthy preterm infants born after 32 weeks gestation; Term infants; Young children 1–4 years
4–18 years Growth and BMI Chart – boys and girls	Children 5–18 years
2–20 years Childhood and puberty close monitoring (CPCM) growth chart Boys and girls	Children and young people whose growth requires close monitoring, or whose measurements are outside the usual centile range

correct term for the area between the centile lines is 'centile space'.

These charts all come in 2 formats:

- A4 which are used mainly in clinical notes;
- A5 for use in the Personal Child Health Record (Growth charts for boys 0–4 years and 2–18 years, and girls 0–4 years and 2–18 years are given in Appendix 2 p. 273–281).

The PCHR, also known as the 'Red Book', is used in the UK to record the health and development of a child. It is given to parents/carers following the birth of every child (Figure 4.2).

BMI centile charts are used for assessing if children aged over 2 years are underweight, normal weight for height, overweight or obese (See Appendix 3 p. 283–287).

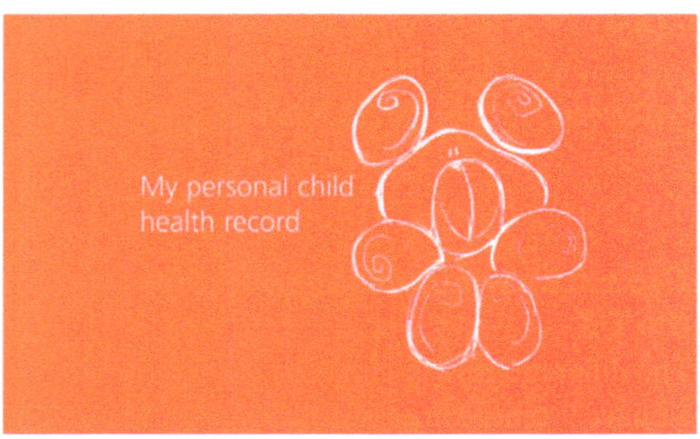

Figure 4.2 Personal Child Health Record used in the UK – also called 'Red Book'

Any other growth charts for normal children are now considered out of date by the Royal College of Paediatrics and Child Health. All recommended charts are produced and printed by Harlow Printing Ltd and can be ordered from them (www.healthforallchildren.co.uk).

There are specialised growth charts for children with:

- Down syndrome;
- Turner syndrome;
- Homozygous sickle cell disease;
- Noonan syndrome;
- Williams' syndrome;
- Cerebral Palsy www.LifeExpectancy.org/articles/GrowthCharts.shtml
- Prader-Willi syndrome;
- Achondroplasia;
- Wolf-Hirschhorn.

Plotting on growth charts

Charts should be plotted in pencil with a dot. Pencil is used because mistakes in plotting are often made and can be corrected more easily if plotted in pencil. The dots should not be joined up with a line, nor emphasised with a circle around them. When several plots are made over a short time it is easier to read the pattern of the dots than crosses which obscure more of the chart.

Age correction for preterm babies

The measurements of preterm babies should be age-corrected when plotting for:

- 1 year for infants born 32–36 weeks gestation;
- 2 years for infants born before 32 weeks gestation.

Age correction adjusts the plot of a measurement to account for the number of weeks a baby was born early. The number of weeks early is equal to 40 weeks minus the gestational age at birth. Hence a baby born at 31 weeks gestation will have been born 9 weeks (40–31 = 9) early and his or her age since birth should be reduced by 9 weeks when plotting measurements taken up until the age of 2 years.

Normal growth patterns

The weight and length/height of infants and children are expected to increase along, or parallel to, the centile lines. However, growth is not usually regular so some small variation over about a centile space is usually seen in normal growth patterns. Growth anywhere between the 2nd and 98th centile lines is considered normal. Growth between the 0.4th and 2nd centile and between the 98th and 99.6th is usually normal and should be interpreted considering the ethnic origin and stature of parents.

Infants and young children may lose weight when they are ill and not eating well but normally regain the weight within a few weeks once they are well and their appetite has returned.

Weight loss after birth

Infants normally lose weight after birth and then regain their birthweight by 3 weeks but more usually 7–10 days. The weight loss is mainly due to a net fluid loss in the first 2–3 days. A weight loss of up to 10 per cent of birthweight is considered normal: more than 10 per cent needs careful assessment to ensure feeding is effective and such infants should be carefully monitored until they have regained their birthweight.

Because of the variability of this neonatal weight loss and gain, there are no centile lines between birth and 2 weeks of age on the growth charts for 0–4 years. However, weights measured at this time should be plotted on the chart and compared with birthweight.

Birthweight centile does not always predict the weight centile later in infancy

The birth weight reflects fetal growth, which is dependent on prenatal nutrition and also any growth restriction or acceleration within the womb. For example, intrauterine growth restriction may occur if the mother is very small in stature, or growth acceleration may occur in fetuses of mothers with diabetes, possibly due to extra insulin produced in response to the hyperglycaemia of the mother and the high glucose level in cord blood.

Within the first 6–8 weeks infants may cross centiles up or down, usually towards the 50th centile, to compensate for either restricted or rapid fetal growth.

Weight gain in infancy

From about 6 to 8 weeks of age infants usually follow along a weight centile line or space but there will normally be some variation above and below it (see Figure 4.3).

Following length centiles in the first 2 years

Some catch-up or catch-down in length centile is usually seen in the first 2 years to compensate for any constraints in intrauterine growth. By 3 years there is good correlation between the height centile and the final height centile to be reached following the pubertal growth spurt.

BMI and body fat differences in girls and boys

BMI varies throughout childhood and this variation is slightly different between boys and girls. Hence there are gender-specific BMI-for-age centile charts. BMI increases during infancy, decreases between 1 and around 5–7 years and then slowly increases throughout the rest of childhood.

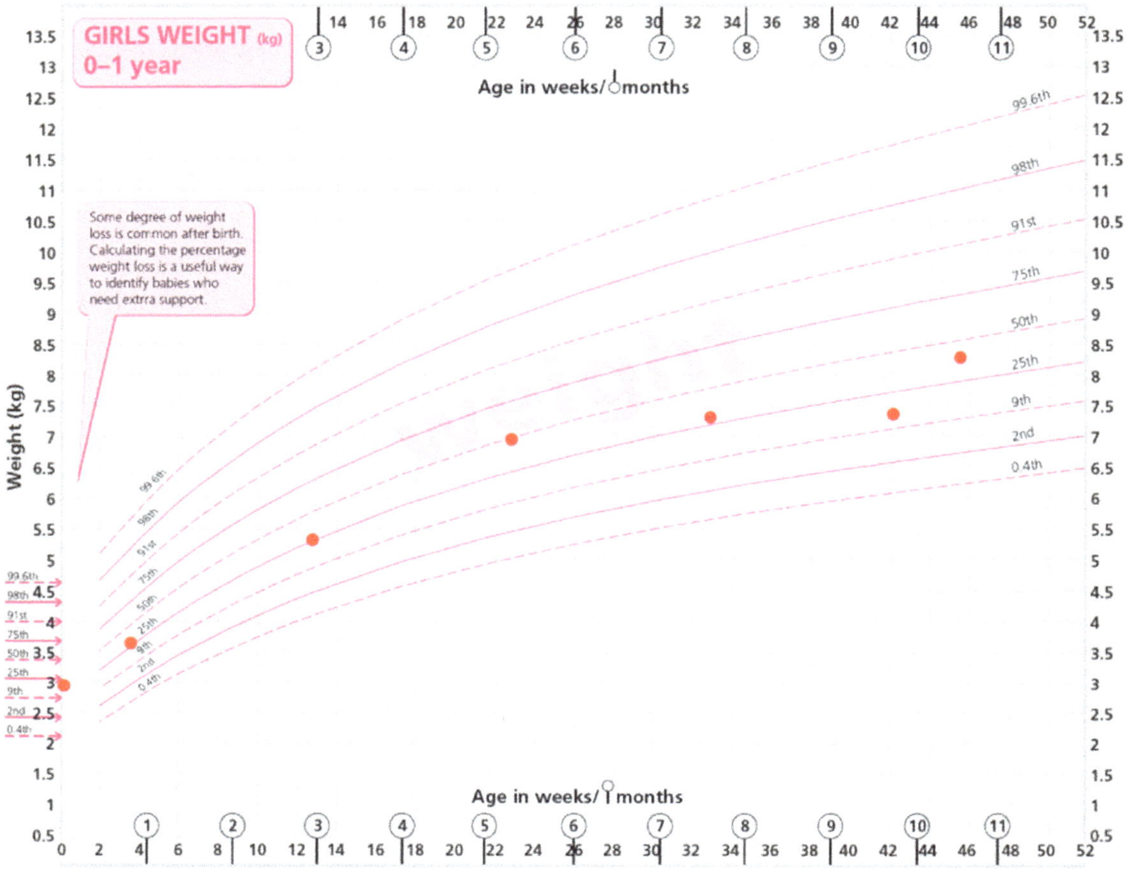

Figure 4.3 Normal growth in an infant girl on an A5 format growth chart

The body fat content is similar in boys and girls at 5–7 years old but thereafter begins to increase along with BMI, with girls gaining fat at a slightly higher rate than boys. This increase in BMI is termed the adiposity rebound. The timing of it is a crucial marker and intervention point for childhood obesity.

Crossing centiles during adolescence

When assessing growth on the weight-for-age and height-for-age centile charts it is quite usual to see centile crossing for both height and weight during the pubertal growth spurt. The growth charts describe an average growth spurt at average ages of the pubertal development but the pubertal growth spurt occurs at different ages. Children who go through their pubertal growth spurt at a younger or older age than the average age will therefore cross centile lines on the chart. This requires consideration when assessing height and weight gain around this time.

Abnormal growth

Poor growth or extremely rapid growth may be the first indication of an underlying medical condition that requires further investigation.

Faltering growth in infancy

NICE Guidelines define faltering growth in infancy after the early days of weight loss and regaining birth weight (National Institute for Health and Care Excellence, Nice Guideline 75, 2017):

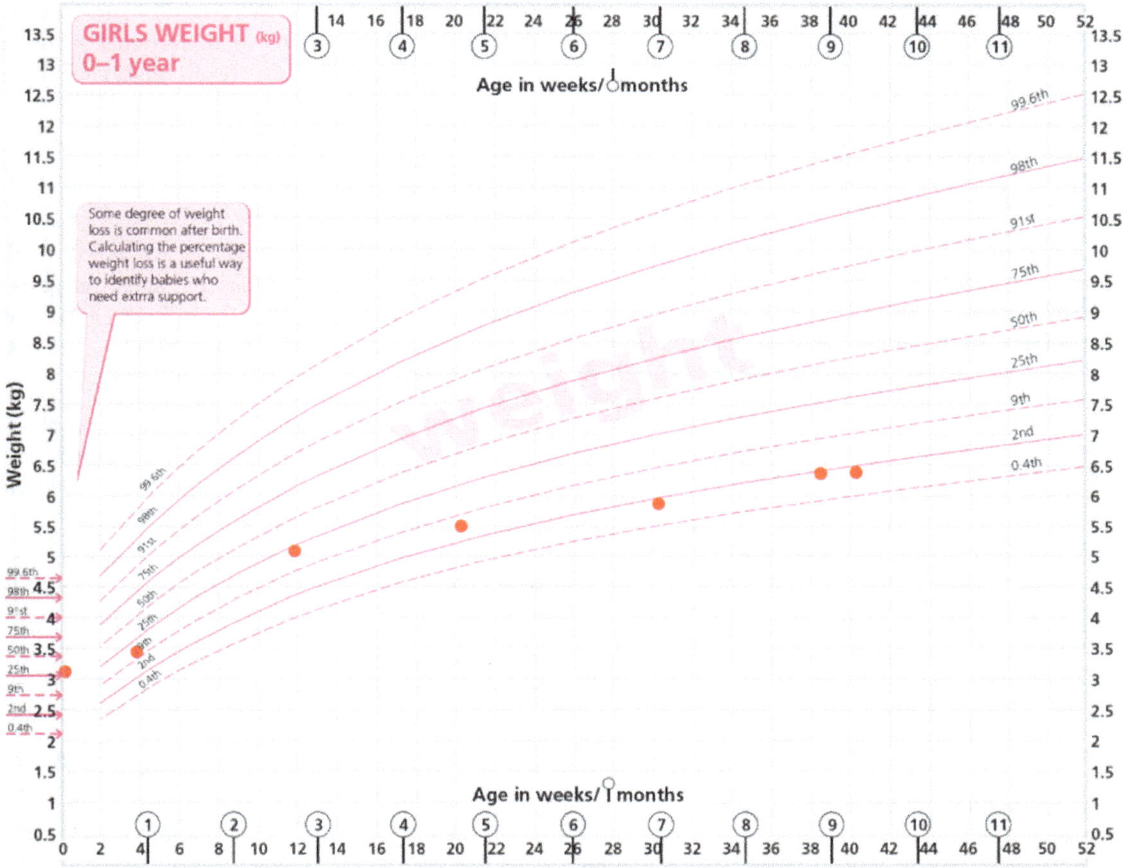

Figure 4.4 Faltering growth in an infant girl showing weight falling through 2 centile spaces. Measurements after 6–8 weeks show a fall across 2 centile spaces

- a fall across 1 or more weight centile spaces, if birthweight was below the 9th centile;
- a fall across 2 or more weight centile spaces, if birthweight was between the 9th and 91st centiles (see Figure 4.4);
- a fall across 3 or more weight centile spaces, if birthweight was above the 91st centile;
- when current weight is below the 2nd centile for age, whatever the birthweight.

Faltering growth in children

is defined as weight or height falling through 2 centile spaces

Weight monitoring

Frequent weight monitoring can cause parental anxiety and National Institute for Health and Care Excellence Nice Guideline 75 2017 recommendations for monitoring weight where there is a concern of faltering growth is for no more often than:

- daily if less than 1 month old;
- weekly between 1–6 months old;
- fortnightly between 6–12 months;
- monthly from 1 year of age.

Referral to a paediatrician should be considered if:

- weight or height is noted, for the first time, to be below the 0.4th centile;
- weight or length/height falls through 2 centile spaces and increasing energy intake from food is not successful in restoring normal growth velocity;
- BMI for age centile is below the 2nd centile.

Rapid growth is defined as crossing centiles upwards on the weight or height for age centile charts. Rapid weight gain is a risk factor for obesity.

Height crossing more than 1 centile space upwards in children over 3 years of age and before puberty may be an indication of excess growth hormone but a referral needs careful consideration as the accuracy of height measurements is often poor. In addition, early puberty is becoming more common.

In children over 2 years, a BMI that is over the 91st centile is considered overweight and a BMI over the 98th centile is considered obese. Families of these children may need to make lifestyle changes to reduce the rate of weight gain in the child (see Chapter 18).

Acknowledgements

Thanks are due to Professor Mehul Dattani, London Centre for Paediatric Endocrinology, University College London and Professor Tim Cole, MRC Centre of Epidemiology for Child Health, University College London.

References and further reading

Baron J, Sävendahl L, De Luca F, Dauber A, Phillip M, Wit JM and Nilsson O (2015 Dec) Short and tall stature: a new paradigm emerges. *Nature Reviews Endocrinology* 11(12): 735–746. doi: 10.1038/nrendo.2015.165. Epub 2015 Oct 6.

Blackwell N, Myatt M, Allafort-Duverger T, Balogoun A, Ibrahim A and Briend A (2015) Mothers Understand And Can do it (MUAC): a comparison of mothers and community health workers determining mid-upper arm circumference in 103 children aged from 6 months to 5 years. *Archives of Public Health* 73(1): 26. doi: 10.1186/s13690-015-0074-z.

Christesen HT, Pedersen BT, Pournara E, Petit IO and Júlíusson PB (2016 Jun 9) Short Stature: Comparison of WHO and National Growth Standards/References for Height. *PLoS One* 11(6): e0157277. doi: 10.1371/journal.pone.0157277. eCollection 2016.

Elliman D (2019) *Health for All Children*, 5th edn. Oxford: Oxford University Press.

Freni-Sterrantino A, Afoakwah P, Smith RB, et al. (2019) Birth weight centiles and small for gestational age by sex and ethnicity for England and Wales. *Archives of Disease in Childhood* **104**: 1188–1192.

McCormack SE, Cousminer DL, Chesi A, et al. (2017) Association Between Linear Growth and Bone Accrual in a Diverse Cohort of Children and Adolescents. *JAMA Pediatrics* 171(9): e171769. doi: 10.1001/jamapediatrics.2017.1769.

National Institute for Health and Care Excellence (November 2014) *Public Health Guidance 11. Improving the nutrition of pregnant and breastfeeding mothers and children in low-income households*. London: NICE.

National Institute for Health and Care Excellence Nice Guideline 75 (September 2017) *Faltering growth: recognition and management of faltering growth in children.*

Public Health England (2020) *National Child Measurement Programme*. https://www.gov.uk/government/collections/national-child-measurement-programme (Accessed March 2020).

Scherdel P, Matczak S, Léger J, Martinez-Vinson C, Goulet O, Brauner R, Nicklaus S, Resche-Rigon M and Chalumeau M (2019 Feb 1), Heude Algorithms to Define Abnormal Growth in Children: External Validation and Head-To-Head Comparison. *The Journal of Clinical Endocrinology and Metabolism* 104(2):241–249.

Scherdel P, Reynaud R, Pietrement C, et al. (2017 Apr 27) Priority target conditions for algorithms for monitoring children's growth: Interdisciplinary consensus. *PLoS One* 12(4): e0176464. doi: 10.1371/journal.pone.0176464. eCollection 2017.

Tasker R, McClure R and Acerini C (2013) *Oxford Handbook of Paediatrics* 2nd Edition Oxford: Oxford University Press.

World Health Organisation (2007) Development of a WHO growth reference for school-aged children and adolescents. *Bulletin of the World Health Organization* 85: 660–667. https://www.who.int/growthref/growthref_who_bull.pdf?ua=1 (Accessed July 2020).

Wright CM, Williams AF, Elliman D, et al. (2010) Using the new UK-WHO growth charts. *British Medical Journal* **340**: c1140.

Resources

Growth charts and BMI charts can be ordered from www.healthforallchildren.co.uk

Growth charts and online training exercises in plotting and interpreting growth charts https://www.rcpch.ac.uk/resources/growth-charts

Self-learning programme: Module 8 Growth and nutrition www.e-lfh.org.uk/healthychild

5

Assessing nutritional intake

Summary

- Dietary intake can be assessed by:
    - estimating or weighing food consumed over 1 or more days and recording this in a food diary or;
    - completing a 24-hour recall of all food and drink consumed or;
    - a food frequency questionnaire (FFQ).
- A recorded food diary can be used to assess energy and nutritional adequacy by either comparison with the principles of healthy eating or by using dietary analysis software containing a database of foods with their energy and nutrient content.
- Parents and older children can be taught how to assess food and drink intake using the principles of a nutritous balanced diet and they can use this to make changes to improve the nutritional adequacy of the diet.
- Nutritional analysis of the diets of large populations of children (e.g. Avon Longitudinal Study of Parents and Children; ALSPAC) have been used to find associations between dietary intakes and later health outcomes.
- The adequacy of the diet is assessed by comparison with Dietary Reference Values (DRV).

As discussed in Chapter 1, a child's diet is considered nutritionally adequate if the nutrient content of the foods, drinks and any supplements consumed meet:

- the Reference Nutrient Intakes (RNIs) for each of the nutrients and;
- the Estimated Average Requirement (EAR) for energy for that child's age and activity level.

In Chapter 2 the principles of a nutritious balanced diet are discussed, and individual diets can be assessed against those principles.

To be able to assess the nutritional adequacy of an individual child's diet knowledge is required of:

- the child's recent or normal consumption of food, drinks and supplements;
- the energy and nutrient content of those foods, drinks and supplements;
- the age, gender and physical activity of the child.

Estimating the recent or usual dietary intake can be done by either taking a dietary history or weighing the food and drink offered and that not consumed over a set period of time. Taking a dietary history is usually done in one of the following ways:

- Food and drink diary: A carer or the child records the food and drinks consumed over 1 or several days – ideally including a mixture of weekdays and weekend days.
- 24-hour recall: The child, parents or carers are asked to remember the quantity of each food and drink the child has consumed in the last 24 hours or on the previous day.
- Food frequency questionnaire: The child or parent or carer reports how often and in what quantity a range of different foods are generally eaten.

There are advantages and disadvantages to each method:

- Recording a dietary diary may not be done accurately and there may be some underreporting of certain foods and over reporting of other foods. This method can be enhanced by a subsequent interview to clarify any anomalies and also to check the validity and accuracy of measurement of any quantities.
- Food frequency questionnaires (FFQ) are less expensive to administer and are therefore used more extensively in large-scale epidemiological studies investigating the relationship between diet and health outcomes. A FFQ records the type of foods eaten and their frequency of consumption. They reflect what the interviewee estimates that they eat but may not be accurate. They also have a use in checking the dietary intake of specific nutrients. In young children they may be used to estimate iron intake by asking how often specific foods with significant iron content are eaten.
- Weighing food and drinks is considered the best estimate of dietary intake but it is time consuming, labour intensive making it expensive and requires training to ensure accuracy. Weighing each food and drink will disrupt the normal flow of meal and snack patterns in the household and consequently may also influence which foods and drinks are offered to the child. Hence the results may not reflect what the child would have eaten had there been no interference to the normal routine. The food and drinks that the child did not consume must also be weighed. A certain amount of the food and drinks offered to infants and young children may be spilt or regurgitated so a weighed intake for this age group may be less accurate than in older age groups.

Assessing nutritional adequacy of a child's diet with a recorded food intake

For assessing individual diets a recorded food diary is a very useful method. Parents of younger children or older children themselves are asked to complete a food diary such as that shown in Figure 5.1.

A dietitan or nutritionist trained in assessing dietary intake can use this information to assess the nutritional adequacy by 1 of 2 methods:

- assessment against the principles of healthy eating using the number of daily servings and portion sizes of the food groups;
- computer software to compare the dietary intake of energy and each nutrient against the RNIs for each nutrient and EAR for energy.

Assessing nutritional adequacy using the food groups

This assessment method is simple and older children and parents can be taught to do it themselves. If the number of portions from the food groups, as described in Table 2.1 and Table 5.1 below is followed then the child can be assumed to be consuming an adequate intake of nutrients.

A chart such as in Figure 5.2 can be used for the assessment of foods from a record of a 24-hour intake. All the food and drinks consumed over a 24-hour period are listed in the left-hand column. A mark is made in the food group columns when a food or drink contributes to a portion from that food group. Whether a mark of 1, 2 or ½ is put in depends on the quantity consumed compared to the appropriate portion size for the child's age.

For example, the food diary could report that the child had eaten the food shown in Figure 5.3.

For breakfast a '1' would be marked in the 'Bread, rice, potato, pasta, other starchy food' column for the bowl of breakfast cereal. Then a '1' in the 'Milk, cheese and yogurt' column for the cup of milk that would have been poured onto the breakfast cereal. If the child leaves half of the milk in the bowl then this could be reduced to a '½'. A '1' in the 'Fruit and vegetable' column would be for the blueberries that were added to the cereal.

The rest of the day's intake would be assessed and marked in the same way. Finally the '1's and '½'s in each food group column would be added up then

Table 5.1 Recommend number of age appropriate portions from each of the food groups

Food group	Recommended number of age-appropriate portions
1. Bread, rice, potatoes, pasta and other starchy foods	Included at each meal – and some snacks 3–5 portions per day
2. Fruit and vegetables	Included at each meal – and some snacks – ideally 3 portions fruit and 3 portions of vegetables per day
3. Milk, cheese and yogurt	3 portions per day
4. Meat, fish, eggs, nuts and beans	2–3 portions per day
5. Oils, butter and fat spreads	Use in food preparation
6. Cakes, biscuits and puddings	1 portion per day
7. Sauces and sweet or savoury spreads	Up to 2 portions per day
Drinks	6–8 per day or 1 with each meal and snack
Vitamin D supplement	10 micrograms vitamin D daily in winter and in summer for those under 5 and those who do not spend time outside with bare skin exposed each day
8. Sweet drinks, confectionery and high fat packet snacks	1 portion per week
Overall	Sweet foods limited to 4 times per day

Daily food and drinks diary					
DATE:					
Time	**Location**	**All food and drinks offered**	**Quantity or weight eaten**	**Time taken**	**Who else was also eating**
7:30	Kitchen table	Bowl Cheerios with full fat milk + 1 tsp sugar 1 slice toast with butter and jam	All milk left All toast eaten	10 minutes	Sister and mother
10:30	School playground	200mL carton apple juice 2 cereal bars	All	15 minutes	Friends
12:00	School canteen	5 tbsp pasta 3 tbsp meat sauce 6 carrot sticks 3 cauliflower florets Bowl apple crumble and custard glass of water	1/2 pasta and meat sauce no carrots or cauliflower All dessert 1/2 water	20 minutes	Friends

Figure 5.1 A daily food and drinks diary

recorded in the row for totals. A comparison can then be made of these figures to the daily recommendations.

An assessment of the intake in Figure 5.3 would be shown as in Figure 5.4.

Date:	Name:								
	Food Groups								Fluid
All food and drinks	Bread, rice, potato, pasta and other starchy foods	Fruit and veg	Milk, cheese, and yogurt	Meat, fish, eggs, nuts and pulses	Oils, butter and fat spreads	Cakes, biscuits and puddings	Sauces, sweet and savoury spreads	Sweet drinks, confectionery and high fat packet snacks	Drinks
Totals:									
Recommended daily portions:	3-5 Or at each meal and some snacks	5-6 Or at each meal and some snacks	3	2-3	Used in food preparation	1	Up to 2	Once per week	6-8

Figure 5.2 Food group chart for 24–hour intake

Case Study

Ellie is now 2 years 9 months and goes to nursery in the morning. She still has a sleep after lunch and her mother is concerned that she eats very poorly at lunchtime. She usually gives her bread and jam just to make sure she has had something. There are no problems with her growth and her mother was asked to write down everything Ellie had eaten the day before: 'Breakfast: cornflakes and milk, orange juice to drink. Milk to drink and fruit at breaktime at nursery. Lunch: jam sandwich and cake. A packet of Wotsits and a carton of a fruit juice drink in the afternoon with her older brother on the way home from school. Fish fingers with chips for tea, milk and a chocalate biscuit for pudding. A bottle of milk on going to bed.'

Ellie's food and drinks in 1 day are shown in Figure 5.5.

Ellie is getting enough calories to keep growing for the time being. She is probably tired when she comes home from her busy morning at nursery which is why she is not eating well at lunchtime. After her afternoon sleep she is hungry and eats well but is given the same snack as her brother, which is not nutritious enough to replace the nutrients she has not had at lunch.

The combination of the food groups is very poor and by comparing the totals to the recommendations you can see she has too much milk and a lot of foods that are high in fat and sugar and not enough foods from food groups 1–5. Consequently Ellie's diet will be low in iron and other minerals. If she continues to eat like this she would become deficient in iron and might get iron-deficiency anaemia.

As the rest of the family do not eat fruit and vegetables, Ellie is not being offered them at home. The only fruit she is having is that which is given for a snack at nursery.

There are several changes that Ellie's mother can make to improve Ellie's diet:

- cut out the bottle of milk before bed as soon as possible;
- change the lunch to a more nutritious sandwich, for example she could try a peanut butter and jam sandwich;
- change the afternoon snack to a more nutritious snack such as carrot sticks with breadsticks which are crunchy like the

Breakfast	Breakfast cereal with milk
	Blueberries
	Water to drink
Mid morning snack	Apple slices
	Cup of milk
Lunch	Lentils in tomato sauce
	Pasta
	Broccoli florets
	Water to drink
	Apple crumble with custard
Midafternoon snack	Crackers with butter and Marmite
	Water to drink
	Fish and potato pie
	Carrot and cucumber sticks
	Plain yogurt with strawberries
Evening meal	Water to drink

Figure 5.3 Example food intake recorded

All food and drinks	Food Groups								Fluid
	Bread, rice, potato, pasta and other starchy foods	Fruit and veg	Milk, cheese, and yogurt	Meat, fish, eggs, nuts and pulses	Oils, butter and fat spreads	Cakes, biscuits and puddings	Sauces, sweet and savoury spreads	Sweet drinks, confectionery and high fat packet snacks	Drinks
Breakfast cereal with milk	1		½						
Blueberries		1							
Water to drink									1
Apple slices		1							
Cup of milk			1						1
Lentils in tomato sauce				1			1		
Pasta	1								
Broccoli florets		1							
Water to drink									1
Apple crumble with custard		1	1			1			
Crackers with butter and Marmite	1				1				
Water to drink									1
Fish and potato pie	1			1					
Carrot and cucumber sticks		1							
Plain yogurt with strawberries		1	1						
Water to drink									1
Extra water during the day									2
Totals:	4	5	3½	2	1	1	1	0	7
Recommended daily portions:	3-5 Or at each meal and some snacks	5-6 Or at each meal and some snacks	3	2-3	Used in food preparation	1	Up to 2	Once per week	6-8

Figure 5.4 Completed assessment of example intake

All food and drinks	Food Groups								Fluid
	Bread, rice, potato, pasta and other starchy foods	**Fruit and veg**	**Milk, cheese, and yogurt**	**Meat, fish, eggs, nuts and pulses**	**Oils, butter and fat spreads**	**Cakes, biscuits and puddings**	**Sauces, sweet and savoury spreads**	**Sweet drinks, confectionery and high fat packet snacks**	**Drinks**
Breakfast Cornflakes and milk Juice to drink	1		1					1	1
At nursery Fruit and milk		1	1						1
Lunch Jam sandwich and milk to drink	1		1		1		1		1
Afternoon Packet of Wotsits Carton of fruit juice drink								1 1	1
Evening meal Fish fingers and chips Chocolate biscuit and milk to drink	1		1	1	2	1			1
Before bed Full bottle of milk			2						2
Totals:	3	1	6	1	3	1	1	3	7
Recommended daily portions:	**3-5 Or at each meal and some snacks**	**5-6 Or at each meal and some snacks**	**3**	**2-3**	**Used in food preparation**	**1**	**Up to 2**	**Once per week**	**6-8**

Figure 5.5 Ellie's food and drinks in 1 day

Wotsits. She could also add in some pieces of cold meat such as ham or cooked chicken to make up for the small lunch that is being eaten.

The whole family needs to begin eating more fruit and vegetables so that they are offered at each meal. This change will take some time but continuing to give fruit juice is detrimental for Ellie's teeth and will not encourage her to learn to like fruit.

If Ellie's mother is able to make these changes then eventually her 1 day's intake would be as shown in Figure 5.6.

A 1-day record of a child's intake may not be indicative of his or her average intake. Young children will often eat well some days and not so well on other days. The eating pattern Monday to Friday may be quite different to the days on the weekend. Days a child goes to nursery, a child minder or school might be quite different to days when he or she stays at home. Birthday party days will also be quite different. Assessing a child's intake over several days or a week is therefore preferable to an assessment of just 1 day.

Total servings from each food group each day can be added together and then divided by 7 to give an average for this food group for the week (Figure 5.7).

In this example, the combination of the food groups over the week is good enough. The average for each food group is very close to the recommendation.

When the combination of the food groups over the week is not ideal then advice can be given by deciding which food groups the child is not having enough of and providing ideas of ways to increase his/her intake of this food group by substituting this food group for another food group he may be having too much of.

Using computer software

Several computer software programmes that calculate the energy and nutrient content of a dietary intake are available. The adequacy of the diet can be assessed by comparison with estimated average energy requirement and RNIs of each nutrient. However, the analysis obtained is only as accurate as:

- the nutrient content of the food database that is in the software – the foods in the database may not match exactly the food that has been bought or prepared;
- the accuracy of the diet history taken – particularly the weight of the foods that the child has consumed;
- the accuracy with which the food and drinks consumed by a child are entered into the software.

Such software can also be used to assess the nutrient contents of menus and individual recipes.

Nutritional assessments for epidemiological data

In the past, weighing food over a 4-day period was the method used in national dietary surveys of children in the United Kingdom (Gregory et al. 1995, 2000) but was an expensive way to collect nationally representative data. The current National Diet and Nutrition Survey (NDNS) is a rolling programme of dietary assessment and uses a 4-day food diary recorded by families and is followed up by an interview to clarify quantities consumed by the family member who is in the study.

Case Study

The food diary record method was used in the Avon Longitudinal Study of Parents and Children (ALSPAC). The data collected has been used in many scientific publications relating health outcomes to dietary intakes in children. Three-day diet records were recorded by parents of a cohort of over 14 000 children, all born in the early 1990s in Avon. A diet record booklet was sent to the parents just prior to them making a clinic visit to have their child weighed and measured at various ages from 4 months to 18 years. The parents were asked to describe everything their child was offered in household measures and to record leftover foods/drinks. The diary was checked through in an interview with the

→

Date:	Name:								
	Food Groups								Fluid
All food and drinks	**Bread, rice, potato, pasta and other starchy foods**	**Fruit and veg**	**Milk, cheese, and yogurt**	**Meat, fish, eggs, nuts and pulses**	**Oils, butter and fat spreads**	**Cakes, biscuits and puddings**	**Sauces, sweet and savoury spreads**	**Sweet drinks, confectionery and high fat packet snacks**	**Drinks**
Breakfast Cornflakes and milk Water to drink	1		½						1
At nursery Fruit and milk		1	1						1
Lunch Jam and peanut butter sandwich and fruit pieces Water to drink	1	1		1	1		1		1
Afternoon Carrot and bread sticks Pieces of cold chicken Milk to drink	1	1	1	1					1
Evening meal Fish fingers and chips And peas Chocolate biscuit and fruit pieces Water to drink	1	1 1		1	2	1			1
Before bed: Extra water to drink									2
Totals:	4	5	2 ½	3	3	1	0	0	7
Recommended daily portions:	**3-5 Or at each meal and some snacks**	**5-6 Or at each meal and some snacks**	**3**	**2-3**	**Used in food preparation**	**1**	**2**	**Once per week**	**6-8**

Figure 5.6 If Ellie's mother is able to make these changes then eventually her 1 day's intake would look like this

All food and drinks	Food Groups								Fluid
	Bread, rice, potato, pasta and other starchy foods	Fruit and veg	Milk, cheese, and yogurt	Meat, fish, eggs, nuts and pulses	Oils, butter and fat spreads	Cakes, biscuits and puddings	Sauces, sweet and savoury spreads	Sweet drinks, confectionery and high fat packet snacks	Drinks
Sunday	5	5	3	2	2	2	3	0	6
Monday	6	4	4	1	3	1	1	0	8
Tuesday	4	6	2	2	1	1	2	0	5
Wednesday	5	3	1	2	2	1	2	0	6
Thursday	3	3	3	3	3	2	0	0	7
Friday	6	4	3	2	2	1	2	1	6
Saturday	4	2	3	1	2	2	4	1	9
Totals for the week:	33	27	19	13	14	9	14	2	47
Average for the week	4.7	3.8	2.7	1.9	2	1.4	2	2 this week	6.7
Recommended daily portions:	**3-5 Or at each meal and some snacks**	**5-6 Or at each meal and some snacks**	**3**	**2-3**	**Used in food preparation**	**1**	**About 2**	**Once per week**	**6-8**

Figure 5.7 Average for each food group for the week

parents by a nutrition fieldworker to improve accuracy. The fieldworker allocated food weights according to the parental description of the portion size using guideline measures for the various foods. For manufactured foods, parents provided packet weights when available. The full details of the methods used and the nutrient and food intakes of the children are described in various papers (Emmett et al. 2002, Cowin and Emmett 2007).

Biochemical measures used for nutritional assessment

Energy and nutrient intake can be measured using biomarkers.

- Doubly-labelled water is used to measure energy expenditure which can be used to validate energy intake from a recorded food diary.
- A 24-hour urine collection can be measured for sodium, potassium, iodine and nitrogen content. Total nitrogen is a measure of protein intake.
- Blood levels of certain nutrients indicate an adequate or inadequate intake (e.g. plasma levels of vitamin C, beta-carotene, folate and vitamin D).

Activity 1

Make a recorded intake of all the food and drinks you have over the next 3 days and analyse it for nutritional adequacy using the food group method described above.

Activity 2

Ask the parents of a child to fill in a 3-day recorded intake and then analyse it in terms of the food groups.

References and further reading

Bush LA, Hutchinson J, Hooson J, et al. (2019) Measuring energy, macro and micronutrient intake in UK children and adolescents: a comparison of validated dietary assessment tools. *BMC Nutrition* **5**: 53. https://doi.org/10.1186/s40795-019-0312-9.

Cowin I and Emmett P (2007) Diet in a group of 18-month-old children in South West England, and comparison with the results of a national survey. *Journal of Human Nutrition and Dietetics* **20**: 254–267.

Emmett P, Rogers I, Symes C and the ALSPAC Study Team (2002) Food and nutrient intakes of a population sample of 3-year-old children in the South West of England in 1996. *Public Health Nutrition* **5**: 55–64.

Food Standards Agency and Public Health England (2018). *Results of the National Diet and Nutrition Survey (NDNS) rolling programme for 2014 to 2015 and 2015 to 2016*. www.gov.uk/government/statistics/ndns-results-from-years-7-and-8-combined Accessed April 2020.

Gregory JR, Collins DL, Davies PSW, Hughes JM and Clarke PC (1995) *National Diet and Nutrition Survey: Children aged* 1½ and 4½ years, Volume 1. Report of the Diet and Nutrition Survey. London: HMSO.

Gregory J, Lowe S, Bates CJ, *et al.* (2000) *National Diet and Nutrition Survey: Young people aged 4–18 years*. London: The Stationery Office.

Resources

Nutritional Analysis Software Packages available in the UK: CompEat – https://www.compeatnutrition.com/

Composition of Foods Integrated Dataset: https://www.gov.uk/government/publications/composition-of-foods-integrated-dataset-cofid

Dietplan (https://www.foresoft.co.uk)

Nutritics https://www.nutritics.com/

Nutrium https://nutrium.io/en

Section 3
Prenatal nutrition

6 Preconception and Fertility

7 Pregnancy

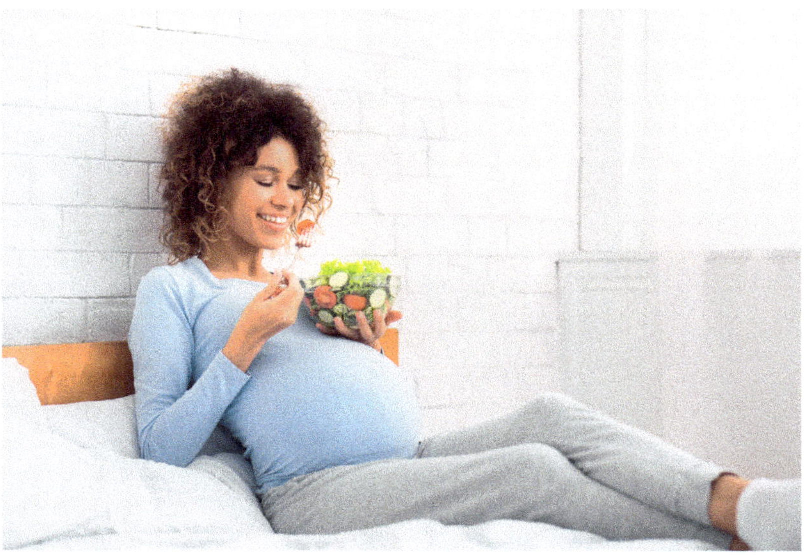

6

Preconception and fertility

Summary

- Nutritional factors affect fertility in both males and females.
- Maternal and paternal nutritional status at conception affects fetal growth and development and has implications for the child's postnatal and long-term health.
- About 50 per cent of pregnancies are unplanned and fetal health and birth outcomes are disadvantaged in a poorly nourished mother.
- Both men and women planning conception should follow a balanced nutritious diet and aim for an ideal body mass index (BMI) within the normal range of 18.5–25 kg/m^2.
- Ideally, overweight and obese women should aim to reduce their weight to this ideal BMI range at least four months prior to conception.
- Women planning a pregnancy should take folic acid and vitamin D supplements and avoid the foods that can cause harm during pregnancy.

The nutritional status of both parents can affect fertility and the chance of conception. Furthermore, maternal and paternal nutritional status, in particular at the time of conception, is an important determinant of fetal growth and development and the foundations of the child's future health. This is thought to occur through epigenetics which are heritable changes in which genes are turned on and off without changing an individual's DNA.

Mothers with a history of poor nutrition before conception may have low nutrient stores and, consequently, the fetus may have reduced access to the nutrients needed for growth and development, particularly in the early stages of gestation. This is particularly important for mothers whose nutritional intake is compromised by nausea and vomiting in the first 3 months.

Women most at risk of poor nutritional status at conception are those who:

- eat a poor or unbalanced diet (this includes many teenagers);
- are trying to lose weight on very low-calorie diets that may be deficient in essential nutrients;
- have had several closely spaced pregnancies.

Nutritional advice preconception

If pregnancies are planned, preconception nutritional status can be improved. However, only about 50 per cent of pregnancies in the United Kingdom are planned, with higher income, better educated and older women more likely to plan than low-income, young and less educated women. Good nutritional status in all women of childbearing age is therefore an ideal.

Those planning a pregnancy should follow a balanced nutritious diet as detailed for pregnancy in Chapter 7. In addition, women should take daily supplements of:

- 400 μg folic acid and;
- 10 μg (400 IU) vitamin D.

A higher dose of 5 mg folic acid/day is recommended for women with:

- spina bifida;
- a history of a previous child with a neural tube defect;
- diabetes.

The 5 mg dose folic acid preparation is available on prescription only.

Preconception, women should also avoid or limit certain foods and drinks as is advised for pregnant women (see Chapter 7, page 89–92).

Optimizing body weight

Women with a BMI above 27 kg/m^2 should be encouraged to lose weight prior to conception as excess maternal body weight combined with the weight of the baby increases the risk of complications such as high blood pressure, gestational diabetes and preterm delivery (Giviziez et al. 2016). The risk of a low-birthweight baby is also higher.

The National Institute for Health and Clinical Excellence (NICE) recommends that women with a BMI over 30 should be informed of the increased risk to themselves and their babies during pregnancy and birth and encouraged to lose weight before becoming pregnant (National Institute for Health and Care Excellence, 2010). It is preferable for weight to be reduced well in advance of conception (at least 3–4 months) to lessen the likelihood of nutritional inadequacy. For pre-pregnancy weight loss NICE recommends providing a structured, tailored programme of ongoing support that combines advice on healthy eating and physical activity and addresses individual barriers to change (National Institute for Health and Care Excellence, 2010). When weight has been lost it is then important to encourage a diet with adequate energy intake and variety to ensure intake of all essential nutrients to prepare for conception.

Women with diabetes

Women with diabetes who are planning to become pregnant should aim to establish good glycaemi control before conception by maintaining their HbAlc below 43 mmol/mol (6.1 per cent) to reduce the risk of congenital malformations. They should be offered an HbA1c measurement on a monthly basis. Diabetic women whose HbAlc is above 10 per cent should be strongly advised to avoid pregnancy until good diabetes control is achieved and sustained (National Institute for Health and Care Excellence, 2015 CG63).

Improving fertility and the chance of conception

Fertility problems affect about 15 per cent of couples and are due to male infertility in about 30–50 per cent of those couples.

Research has shown several key nutritional influences that can decrease fertility and the chance of a woman conceiving:

- body weight;
- weight loss and undernutrition;
- eating disorders;
- poor iron stores;
- extreme levels of exercise;
- caffeine;
- alcohol.

Body weight

Women with a BMI of 20–25 kg/m^2 have been shown to have a higher rate of conceiving than those with a BMI higher than 25 kg/m^2 or lower than 20 kg/m^2 (Giviziez et al. 2016).

Overweight and obesity with or without polycystic ovary syndrome

Being overweight does not prevent all women from conceiving but overweight and obesity can affect ovulation and also the response to fertility treatment.

Obesity with or without the problem of polycystic ovary syndrome (PCOS) is associated with a doubling in the rate of ovulatory infertility. In both

PCOS and simple obesity weight reduction is associated with a return of ovulation, menstruation and fertility in many cases. Chances of in vitro fertilization are also improved.

Excessive body fat especially central obesity

Central body obesity, indicated by a waist circumference >90 cm (35 inches), is a risk factor for infertility as it takes women with high central obesity longer to become pregnant than women with low central obesity. Excess subcutaneous abdominal fat rather than intra abdominal fat is associated with a higher risk.

Underweight

Conception can occur in women well below average or ideal weight. However, women who have a low BMI (BMI < 20 kg/m^2) are less likely to conceive.

A study in the 1990s in the United States showed that an improved nutritional status in adolescent girls was associated with an increasingly early date of menarche signalling the onset of fertility (Frisch 1994). The mean body weight at which menarche occurred in US girls was 48 kg with a mean height of 1.59 m at 12.9 years. Of the mean body weight at the completion of growth (16–18 years) 16 kg was fat, representing an energy reserve for reproduction of 602 MJ (144, 000 kcal). Such an energy reserve would provide the theoretical energy requirements of both pregnancy and 3 months of lactation. Frisch's observation was that body fat proportion of less than 22 per cent of body weight was associated with the absence of ovulation and that healthy fertile women who were ovulating on a monthly basis had an average body fat proportion of 28 per cent.

Weight loss and undernutrition

In normal weight women, weight loss of 10–15 per cent causes hormonal disruption, resulting in amenorrhoea and anovulation. About 30 per cent of impaired fertility cases are related to weight loss. Weight gain is the recommended treatment for amenorrhoea related to low body weight.

Eating disorders

Both anorexia nervosa and bulimia nervosa are related to amenorrhoea, anovulation and infertility.

Extreme levels of exercise

High levels of exercise together with a low energy intake in young women (energy intake <30 per cent of requirements) can result in a condition known as the 'female athlete triad' with 3 symptoms: disordered eating, amenorrhoea and osteoporosis (Mehta et al. 2018). The latter is as a result of low oestrogen production.

Poor iron stores

Iron status prior to pregnancy is related to fertility and those susceptible to iron deficiency anaemia benefit from an improved iron intake (Hahn et al. 2019).

Alcohol, smoking and drug misuse

Although lifestyles involving alcohol, smoking and drug misuse are detrimental to fetal and infant development and health, it is not clear if they affect fertility in women as most evidence is from animal studies. The Department of Health advises the safest approach is to avoid alcohol altogether, particularly during the first 3 months gestation, which includes the time before a mother knows she is pregnant, as definite evidence on whether small amounts of alcohol increases risks of miscarriage, premature birth and low birthweight is still uncertain (NHS Choices 2020).

Male infertility

The causes of male infertility remain largely unknown as it is difficult to identify the role of single factors, and various studies have shown conflicting data. Lifestyle factors such as smoking, alcohol and diet, environment and socio-economic factors may affect sperm motility, fertility or pregnancy outcomes.

Obesity, poor dietary habits particularly high fat diets and low intakes of fruit and vegetables

Table 6.1 Nutritional influences that decrease fertility

Nutritional influences that can decrease fertility	In females	In males
Weight loss >15% of normal weight	✓	✓
Negative energy balance	✓	✓
Inadequate body fat	✓	✓
Obesity	✓	✓
Excessive body fat especially central adiposity	✓	✓
High fat, low protein diet		✓
Extreme levels of exercise	✓	✓
High alcohol intake		✓
Eating disorders	✓	
High-fibre/low-fat diets	✓	
Poor iron stores	✓	
Coeliac disease	✓	
Diabetes mellitus	✓	
Inadequate zinc status		✓
Inadequate antioxidant status		✓
Heavy metal exposure		✓
Exposure to halogens (pesticides), glycol (antifreeze) and environmental oestrogen-like chemicals (DDT and PCB)		✓

have been associated with low sperm counts. Zinc, selenium and vitamin C may be particularly important in sperm production (Tas et al. 1996).

Exposure to heavy metals, halogens (pesticides), glycol (antifreeze) and oestrogen-like chemicals (DDT and PCB) in the environment have also been shown to reduce male fertility. The oestrogen-like chemicals reduce the activity of the androgen hormones (e.g. testosterone).

The most prudent advice for men is to:

- consume a balanced and varied diet based on the food groups, ensuring adequate fruit and vegetable intake;
- limit themselves to a moderate alcohol intake of less than 3–4 units per day;
- aim for a healthy body weight – very underweight men should gain weight and obese men should lose weight.

Nutritional influences that decrease fertility are summarized in Table 6.1.

Activity 1

List the nutritional topics you would discuss with the following in a clinic for couples who are failing to conceive:

a. an underweight woman;
b. an overweight couple;
c. a couple both of normal weight.

Activity 2

What advice would you give to a diabetic woman planning a pregnancy?

References and further reading

Balen AH, Morley LC, Misso M, Franks S, Legro RS, Wijeyaratne CN, Stener-Victorin E, Fauser BC, Norman RJ Teede H(2016> <Nov) The management of anovulatory infertility in women with polycystic ovary syndrome: an analysis of the

evidence to support the development of global WHO guidance. *Human Reproduction Update* **22**(6): 687–708. Epub 2016 Aug 10.

Frish R (1994) The right weight: body fat, menarcheand fertility. *Proceedings of the Nutrition Society* **53**: 113–129.

Giahi L, Mohammadmoradi S, Javidan A, Sadeghi MR (2016 Feb) Nutritional modifications in male infertility: a systematic review covering 2 decades. *Nutrition Reviews* **74**(2): 118–130. doi: 10.1093/nutrit/nuv059. Epub 2015 Dec 24.

Giviziez CR, Sanchez EG, Approbato MS, Maia MC, Fleury EA, Sasaki RS (2016 Dec 1) Obesity and anovulatory infertility: A review. *JBRA Assisted Reproduction* **20**(4): 240–245. doi: 10.5935/1518-0557.20160046. Review.

Hahn KA, Wesselink AK, Wise LA, Mikkelsen EM, Cueto HT, Tucker KL, Vinceti M, Rothman KJ, Sorensen HT, Hatch EE (2019 Sep 1) Iron Consumption Is Not Consistently Associated with Fecundability among North American and Danish Pregnancy Planners. *Journal of Nutrition* **149**(9): 1585–1595. doi: 10.1093/jn/nxz094.

Kuchenbecker WK, Groen H, Zijlstra TM, Bolster JH, Slart RH, van der Jagt EJ, Kobold AC, Wolffenbuttel BH, Land JA, Hoek A (2010 May) The subcutaneous abdominal fat and not the intraabdominal fat compartment is associated with anovulation in women with obesity and infertility. *The Journal of Clinical Endocrinology and Metabolism* **95**(5): 2107–2112. doi: 10.1210/jc.2009-1915. Epub 2010 Mar 3.

Kudesia R, Wu H, Hunter Cohn K, Tan L, Lee JA, Copperman AB, Yurttas Beim P (2018 Nov) The effect of female body mass index on in vitro fertilization cycle outcomes: a multi-center analysis. *Journal of Assisted Reproduction and Genetics* **35**(11): 2013–2023. doi: 10.1007/s10815-018-1290-6. Epub 2018 Aug 21.

Lassi ZS, Imam AM, Dean SV, Bhutta ZA (2014 Sep 26) Preconception care: caffeine, smoking, alcohol, drugs and other environmental chemical/radiation exposure. *Reproductive Health* **11** Suppl 3: S6. doi: 10.1186/1742-4755-11-S3-S6. Epub 2014 Sep 26.

Mehta J, Thompson B, Kling JM (2018) The female athlete triad: It takes a team. *Cleveland Clinic Journal of Medicine* **85**(4): 313-320. doi: 10.3949/ccjm.85a.16137.

Mishra GD, Waller M, Gete DG (2020) Prepregnancy dietary patterns and risk of preterm birth and low birth weight: findings from the Australian Longitudinal Study on Women's Health. *The American Journal of Clinical Nutrition*. DOI: 10.1093/ajcn/nqaa057.

NHS Choices (2011) Alcohol and drugs during pregnancy. https://www.nhs.uk/conditions/pregnancy-and-baby/alcohol-medicines-drugs-pregnant/ (accessed July2020).

National Institute for Health and Care Excellence (November 2014) *Public Health Guidance 11. Improving the nutrition of pregnant and breastfeeding mothers and children in low-income households*. London: NICE.

National Institute for Health and Care Excellence (February 2015) *Clinical Guidance 63. Diabetes in pregnancy: management of diabetes and its complications from preconception to the postnatal period*. www.nice.org.uk/Guidance/CG63 (accessed April2020).

National Institute for Health and Care Excellence (2010) *Public Health Guidance 27. Weight management before, during and after pregnancy*. July 2010. www.nice.org.uk/PH27 (accessed April2020).

Ricci E, Al-Beitawi S, Cipriani S, Alteri A, Chiaffarino F, Candiani M, Gerli S, Viganó P, Parazzini F (2018 Jan) Dietary habits and semen parameters: a systematic narrative review. *Andrology* **6**(1): 104–116. doi: 10.1111/andr.12452. Epub 2017 Dec 20.

Tas S, Lauwerys R and Lison D (1996) Occupational hazards for the male reproductive system. *Critical Reviews in Toxicology* **26**: 261–307.

Yoshida K, Maekawa T, Hong Ly N, et al. (2020) ATF7-Dependent Epigenetic Changes Are Required for the Intergenerational Effect of a Paternal Low-Protein Diet. *Molecular Cell*. doi: 10.1016/j.molcel.2020.02.028.

Resources

NHS Choices: https://www.nhs.uk/conditions/pregnancy-and-baby/planning-pregnancy/ (Accessed April 2020)

7

Pregnancy

Summary

- During pregnancy, the maternal diet must provide sufficient energy and nutrients to meet the mother's usual requirements as well as those of the growing fetus and stores for use during lactation.
- A balanced nutritious diet for pregnancy is based on the food groups with additional supplements of folic acid and vitamin D.
- Common nutrient deficiencies in UK women prior to conception and during pregnancy include iron, iodine, folate and vitamin D.
- Populations at risk of poor pregnancy outcomes due to inadequate nutritional status and/or intake during pregnancy include teenagers, women from low-income groups, vegetarian and vegan women and under- or overweight women.
- More care needs to be taken with food hygiene during pregnancy as fetal development can be adversely affected by food-borne organisms and pollutants.

The nutritional status of a woman during pregnancy influences:

- the growth and development of her fetus and forms the foundations for her child's later health;
- the mother's own health, both in the short and long term.

Poor nutrition during pregnancy has been linked to an increased risk of having a baby with a low birthweight. The link between low birthweight and infant mortality remains strong and, if they survive, low-birthweight babies suffer from higher rates of childhood illness and conditions such as hearing and visual impairment, neurodevelopmental delay and behavioural disorders. Several studies of school age children who had a low birthweight have shown less well-developed language and social skills, more behavioural and attention span problems, and lower IQ, cognitive ability and academic achievement (Dahl et al. 2006).

Poor rates of fetal and infant growth have also been linked to higher rates of premature death among adults and higher rates of cardiovascular disease and other conditions such as diabetes and high blood pressure. This fetal programming of later disease development is by epigenetic changes which are heritable and passed to future generations (Langley-Evans 2015).

Healthy eating for pregnancy

Pregnant women require slightly higher amounts of certain nutrients than non-pregnant women. Most nutrients can be met by eating a balanced nutritious diet based on the five food groups in the 'Eatwell Guide' shown in Figure 2.1 (page 21). The nutrients that will not be met even with a balanced nutritious diet are folic acid and vitamin D. A dietary supplement of both these is recommended (National Institute for Health and Care Excellence 2014, 2008).

Table 7.1 Recommended daily intake for women during pregnancy

Food groups	Recommended daily intake
1: Bread, rice, potatoes, pasta and other starchy foods	Base each meal and some snacks on these foods. Use wholegrain varieties as often as possible
2: Fruit and vegetables	Include 1 or more of these at each meal and aim for at least 5 portions per day
3: Milk, cheese and yogurt	2–3 portions of milk, cheese, yogurt. Use low-fat varieties if weight gain needs to be limited
4: Meat, fish, eggs, nuts and pulses	2–3 portions. 2 servings of fish per week are recommended, 1 of which should be oily fish
5: Oils butter and fat spread	Use in food preparation. For those trying to lose weight limit them to about 2 small portions per day
Fluids	About 6–8 drinks per day (litres) will provide adequate fluid to prevent dehydration. This includes all drinks: water, tea, coffee, milk and soups. More drinks may be needed in hot weather and after physical activity

Recommended daily intakes for women during pregnancy are outlined in Table 7.1.

Key nutrients during pregnancy

Certain key nutrients are commonly low in UK women and they need extra consideration during pregnancy to ensure good pregnancy outcomes. They are:

- folate;
- vitamin D;
- iron;
- iodine;
- omega 3 fatty acids;
- calcium;
- vitamin B12.

Folate, folic acid and neural tube defects

Research has shown a link between low folic acid/folate intakes and the development of neural tube defects (NTDs) (Medical Research Council Vitamin Study Group 1991). To reduce the risk of NTDs, supplementation with folic acid prior to conception and during the first 12 weeks of pregnancy is recommended. There are two dose levels:

- 5 mg/day (prescription only) for women with spina bifida, with a history of a previous child with an NTD or with diabetes, coeliac disease or sickle cell disease or on anti-epileptic medication;
- 400 μg (0.4 mg)/day for all other women. These supplements are available over the counter and on prescription.

The blood analyses from the NDNS Years 1–9 show that in 2016/17 almost 90 per cent of women of childbearing age have red blood cell folate concentration indicating increased risk of neural tube defect-affected pregnancies.

Mandatory fortification of flour with folic acid has been debated in the United Kingdom but has not been recommended despite the example of a fall in NTD rates of up to 40 per cent in the United States and Canada where flour has been fortified with folic acid for over 15 years.

Dietary folates

Folate is the form of folic acid found in food and the content decreases with long storage times and heat. Cooking may cause a considerable reduction. As the current average intake from diets is about 200 μg per day, women who may become pregnant should aim to increase their dietary intake of folate, in addition to the folic acid supplement, by:

- eating more folate-rich foods;
- avoiding overcooking folate-rich foods;
- choosing breads and breakfast cereals fortified with folic acid.

Foods rich in folate include:

- yeast extract;
- pulses – peas, lentils and beans;
- oranges;
- green leafy vegetables (brussels sprouts, spinach and broccoli);
- potatoes.

Liver is a rich source of folate but is not recommended during pregnancy because it has very high levels of the retinol form of vitamin A.

Vitamin D

The RNI of 10 μg/day applies to pregnant women as it does for all adults (Scientific Advisory Committee on Nutrition 2016). SACN recommend adults should consider taking a supplement to achieve this, particularly September to March when cutaneous synthesis of vitamin D does not occur in the United Kingdom. As mean intakes from food sources for women of childbearing age are around 2 μg/day, it is advisable that women likely to become pregnant should take this supplement before and during pregnancy all year.

Groups of women who are particularly at risk of low vitamin D status are:

- those with black or coloured skin (e.g. of Asian, African, Caribbean and Middle Eastern origin);
- those who have limited skin exposure to sunlight (e.g. those who remain covered when outside or who are housebound);
- obese women – those with a body mass index (BMI) >30 kg/m^2.

During pregnancy, lack of vitamin D may adversely affect fetal bone mineralisation and the accumulation of vitamin D stores for the early months of life. Babies born to women with low vitamin D levels are at higher risk of:

- seizures (hypocalcaemic fits) and breathing problems as young infants;
- rickets and growth delay as older infants and toddlers;
- cardiomyopathy.

In addition, children born to mothers with low vitamin D levels during pregnancy have been found to be more likely to have lower levels of bone minerals at 9 years of age than children born to mothers with normal vitamin D levels (Javaid et al. 2006).

Iron

Women with good iron status prior to conception and who eat a balanced nutritious diet will not need extra iron during pregnancy because the rising demands of iron by the growing fetus are met by:

- diminished losses from the mother as menstrual bleeding is absent during pregnancy;
- increased iron absorption during pregnancy – the level of absorption increases progressively as pregnancy advances. Also, a greater percentage increase in absorption will occur in anaemic than in non-anaemic women.

The fetus accumulates most of its iron during the last trimester, laying down stores for about the first 4–6 months of life.

Routine iron supplementation is not recommended for all women (National Institute for Health and Care Excellence 2008) and is usually only recommended for those with a history of anaemia who are likely to have low iron stores or who develop clinical signs of anaemia during pregnancy. Women at risk of deficiency during pregnancy are those that start their pregnancy with low iron stores, perhaps due to large menstrual losses and/or low intakes. Iron supplementation may have side-effects such as constipation or nausea.

Iron-rich foods to include are:

- meat, especially red meat, such as beef, lamb, pork dark poultry meat;
- oily fish – limit to two servings per week (see page 83);
- pulses (peas, beans and lentils);
- iron-fortified breakfast cereals;
- green vegetables;
- dried fruit (e.g. apricots, prunes, raisins).

Note: Liver is high in iron but is not recommended during pregnancy because of its high retinol content.

Women following a vegetarian diet and those who eat little meat can increase their iron absorption from cereal and vegetable sources by:

- having food or a drink containing vitamin C with a meal (e.g. orange after baked beans on toast);
- avoiding drinking tea at mealtimes as the tannins present in tea bind with the iron, reducing its absorption.

Iodine

This essential nutrient is required for the biosynthesis of thyroid hormones, which are responsible for regulating growth, development and metabolism. Although the United Kingdom does not recommend a higher intake of iodine during pregnancy than the RNI for adults of 140 µg/day, other scientific organisations do:

- European Food Safety Authority recommend 200 µg/day (European Food Safety Authority 2014);
- The US RDA is 220–250 µg/day.

Women who do not eat fish and eggs and do not have three servings of cows' milk, cheese or yogurt per day are unlikely to reach either of these recommendations. Hence vegan women and those avoiding dairy products are particularly at risk of deficiency. The consequences of poor iodine intake can compromise brain development in the fetus and consequently IQ levels in childhood and later life. A supplement suitable for pregnancy should be considered for women who do not consume iodine-rich foods. However excess iodine intake is also detrimental so kelp and seaweed supplements, which are not regulated and may contain very high levels of iodine causing thyroid problems, should not be taken.

Omega 3 fats

Docosahexaenoic acid (DHA) and eicosapentaenoic acid (EPA) are the long-chain polyunsaturated (LCP) omega-3 fats that are vital for brain growth, visual and neurological development in the fetus and young infant. Women who do not eat fish may not get enough of these fats.

The International Society for the Study of Fatty Acids and Lipids (ISSFAL) recommends that pregnant women should consume:

- 200 mg DHA/day as is recommended for the general adult population (Koletzko et al. 2007);
- >500 mg/day of DHA + EPA.

This can be achieved by eating one or two portions of oily fish a week. A portion is about 100 g cooked weight. Oily fish includes salmon, trout, mackerel, sardines, pilchards, herring, kippers, eel, whitebait and fresh tuna. Canned tuna does not count as an 'oily fish' as the fat content is reduced prior to canning.

Pregnant women who do not eat oily fish may choose to take supplements of omega 3 fats to ensure an adequate intake of long-chain omega 3 fats. Supplements containing:

- 200 mg-1 g DHA/day and;
- 500 mg-2.7 g in total of omega 3 LCPs (DHA + EPA).

have not caused harm in pregnant women (Koletzko et al. 2007).

Women should look for a suitable preparation which provides quantities within the range above but without the retinol form of vitamin A. Fish oils supplements usually contain retinol and are not suitable.

Calcium

Despite high fetal requirements for calcium, additional calcium is not usually needed as the mother's calcium absorption increases during pregnancy. However, some women, particularly teenagers, avoid dairy products and have low calcium intakes. Care should be taken that during pregnancy adequate calcium is consumed by eating 2–3 servings daily of any of the following:

- milk: 1 glass (200 ml);
- cheese: 30–45 g;
- yogurt: 150–200 g;
- tofu: 50 g.

Pregnant adolescents have higher needs, however, as they will not have achieved their own peak bone mass and should be encouraged to eat at least three servings of these calcium-rich foods each day.

Women who do not consume dairy products or calcium-enriched drinks such as plant based alternatives to milk should be advised to take a calcium supplement of about 700 mg calcium to ensure an adequate calcium intake. Plant based alternatives to milk may be enriched with calcium but are not always enriched with iodine making them unsuitable as a direct substitute for milk during pregnancy.

Supplements for pregnant women

Recommendations and the availability and relative costs of suitable supplements for women who may become pregnant and who are pregnant are listed in Tables 7.2 and 7.3.

Table 7.2 Folic acid and vitamin D supplement recommendations

Vitamin	Daily dose	Recommendation
Folic acid	400 µg	For any women and adolescent girls who may become pregnant and up to the 12th week of pregnancy. This supplement can safely be taken throughout the whole of the pregnancy and while breastfeeding
	5 mg	For women at high risk of having an NTD-affected pregnancy. GPs should prescribe for women who are planning a pregnancy, or are in the early stages of pregnancy, if they: • (or their partner) have an NTD • have had a previous baby with an NTD • (or their partner) have a family history of NTD • have diabetes • have coeliac disease • have sickle cell anaemia • are taking anti-epileptic drugs • are overweight
Vitamin D	10 µg	For all women and adolescent girls who may become pregnant, and for those who are pregnant

NTD, neural tube defect.

Table 7.3 Suitable supplements for pregnant women and for women who may become pregnant

Supplement	Content	Availability	Relative cost
NHS Healthy Start vitamins for women	400 µg folic acid 10 µg vitamin D3 70 mg vitamin C	NHS outlets only and some children's centres	Relatively inexpensive
Simple vitamin D supplements	Vitamin D only – dose varies 10–25 µg	Some retail pharmacies*	Relatively inexpensive
Simple Folic acid supplements	400 µg folic acid	Some retail pharmacies*	Relatively inexpensive
Branded supplements for preconception and pregnancy	Folic acid, vitamin D and a wide range of other nutrients including iron, iodine and omega 3 fats.	Retail pharmacies, supermarkets*	Relatively expensive

* Only brands sold in pharmacies should be used as vitamin and mineral supplements are not regulated and pharmacies only sell brands with good quality control.

Appropriate weight gain during pregnancy

Additional energy is needed during pregnancy to support the growth of the fetus and to enable fat to be deposited in the mother's body for later use during lactation. However reductions in metabolic rate compensate for the increased energy needs during the first two trimesters and pregnant women only need to increase their energy intake during the last trimester when an extra 200 kcal per day is recommended (e.g. two slices of buttered bread provide 200 kcal). They should be strongly advised against 'eating for two'.

Physical activity during pregnancy is encouraged for both maternal and fetal health and most women reduce their activity in the third trimester.

There are currently no UK evidence-based recommendations on appropriate weight gain during pregnancy. However, the American Institute of Medicine (IOM) recommends the weight gains listed in Table 7.4.

Women who gain weight within the IOM ranges are more likely to have better maternal and infant outcomes than those who gain more or less weight (Kominiarek et al. 2018):

- Gaining too little weight is associated with preterm birth and low birthweight term infants.
- Excess gestational weight gain is associated with gestational diabetes, pre-eclampsia, macrosomia, neonatal hypoglycaemia, caesarean delivery and difficulties during delivery such as shoulder dystocia. It is also associated with postpartum weight retention in the short, intermediate and long term and risk of childhood obesity for the fetus.

Overweight and obese women

In the Health Survey for England in 2018, 20–30 per cent of women of childbearing age were obese which causes dyslipidaemia, hyperleptinaemia, hyperinsulinaemia and an exaggerated systemic inflammation. It is associated with health inequalities, particularly socio-economic deprivation, inequalities within ethnic groups and poor access to maternity services (Heslehurst et al. 2007).

National Institute for Health and Care Excellence (2014) recommends that obese women are referred to a registered dietitian for assessment and advice and that overweight and obese pregnant women should be advised:

- not to lose weight during pregnancy as this may compromise their nutrient intake and that of the fetus;
- to limit the amount of weight gained in pregnancy;
- to take regular physical activity to help limit their weight gain, as studies have shown that exercise in pregnancy is safe and reduces their risk of gestational diabetes.

Underweight women

Women with a low BMI at the start of pregnancy need to increase their food intake to provide more energy and nutrients for both themselves and their fetus.

Table 7.4 Appropriate weight gains during pregnancy

Pre-pregnancy weight	Pre-pregnancy BMI (kg/m^2)	Appropriate weight gain during pregnancy (kg)
Normal weight	18.5–24.9	11.5–16
Overweight	25–29.9	7–11.5*
Obese	>30	5–9*
Underweight	<18.5	12.5–18

* or less if the fetus is growing well.

Adapted from American College of Obstetrics and Gynecology 2013.

Women at increased nutritional risk during pregnancy

Women with pre-existing medical conditions

Women with pre-existing conditions, such as diabetes mellitus, food allergies and malabsorption syndromes, should be referred to a dietitian prior to pregnancy and have their nutritional status monitored closely throughout the pregnancy.

Diabetes

Women with diabetes account for 2–5 per cent of pregnancies in England and Wales. About 90 per cent of these are due to gestational diabetes, while the remainder have become pregnant with pre-existing diabetes. Both forms of diabetes in pregnancy are associated with health risks to both the woman and the developing fetus.

The following conditions are more common during pregnancy in women with pre-existing diabetes (National Institute for Health and Care Excellence 2015):

- miscarriage;
- pre-eclampsia;
- deteriorating diabetic retinopathy;
- preterm labour;
- stillbirth;
- congenital malformations;
- macrosomia (abnormally large body size);
- birth injury;
- perinatal mortality;
- postnatal adaptation problems such as hypoglycaemia.

Hyperglycaemia during pregnancy is associated with an increased risk of childhood obesity.

Gestational diabetes

The risk factors for gestational diabetes are:

- BMI >30 kg/m^2;
- previous macrosomic baby (birthweight of 4.5 kg or above);
- previous gestational diabetes;
- family history of diabetes (first-degree relative with diabetes);
- family origin with a high prevalence of diabetes, such as South Asian (specifically women whose country of family origin is India, Pakistan or Bangladesh), black Caribbean or Middle Eastern (specifically women whose country of family origin is Saudi Arabia, United Arab Emirates, Iraq, Jordan, Syria, Oman, Qatar, Kuwait, Lebanon or Egypt).

Women with any one of these risk factors should be offered testing for gestational diabetes (National Institute for Health and Care Excellence 2008).

In most women, gestational diabetes will respond to changes in diet and physical activity. National Institute for Health and Care Excellence (2015) recommend that women with gestational diabetes:

- should receive dietary advice including choosing low glycaemic index carbohydrates;
- take moderate exercise of at least 30 minutes daily;
- are advised to restrict calorie intake (to 25 kcal/kg/day or less) if their pre-pregnancy BMI is above 27 kg/m^2 (a registered dietitian can give this advice);
- should aim to keep fasting blood glucose between 3.5 and 5.9 mmol/L and one-hour postprandial blood glucose below 7.8 mmol/L. Oral hypoglycaemic agents or insulin may be required. Maintaining these levels throughout pregnancy will reduce the risk of miscarriage, congenital malformation, stillbirth and neonatal death. It is important to explain that risks can be reduced but not eliminated (National Institute for Health and Care Excellence 2015).

Adolescents

Studies have shown that teenage pregnancy is associated with:

- lower gestational weight gain;
- an increased risk of low birthweight;

- pregnancy-induced hypertension (PIH);
- preterm labour;
- iron-deficiency anaemia;
- maternal mortality.

Nutritional status at conception is more likely to be suboptimal as the diets of teenagers in the United Kingdom are poor (See Chapter 16). The National Diet and Nutrition Surveys have shown that a large percentage of teenage girls have inadequate intakes of vitamin A, riboflavin, folate, calcium, iodine, iron and zinc. Blood tests showed low blood levels of iron, folate and vitamin D (Public Health England 2018).

Factors influencing poor dietary intakes in teenage girls include:

- making own independent food choices;
- finalising their autonomy and rejecting family meals and family food values;
- high intake of high-calorie, low-nutrient foods such as sweet drinks and junk foods;
- dieting to manage weight;
- following vegetarian or vegan diets without substituting alternative sources of iron when meat is eliminated;
- low intake of milk and milk products.

Adolescent girls may have increased nutritional requirements because they need to complete their own growth as well as providing for the fetus. The shorter the length of time between the onset of menarche and pregnancy, the greater the nutritional risk. In particular, teenagers will not have achieved their peak bone mass and should be encouraged to eat at least three servings of calcium-rich foods each day, such as milk, cheese, yogurt and calcium and iodine enriched plant-based alternatives to milk.

Around 75 per cent of adolescent pregnancies are unplanned and teenagers are therefore unlikely to be taking folic acid and vitamin D supplements prior to conception or in early pregnancy.

Pregnant teenage girls under the age of 18 years are eligible to join the Healthy Start scheme regardless of their financial circumstances (www.healthystart.nhs.uk). If they join, they are entitled to receive free vitamin supplements of folic acid and vitamin D along with vouchers to purchase milk, fruit and vegetables.

Vegetarian and vegan women

Many vegetarian women have significantly better diets than those of non-vegetarian women, but those particularly at risk are:

- those, often adolescents, who have decided to avoid meat and other animal foods without taking care to ensure alternative sources of nutrients;
- recent immigrants who may not be able to access the foods they would have eaten in their country of origin.

A study of pregnant vegetarian women of Asian background living in the United Kingdom in the 1990s found (Reddy et al. 1994):

- shorter duration of pregnancy;
- more emergency caesarean sections;
- lower birthweight;
- shorter body length;
- smaller head circumference.

Before and during pregnancy, more care needs to be taken to ensure adequate intakes of iron, iodine, omega 3 fats, riboflavin, calcium and vitamin B12.

Vegetarian women who avoid red meat need to eat three servings of foods from food group 4 (see page 82) to make sure they are eating enough iron. Vegetarian women eating two servings of fish per week and three servings daily of milk, cheese and yogurt will have adequate iodine, calcium, vitamin B12 and omega 3 intakes.

Pregnant women who follow a vegan diet normally avoid all sources of animal foods, including milk and milk products, eggs, meat and fish. They should take care to ensure that they consume sufficient:

- iodine from a supplement suitable for pregnancy;
- iron from good sources such as nuts, pulses and fortified breakfast cereals;

- vitamin B12 from good sources such as fortified yeast extracts, fortified milk substitutes, fortified textured soya protein and fortified cereals (if these are not included in the diet a vitamin B12 supplement may be needed);
- omega 3 – by including walnuts and walnut or rapeseed oil on a daily basis or taking an omega 3 supplement (see page 84);
- calcium from enriched plant alternatives to milk each day or taking a calcium supplement.

They should also be advised that children who are raised on a vegan diet will not grow to their genetically inherited optimal height (see page 24)

Women who have previously had a low-birthweight baby

It is important to ascertain whether or not the cause of the reduced birthweight in a previous pregnancy had a nutritional component such as poor gestational weight gain and/or a reduced food intake. Short birth intervals predispose to lower birthweights because women may not have had time to replenish their nutrient stores between pregnancies, particularly if they have breastfed their babies.

Women who are homeless, living in bed and breakfast accommodation or on low incomes

These women may have the combined difficulty of living on state benefits and may be living with limited cooking facilities. Nutritional risk factors more common in low-income pregnant women are:

- maternal obesity and weight retention after birth;
- low iron stores;
- not taking folic acid or vitamin D supplements prior to pregnancy and during pregnancy;
- poor diet sometimes associated with use of drugs or excess alcohol.

Outcomes more likely are Caesarean delivery, preeclampsia, preterm delivery, stillbirth, obstetrical haemorrhage and low birthweight <2.5 kg and consequently an increased risk of neonatal morbidity and mortality (Kim et al. 2018).

Recent immigrants

Recent immigrants to the United Kingdom may not be able to access the foods they would have eaten in their country of origin and may not eat a sufficiently nutritious diet here. They may have poor nutritional status if they have been subjected to famine, food insecurity which happens during wars and/or parasitic infections.

Women with alcohol or drug problems or eating disorders

Women who have alcohol or drug problems are less likely to eat a balanced diet.

Women who give up smoking should take care not to snack on high-calorie foods in place of smoking, as this would put them at risk of gaining excess weight.

Pregnant women with past or current eating disorders such as anorexia nervosa, bulimia nervosa or binge eating disorder should be viewed as being at high risk and monitored closely both during and after pregnancy to optimise maternal and fetal outcomes (Watson et al. 2017).

Women who are restricting their food intake for reasons such as slimming or self-diagnosed food allergies may cut out whole food groups without advice from a registered dietitian and may be omitting important nutrient sources (National Institute for Health and Care Excellence 2014).

Food, drinks and supplements to avoid or limit

Vitamin A

There are two dietary forms of vitamin A:

- retinol from animal sources;
- beta carotene from plant sources – particularly brightly coloured vegetables and fruit.

Both forms are found in a nutritious balanced diet and are important during pregnancy. However, high doses of retinol are associated with teratogenesis (malformations in the fetus).

High retinol foods to avoid are:

- vitamin supplements containing retinol;
- cod liver oil supplements and other fish oil supplements containing vitamin A;
- liver and liver products such as liver paté as liver contains very high amounts of retinol.

Oily fish

Oily fish should be eaten once or twice per week because it is a good source of iodine, vitamin D and omega 3 fats for both fetus and mother. It is limited to two servings per week because some of these fish contain dioxins and PCBs (polychlorinated biphenyls) that might affect the nervous systems of the fetus.

Tuna should also be limited to four medium sized cans of tuna a week (with a drained weight of about 140 g per can) or fresh tuna steaks (weighing about 140 g when cooked or 170 g raw).

Large fish such as swordfish, marlin and shark should be avoided due to the possibility of high mercury levels.

Alcohol

Alcohol intoxication should be avoided at any stage of pregnancy and especially in the early weeks where it is associated with teratogenesis and may cause miscarriage.

The advice around limiting or avoiding alcohol intake during pregnancy varies and although there is no overall consensus opinion, there is evidence that:

- the alcohol in the mother's bloodstream crosses the placenta into the bloodstream of the fetus;
- the safest approach in pregnancy is to choose not to drink at all;
- small amounts of alcohol during pregnancy (not more than one or two units, not more than once or twice a week) have not been shown to be harmful;
- regular binge drinking (five or more units of alcohol on one occasion) around conception and in early pregnancy is particularly harmful to a woman and her baby;
- drinking heavily throughout pregnancy (more than ten units per day) is linked with an increased risk of fetal alcohol syndrome;
- fetal alcohol syndrome is characterised by reduced birthweight and length, a small head size with characteristic facial appearance and a variety of congenital abnormalities;
- alcohol has a detrimental effect on the absorption and utilisation of folate, thus compounding the problem in women who do not take folic acid supplements.

NICE recommends that pregnant women avoid alcohol but women who do choose to drink should consume no more than one or two units of alcohol, once or twice a week (National Institute for Health and Care Excellence 2008).

Alcohol units are defined in Table 7.5.

Caffeine

A limit of 200 mg/day of caffeine intake is currently recommended for pregnant women because high levels of caffeine are suspected of causing miscarriage or low birthweights.

Table 7.5 Alcohol units

Units of alcohol	Alcoholic drinks
1	Half a pint of ordinary strength beer, lager or cider (3.5 per cent alcohol by volume ABV) A 125 ml glass of wine (9 per cent ABV) A 25 ml measure of spirits (40 per cent ABV)
1.5	A 125 ml glass of wine at 11 per cent or 12 per cent ABV 1 bottle of 'alcopop'
2	A 175 ml glass of wine at 11 per cent or 12 per cent ABV

The caffeine content of drinks and chocolate is as follows:

1 shot of espresso coffee	140 mg
1 mug of filter coffee	140 mg
1 mug of instant coffee	100 mg
1 cup of brewed coffee	100 mg
1 mug of tea	75 mg
1 cup of tea	50 mg
1 mug of decaffeinated coffee or tea	about 10mg
1 can (330 mls) of cola	up to 40 mg
1 can (250 mls) of 'energy' drink	up to 80 mg
1 bar (50 g) of plain chocolate	up to 25 mg
1 bar (50 g) of milk chocolate	up to 10 mg

Certain cold and flu remedies also contain caffeine.

Food safety

General food hygiene should be followed carefully but extra care should be taken:

- when buying unwrapped foods (e.g. cooked meats and prepared salads) – if scrupulous food handling guidelines have not been followed, these foods can easily become contaminated;
- with cook-chill foods – these are ready cooked foods sold chilled and should not be eaten cold, but heated until piping hot right through. They should be heated once only, and the leftovers discarded.

Certain food-borne illnesses can cause miscarriage, stillbirth, abnormalities in the developing fetus or severe illness in the newborn (Table 7.6).

Raw shellfish (e.g. prawns, cockles and mussels) can cause food poisoning and should only be eaten if they are bought packaged and stamped with a 'use-by' date.

Foods that are safe to eat during pregnancy include:

- cooked shellfish, including prawns that are part of a hot meal and have been cooked thoroughly;
- live or bio yogurt;
- probiotic drinks;
- fromage frais;
- crème fraîche;
- soured cream;
- spicy food;
- eggs with the British Lion mark can be eaten raw or under cooked;
- mayonnaise, ice cream and salad dressing made with pasteurised egg or home-made versions made with eggs with the British Lion mark;
- honey may be eaten during pregnancy, but is not suitable for infants until over 12 months of age;
- many cheeses including hard cheese such as cheddar and parmesan, feta, ricotta, mascarpone, cream cheese, mozzarella, cottage cheese, processed cheese such as cheese spreads.

Allergy prevention advice

Avoiding any particular foods during pregnancy will **not** reduce the risk of the fetus developing a food allergy following birth or later in life.

Common dietary problems during pregnancy

Nausea and vomiting

Nausea in pregnancy is reported in 50–80 per cent of pregnant women; 52 per cent of pregnant women experience symptoms of both nausea and vomiting during early pregnancy, and 28 per cent experience nausea only.

Symptoms commonly start 4–7 weeks after the last menstrual period and cease by 12 weeks in 60 per cent of affected women. About 9 per cent of affected women have symptoms that persist beyond 16 weeks and may persist until 22 weeks of gestation. Symptoms often come and go and can

Table 7.6 Food-borne illnesses

Food-borne illness	Foods/materials to avoid	Precautions to take
Listeriosis – a flu-like illness caused by the bacteria *Listeria monocytogenes*	Pâté – meat, fish or vegetable unless tinned or pasteurised Mould-ripened soft cheeses (e.g. Brie, Camembert, soft blue-veined cheeses) Unpasteurised/raw milk and milk products (from cow, goat sheep etc.) Ready meals especially those containing chicken that are not reheated before consumption	Avoid pâté, soft cheeses and unpasteurised milk products Reheat ready meals to piping hot right through Avoid Sushi made with raw fish
Salmonella – a bacteria which is the major cause of food poisoning in the UK	Raw or partially cooked eggs that do not have the British Lion Mark and foods containing them such as mayonnaise and mousse Undercooked poultry and other meat	Meat including poultry should be thoroughly defrosted in the fridge and cooked until piping hot right through. Eggs should be cooked so both white and egg are solid
Toxoplasmosis – a disease caused by the parasite *Toxoplasma gondii* found in raw meat, soil and cat faeces	Raw or undercooked meat Unpasteurised/raw milks and milk products (from cow, goat sheep etc.) Soil Cat litter trays	Wash vegetables and salad thoroughly to remove any soil or dirt Wash hands after handling raw meat Thoroughly cook meat Wear rubber gloves when emptying cat litter trays Wash hands after handling cats
Campylobacter – a bacteria that commonly causes food poisoning in the UK	Undercooked poultry Unpasteurised/raw milks and milk products (from cow, goat sheep etc.) Untreated water Domestic pets Soil	Wear gloves while gardening Do not help with lambing or milking ewes that have recently given birth

occur at any time during the day. Typical symptoms include nausea, vomiting, fatigue, loss of appetite and weight loss (usually around 5 per cent of pre-pregnancy body weight).

Hyperemesis gravidarum is the most severe form of persistent nausea and vomiting, leading to dehydration, ketonuria, electrolyte imbalance and weight loss greater than 5 per cent of pre-pregnancy weight. It affects between 0.3 per cent and 2 per cent of all pregnant women and they need extra medical care.

The cause of nausea is thought to be the changing pregnancy hormone levels and it can occur at any time of day or night – not just in the mornings. It is often triggered by certain foods, like coffee and fried or spicy foods, or smells, such as perfumes, cigarette smoke or petrol. It can also be caused by hunger.

Advice to be given that may help includes:

- eating small, frequent meals based on starchy foods, once every two hours or so throughout the day, including foods such as bread, toast, plain biscuits or ginger biscuits, banana and breakfast cereals;
- eating plain or ginger biscuits about 20 minutes before getting out of bed in the morning
- eating cold meals rather than hot meals, which may prevent any smell-related nausea, as cold food gives off less smell than hot food;
- taking glucose tablets to possibly help prevent blood sugar levels from dropping (low blood sugar levels may cause nausea);
- avoiding any foods or smells that trigger symptoms;
- avoiding drinking cold, tart or sweet beverages;
- avoiding caffeine and alcohol;
- having lots to drink to avoid dehydration but drinking little and often rather than large amounts to prevent vomiting.

Cravings and taste changes

Changes in taste, cravings and appetite may also be related to hormonal changes or due to the removal of energy substrates from maternal blood by the fetus. Unless they alter the balance of a nutritious diet they do not present a problem. Pica is a term given to the craving of non-food substances, such as soap, chalk and coal.

Heartburn/oesophageal reflux

This is generally more common in multiple pregnancies and during the last three months of single pregnancies when pressure from the baby in the uterus can cause acid to be pushed back up from the stomach. The following changes may help:

- smaller, more frequent meals;
- sitting up straight when eating to relieve the pressure;
- not lying down flat after eating;
- sleeping propped up by extra pillows if it occurs at night;
- avoiding any foods that cause discomfort.

Constipation

This is common at all stages of pregnancy and can be relieved by increasing the amount of high-fibre foods, such as fruit, vegetables, pulses, nuts and wholegrain cereals. An increase in fluid intake to 6–8 drinks per day or about 2 litres of all drinks may help. Iron supplements tend to exacerbate constipation.

Promoting breastfeeding antenatally

NICE recommends that:

> Pregnant women should be offered opportunities to attend participant-led antenatal classes, including breastfeeding workshops. Before or at 36 weeks gestation they should receive breastfeeding information, including technique and good management practices, such as detailed in the UNICEF 'Baby Friendly Initiative' (https://www.unicef.org.uk/babyfriendly/) (National Institute for Health and Care Excellence 2008).

Activity 1

Develop a plan for a session with pregnant teenage girls. Include five key recommendations.

Activity 2

Write a one-day menu including the appropriate number of servings from each food group to provide a balanced, nutritious diet and appropriate supplements for a woman eating entirely from commercially prepared foods.

Activity 3

What are the messages to communicate to avoid food-borne risks?

References and further reading

American College of Obstetrics and Gynecologists (2013) Weight Gain During Pregnancy. Committee Opinion No. 548. *Obstetrics & Gynecology* **121**: 210–212.

Bauer I, Hartkopf J, Kullmann S, et al. (2020) Spotlight on the fetus: how physical activity during pregnancy influences fetal health: a narrative review. *BMJ Open Sport & Exercise Medicine* **6**(1): e000658. Published 2020 Mar 16. doi:10.1136/bmjsem-2019-000658.

Berti C, Cetin I, Agostoni C, et al. (2016) Pregnancy and Infants' Outcome: Nutritional and Metabolic Implications. *Critical Reviews in Food Science and Nutrition* **56**(1): 82–91.

British Dietetic Association (2019) Food Fact Sheet Iodine. https://www.bda.uk.com/resource/iodine.html.

Choi KH, Martinson ML (2018 Oct) The relationship between low birthweight and childhood health: disparities by race, ethnicity, and national origin. *Annals of Epidemiology* **28**(10): 704–709.e4. doi: 10.1016/j.annepidem.2018.08.001. Epub 2018 Aug 9.

Dahl LB, Kaaresen PI, Tunby J, Handegård BH, Kvernmo S and Rønning JA (2006) Emotional, behavioral, social, and academic outcomes in adolescents born with very low birth weight. *Pediatrics* **118**: e449–e459.

Delange F (2007) Iodine requirements during pregnancy, lactation and the neonatal period and indicators of optimal iodine nutrition. *Public Health Nutrition* **10**: 1571–1580.

Department of Health (1992) Folic Acid and the Prevention of Neural Tube Defects. Report of an Expert Advisory Group for the Department of Health. London: HMSO.

Emmett PM, Louise Jones L & Golding J (2015) Pregnancy diet and associated outcomes in the Avon Longitudinal Study of Parents and Children. *Nutrition Reviews* **73**(suppl 3): 154–174. DOI: 10.1093/nutrit/nuv053

European Food Safety Authority (2014) Scientific Opinion on Dietary Reference Values for iodine. *EFSA Journal* **12**(5): 3660.

Finkelstein JL, Guillet R, Pressman EK, et al. (2019) Vitamin B_{12} Status in Pregnant Adolescents and Their Infants. *Nutrients* **11**(2): 397. Published 2019 Feb 13. doi:10.3390/nu11020397

Harding KB, Peña-Rosas JP, Webster AC, et al. (2017 Mar 5) Iodine supplementation for women during the preconception, pregnancy and postpartum period. *Cochrane Database Syst Rev* **3**: CD011761. doi: 10.1002/14651858.CD011761.pub2.

Heslehurst N, Ellis LJ, Simpson H, Batterham A, Wilkinson JR and Summerbell CD (2007) Trends in maternal obesity incidence rate, demographic predictors, and health inequalities in 36,821 women over a 15-year period. *British Journal of Obstetrics and Gynaecology* **114**(2): 187–194.

Hoffman DJ, Reynolds RM, Hardy DB (2017 Dec 1) Developmental origins of health and disease: current knowledge and potential mechanisms. *Nutrition Reviews* **75**(12): 951–970. doi: 10.1093/nutrit/nux053.

Javaid MK, Crozier S, Harvey N, *et al.* (2006) Maternal vitamin D status during pregnancy and childhood bone mass at age 9 years: a longitudinal study. *Lancet* **367**: 36–43.

Kim, M, Lee, S, Bae, S *et al.* (2018) Socioeconomic status can affect pregnancy outcomes and complications, even with a universal healthcare system. *International Journal for Equity in Health* **17**, 2. https://doi.org/10.1186/s12939-017-0715-7

Koletzko B, Cetin I and Brenna JT (2007) Dietary fat intakes for pregnant and lactating women. *British Journal of Nutrition* **98**: 873–877.

Kominiarek MA, Saade G, Mele L, et al. (2018 Oct) Eunice Kennedy Shriver National Institute of Child Health and Human Development (NICHD) Maternal-Fetal Medicine Units (MFMU) Network. Association Between Gestational Weight Gain and Perinatal Outcomes. *Obstetrics & Gynecology* **132**(4): 875–881. doi: 10.1097/AOG.0000000000002854

Langley-Evans SC (2015 Jan) Nutrition in early life and the programming of adult disease: a review. *Journal of Human Nutrition and Dietetics* **28** Suppl 1: 1–14. doi: 10.1111/jhn.12212. Epub 2014 Jan 31

LifeCycle Project-Maternal Obesity and Childhood Outcomes Study Group, Voerman E, Santos S, Inskip H, et al. (2019 May 7) Association of Gestational Weight Gain With Adverse Maternal and Infant Outcomes. *JAMA* **321**(17): 1702–1715. doi: 10.1001/jama.2019.3820.

Medical Research Council Vitamin Study Group (1991) Prevention of neural tube defects: results research council vitamin study. *Lancet* **238**: 131–177.

National Institute for Health and Care Excellence (November 2014) Public Health Guidance 11. *Improving the nutrition of pregnant and breast-feeding mothers and children in low-income households*. London: NICE (accessed April 2020).

National Institute for Health and Care Excellence (2008) *Clinical Guidance 62. Antenatal care: routine care for the healthy pregnant woman.* Currently being updated with publication expected April 2021.

National Institute for Health and Care Excellence (February 2015) *Clinical Guidance 63. Diabetes in pregnancy: management of diabetes and its complications from preconception to the postnatal period.* www.nice.org.uk/Guidance/CG63 (accessed April 2020).

National Institute for Health and Care Excellence (July 2010) *Public Health Guidance 27. Weight management before, during and after pregnancy.* www.nice.org.uk/PH27 (accessed April 2020).

Public Health England (2018) Results of the National Diet and Nutrition Survey (NDNS) rolling programme for 2014 to 2015 and 2015 to 2016.

Reddy S, Sanders TA, & Band Obeid O (1994) The influence of the maternal vegetarian status on the essential fatty acid status of the newborn. *European Journal of Clinical Nutrition* **48**, 358–36.

Scientific Advisory Committee on Nutrition (2016 July) Vitamin D and Health. London: Public Health England.

Sebastiani G, Herranz Barbero A, Borrás-Novell C, et al. (2019) The Effects of Vegetarian and Vegan Diet during Pregnancy on the Health of Mothers and Offspring. *Nutrients* **11**(3): 557. Published 2019 Mar 6. doi:10.3390/nu11030557

Tarrade A, Panchenko P, Junien C, Gabory A (2015 Jan 1) Placental contribution to nutritional programming of health and diseases: epigenetics and sexual dimorphism. *The Journal of Experimental Biology* **218**(Pt 1): 50–58. doi: 10.1242/jeb.110320.

Velasco I, Bath SC, Rayman MP (2018 Mar 1) Iodine as Essential Nutrient during the First 1000 Days of Life. *Nutrients* **10**(3). pii: E290. doi: 10.3390/nu10030290

Watson HJ, Zerwas S, Torgersen L, et al. (2017 Jul) Maternal eating disorders and perinatal outcomes: A three-generation study in the Norwegian Mother and Child Cohort Study. *Journal of Abnormal Psychology* **126**(5): 552–564. doi: 10.1037/abn0000241.

Section 4
Infants: 0–12 months

8 Milk Feeding

9 Complementary Feeding

10 Common Feeding Problems in Infancy

11 Preterm Infants

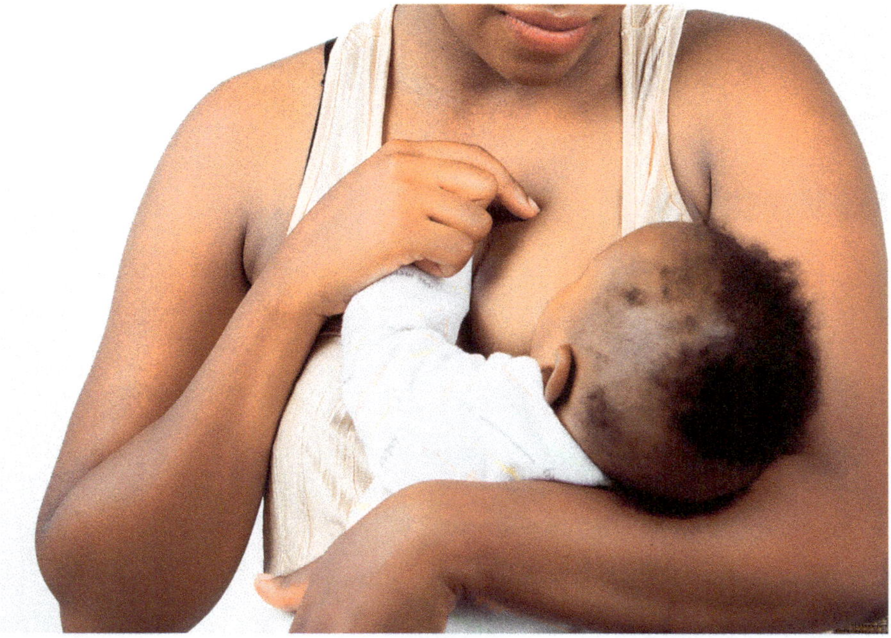

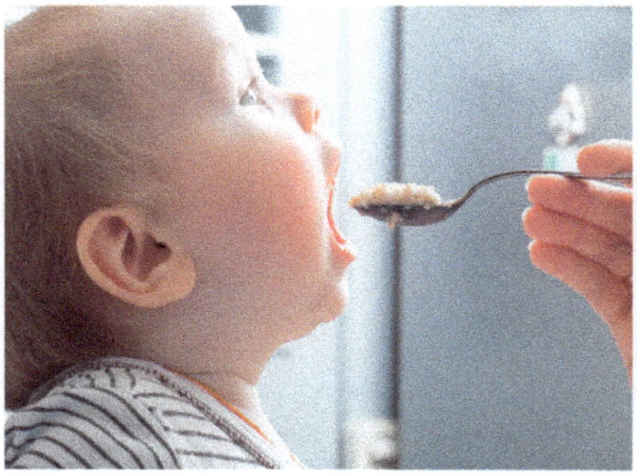

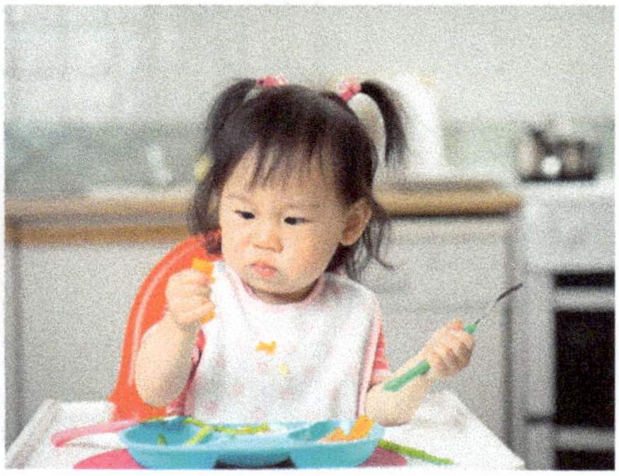

8

Milk feeding

Summary

- Breast milk is the optimal milk feed for infants because along with a vitamin D supplement it is nutritionally adequate for about the first 4–6 months of life and reduces the risk of illness in infants.
- Breastfeeding mothers may need support to overcome any problems and help them to continue to breastfeed for as long as they wish to.
- Infant formula is the only alternative to breast milk for the first 6 months. Along with a vitamin D supplement, it is nutritionally adequate but does not provide the same protection against illness. It also carries a risk of contamination.
- Follow-on formula can be used in place of infant formula after 6 months but this change is not necessary.
- There are minor differences between brands and types of infant formulas.
- All bottles, teats, pumps and containers must be washed and sterilised before being used for expressed breast milk or infant formula until the infant is 12 months old.

Nutritional requirements of infants 0–6 months

The nutritional requirements of term infants from birth to 4–6 months (see Chapter 1) can be satisfied by exclusive breastfeeding and a vitamin D supplement. Infant formula is the only breast milk substitute suitable during this time.

Choice of milk feeding

Exclusive breastfeeding is the optimal way to feed infants until complementary feeding with solid food begins at 4–6 months of age. It provides:

- the complete nutritional requirements;
- protection against illness.

Ideally, the main milk drink should continue to be breast milk alongside complementary foods and beyond for as long as the mother wishes to continue breastfeeding. About 95 per cent of women are able to produce sufficient milk and, therefore, less than 1 in 20 women will have primary lactation insufficiency (Neifert 2001).

The contraindications to breastfeeding are:

- the baby has classical galactosaemia, a long chain fatty acid oxidation defect or glucose-galactose malabsorption;
- the mother is taking certain medications, receiving radiotherapy or chemotherapy, is a drug abuser or takes excessive alcohol;
- HIV positive status of the mother as HIV transmission from mother to infant can occur via breastmilk.

Infant formula is the only nutritionally adequate alternative to breast milk during the first 6 months for term infants. Even though it does not provide immunity to protect infants from illness, it is a socially acceptable way to feed infants. The last UK Infant Feeding Survey in 2010 reported that 81 per cent of mothers initiate breastfeeding soon after birth; however, exclusive breastfeeding declines rapidly with only 46 per cent mothers doing so at the end of the first week, 23 per cent at six weeks and 1 per cent at six months (McAndrew et al. 2012). Higher hospital admission rates are seen in formula fed infants compared to breastfed infants and estimates are that if all UK infants were exclusively breastfed, the number hospitalised each month with diarrhoea would be halved, and the number hospitalised with a respiratory infections would be cut by a quarter (Quigley et al. 2007).

When parents have access to reliable advice and information, they can make an informed choice on how to feed their infants. Maternity units that follow the World Health Organization 'Ten Steps to Successful Breastfeeding' have higher numbers of mothers breastfeeding on discharge from the unit. The ten steps are:

Critical management procedures

1a Comply fully with the *International Code of Marketing of Breast-milk Substitutes* and relevant World Health Assembly resolutions.
1b Have a written infant feeding policy that is routinely communicated to staff and parents.
1c Establish ongoing monitoring and data-management systems.
2. Ensure that staff have sufficient knowledge, competence and skills to support breastfeeding.

Key clinical practices

3. Discuss the importance and management of breastfeeding with pregnant women and their families.
4. Facilitate immediate and uninterrupted skin-to-skin contact and support mothers to initiate breastfeeding as soon as possible after birth.
5. Support mothers to initiate and maintain breastfeeding and manage common difficulties.

Key clinical practices

6. Do not provide breastfed new-borns any food or fluids other than breast milk, unless medically indicated.
7. Enable mothers and their infants to remain together and to practise rooming-in 24 hours a day.
8. Support mothers to recognise and respond to their infants' cues for feeding.
9. Counsel mothers on the use and risks of feeding bottles, teats and pacifiers.
10. Coordinate discharge so that parents and their infants have timely access to ongoing support and care.

When her decision on how to feed her infant is made, a mother needs to be supported and advised on safe feeding. Breastfeeding mothers often need support to overcome any difficulties and problems that arise, as without appropriate support many give up breastfeeding before they wish to. Mothers choosing to formula feed need to be shown how to sterilise feeding equipment and make up formula feeds safely.

Milk feeding choices for mothers with HIV

In the United Kingdom, women known to be HIV antibody positive, should be advised not to breastfeed but to use infant formula for feeding their baby as the HIV virus can be passed to the infant via breast milk. Mixed feeding – offering both breast milk and infant formula – carries the highest risk of HIV transmission to the infant. Where HIV-positive mothers do not have facilities to make up infant formula safely, they are advised to breastfeed exclusively to reduce the risk of death through gastroenteritis from bacterial contamination of infant formula not made up hygienically. The WHO recommends that HIV-positive mothers or their infants take antiretroviral drugs throughout the period of breastfeeding and until their infant is 12 months old.

Table 8.1 Average energy and macronutrient composition of breastmilk stages compared to formula milks (Hester et al. 2012)

	Energy (kcal/100 ml)	Protein (g/100 ml)	Fat (g/100 ml)	Carbohydrate (g/100 ml)
Colostrum 1–5 days	53.6 ± 2.5	2.5 ± 0.2	2.2 ± 0.2	5.6 ± 0.6
Transition breastmilk 3 –14 days	57.7 ± 4.2	1.7 ± 0.1	3.0 ± 0.1	5.9 ± 0.4
Mature breastmilk from about 14 days	65.2 ± 1.1	1.3 ± 0.1	3.8 ± 0.1	6.7 ± 0.2
Infant formula(average various UK brands)	67	1.3	3.4	7.4

Breastfeeding

Breastfeeding is the natural way of providing nutritional, emotional and social care for the infant. There are also environmental benefits in that no transport or bottle and teat manufacturing costs are involved.

Benefits of breast milk for the infants and their mothers

The health of both mother and child benefit, in the short and long term, and the longer the duration of breastfeeding, the greater the health benefits to both. Exclusive breastfeeding until complementary feeding begins and then continued breastfeeding alongside complementary foods provides maximum health benefits to infants.

For the infant (Ip et al. 2009; Scientific Advisory Committee on Nutrition 2018):

- reduced incidence of non-specific gastroenteritis and lower severe respiratory infections;
- reduced risk of otitis media;
- fewer visits to the doctor in the first 2 years of life.

For the mother:

- delay in return to menstruation allowing maternal iron stores to replenish following pregnancy and childbirth;
- reduced risk of breast and ovarian cancer;
- lower risk of postnatal depression;
- lower incidence of osteoporosis and hip fractures when over 65 years.

Evidence is controversial around whether breastfeeding reduces the risk of asthma and obesity in the child.

Stages of breast milk

The composition of breast milk changes at different stages of infant development. The identifiable stages are colostrum, transitional milk and mature milk. Differences are shown in Table 8.1.

Colostrum

During pregnancy the glandular tissue of the breast proliferates and can produce colostrum from mid-pregnancy. It is ready in the breasts when the baby is born and has the following properties:

- a high-density, low-volume milk, which is ideal for the newborn infant;
- less fat, lactose and water-soluble vitamins than mature milk, but more protein, zinc and fat-soluble vitamins A and K;
- a laxative effect to aid the passage of an infant's first stool (meconium);
- rich in antibodies and immunoglobulins which provide protection against bacteria and viruses.

Over the first 2½ days, infants may be quite sleepy and feed infrequently. Very small volumes of colostrum (10–13 ml/kg per day) are taken and are adequate (Dollberg et al. 2001). Supply is under hormonal control and will not increase with more frequent feeding. A net body weight loss occurs, which is mainly fluid as infant's blood volume decreases by about 25 per cent over this time. A weight loss of up to about 10 per cent of birthweight is considered normal.

However, blood glucose testing at 2–4 hours after birth should be carried out routinely in infants of women with diabetes. They should also feed as soon as possible after birth (within 30 minutes) and then at frequent intervals (every 2–3 hours) until feeding maintains pre-feed blood glucose levels at a minimum of 2.0 mmol/L (National Institute for Health and Care Excellence 2015).

Transitional milk

Transitional milk is colostrum diluted with mature milk and is produced from around the third day after delivery. It is a less concentrated feed than colostrum, having a higher water content. Colostrum production gradually diminishes and transitional milk gradually changes into mature milk by about the 14th day.

Mothers may experience breast discomfort on day 2 or 3 as the blood and lymph flow increases in the breast in preparation for the higher volumes of transitional milk. Breasts may feel full and heavy and the infant begins to demand feeds more frequently. Company and support from another adult will be beneficial as a mother may need to feed very frequently throughout that 24 hours. Mothers can be reassured that although they may have an uncomfortable 24 hours, over that time the volume of milk produced will eventually equal the amount that their infant is demanding and their breasts will become more comfortable again.

Over the subsequent few days infants begin to take larger volumes at each feed and settle into a routine of feeding less frequently. Some feed about every 3–4 hours, however, other babies prefer more frequent feeds until they are older.

More skin-to-skin contact between a mother and her infant is recommended for newborn infants who do not feed well.

Mature milk

Mature milk production is controlled by hormones and feedback mechanisms. Removal of milk from the breast is essential for continued production.

Throughout each feed the composition of the milk changes:

- At the beginning of the feed the milk has a high water content and low fat content satisfying the infant's thirst.
- As the feed progresses the fat content increases, increasing the energy content of the milk and satisfying the infant's hunger.

Allowing infants to finish feeding from 1 breast before being offered the other breast ensures that both low fat and high fat milks are taken, providing the correct balance of energy and nutrients. Some infants demand feeds frequently while others take larger volumes less frequently, but the total daily fat intake is not affected by the frequency of feeding nor whether 1 or both breasts are suckled at each feed (Kent et al. 2006).

No other food or fluids need to be offered, unless medically indicated, until complementary feeding begins. Even in hot weather additional water is unnecessary as breastfeeding on demand will satisfy infants' fluid requirements as they take shorter, more frequent feeds to satisfy any increased thirst.

Mature milk will provide all the nutrients an infant needs until 4–6 months except for vitamin D.

Vitamin D supplementation

Breast milk is very low in vitamin D and Public Health England, the European Food Safety Authority and The European Society for Paediatric Endocrinology recommend that all infants should begin a vitamin D supplement from birth (Braegger et al. 2013, Munns et al. 2016). Infants whose mothers were vitamin D deficient during pregnancy are born with inadequate stores and are at risk of tetanic seizures and cardiomyopathy due to vitamin D deficiency.

Table 8.2 Variability of frequency and length of breastfeeds

Age of baby	Frequency of feeds	Length of feeds
First 48 hours	Infrequent and as few as 3 feeds in first 24 hours	Variable
From day 3 to 7	Increase in frequency on day 3 to up to 12 feeds in 24 hours and then slowly decreasing in frequency	Very variable, both between babies and from feed to feed
After 7 days	Variable between infants but most feed about 6–8 times in 24 hours	Still variable but each baby will begin to develop an individual pattern over a 24-hour period

Supporting mothers to start and continue breastfeeding

When infants are delivered onto the mother's bare skin the period of skin-to-skin contact triggers the onset of lactation, stimulates instinctive feeding behaviour and facilitates bonding. Infants should be offered a breastfeed soon after birth – ideally within the first hour (World Health Organization 2002).

Breastfeeding is a skill that mothers and their babies learn together. Reassurance and consistent advice on correct positioning and attachment for breastfeeding will help mothers to breastfeed successfully and overcome problems.

A mother needs to learn the cues her infant gives her to show he or she is hungry. Most newborn infants show the rooting reflex when hungry, turning the head from side to side and making sucking movements. Infants who remain close to their mother can be fed on demand throughout the day and night.

Offering both breasts at each feed is ideal and when mothers develop a routine for each feeding session, the baby learns what to expect at each feed and will be more relaxed during feeding sessions.

Example of a feeding session routine

Offer the first breast and allow the infant to feed for as long as he or she wishes, allowing the baby to come off the breast when he or she has had enough. Give the baby a cuddle, holding him or her upright to wind. Next change the nappy and then offer the second breast, allowing the baby to feed for as long as he or she wishes and again to come off this breast when he or she has had enough or falls asleep.

By feeding correctly and on demand a good milk supply should be ensured for at least 95 per cent of mothers.

The frequency and length of breastfeeds will vary from infant to infant and changes with age. Some guidance is given in Table 8.2.

Positioning and Attachment

Positioning

Infants should be held:

- close to the mother and the angle of the breast will determine which position is best for the infant to effectively milk the breast – the mother can be sitting or lying. Some mothers like a pillow to support their back and another on their lap to support the infant. Following a caesarean section the underarm method or 'rugby ball hold' may be more comfortable.
- with the infant's back, shoulders and neck supported allowing the head to easily tilt backwards.
- with the infant's ear, shoulder and hip in a line to ensure the neck is not twisted during feeding.

Attaching onto the breast

1. The infant should be brought towards the breast with his or her nose level with the mother's nipple, with the chin and lower lip reaching the breast first.
2. As the infant comes close to the breast and

touches it, the mouth will gape open. This gape can be encouraged by stroking the top lip with the nipple.

3. The infant will usually tilt his or her head back bringing the chin to the breast first. At the height of the gape, the infant's mouth should be brought onto the nipple and areola with as much of the areola below the nipple being taken into the mouth as possible.
4. Once attached to the breast there should be more areola visible above the baby's top lip than the lower lip; the lower lip should be turned out and the tongue under the mother's nipple; the chin can be indented into the breast and the nose must be free for breathing.
5. If the infant is correctly positioned it will not be necessary to press the breast away from the infant's nose and the infant should be able to see the mother's face with his or her top eye.
6. When the infant has fed successfully he or she will come off the breast spontaneously, leaving a round, soft nipple.

Indicators of good attachment

- the infant's mouth is wide open while feeding;
- the infant's chin is touching the breast;
- the infant's cheeks are full – baby has a great big mouthful of breast;
- more of the mother's areola can be seen above the baby's upper lip;
- the infant's cheeks stay rounded during sucking;
- the infant rhythmically takes long sucks and swallows – although it is normal for the baby to pause from time to time.

Although painless feeding may not be a reliable sign of good attachment, breastfeeding should not hurt after the first few sucks. If discomfort continues, the mother should take the infant off the breast and attach him or her to the breast again, aiming to improve the attachment.

Indicators of poor attachment

- the infant's lips are pursed;
- the infant's mouth is not open wide;
- the infant's cheeks are sucked in with each jaw movement;
- there is a gap between the infant's chin and the mother's breast;
- the infant has not got a big mouthful of breast;
- the infant's mouth is central or uppermost on the mother's areola;
- nipple pain continues throughout the breastfeed;
- the nipple is pointed, flattened, lined or wedge shaped after feeding.

Problems that suggest poor attachment include:

In mothers	In infants
• Breast pain while feeding • Sore or cracked nipples, engorgement • Too little milk • Mastitis or breast abscess	• Generally unhappy/ unsettled • Slow weight gain • Faltering growth • Explosive or green stools

Progression of a breastfeed

- When correctly attached, sucking will start immediately.
- The sucking action will change from short shallow sucks to long deep sucks.
- Infants will pause from time to time.
- Infants become more relaxed as the feed progresses.
- The feed should be quiet, swallowing may be heard, but any noisy gulping, clicking or kissing sounds may indicate that optimal attachment has not occurred.
- The length of feeds will vary according to the infant's needs in the early days. Feeds may be long but will probably become shorter as baby becomes more efficient at sucking through practice and oral development.
- Infants usually let go of the breast spontaneously on finishing the feed.

- The mother's nipple should be the same shape as it was before the feed – any changes in shape or colour indicate that the nipple should be further back in the baby's mouth.

Breastfeeding twins and multiples

In the same way that mothers make enough milk for 1 infant, it is possible to breastfeed multiples.

Mothers approach this in different ways but most start by feeding each baby separately until they are confident with positioning and attachment. Once that has been achieved, feeding 2 twins together will shorten overall feeding times. The underarm hold will probably be the easiest to manage both twins at the same time in the early days. The twins should swap breasts at alternate feeds to ensure both breasts are equally stimulated, as 1 twin may suck more efficiently than the other.

For triplets or more infants, mothers need more individual help. If a mother wishes to give some formula, giving breast milk as well to her infants will benefit them.

Monitoring breastfed infants

Frequent weighing of breastfed infants is no longer recommended as small or no discernible weight gain can be distressing for parents and cause them to give up breastfeeding. Small gains in weight can easily be masked by a change in fluid content: an infant with a full bladder can weigh up to 200 g more than after emptying his or her bladder.

A breastfed infant who is feeding adequately will:

- be alert, responsive and healthy in appearance;
- take a minimum of six feeds in 24 hours during the day and night in the first few weeks;
- have at least six wet nappies in 24 hours;
- have at least 2 yellow stools daily.

Overcoming breastfeeding problems and difficulties

Many mothers need support to continue breastfeeding and when discharged from the maternity unit they should be given (National Institute for Health and Care Excellence 2014):

- contact details of breastfeeding counsellors they can contact for help and support with breastfeeding in case they encounter problems;
- information on local peer support groups since it has been shown that breastfeeding mothers who are in contact with other breastfeeding mothers continue breastfeeding for longer.

The majority of breastfeeding problems are directly or indirectly attributable to incorrect attachment of the infant to the breast. Even if the attachment appears good, it can usually be improved.

To assess breastfeeding problems the healthcare practitioner should:

- take a breastfeeding history – going back to the birth if necessary;
- ask about a typical feed;
- ask about a typical day, including feed frequency, behaviour in between feeds, including the sleep pattern;
- examine the infant, noting general appearance, including the tongue;
- check the infant's weight gain and growth chart;
- take note of the number of wet nappies and stool frequency and colour;
- observe a feed and assess positioning and attachment, noting jaw action, swallow, length of feed and infant's behaviour, and listening for audible swallowing;
- examine the mother;
- ask about family life and the mother's responsibilities in addition to her infant.

Sore or cracked nipples

Sore nipples are usually due to poor attachment and the pain should decrease when attachment is improved. However, in some instances sore nipples may be due to:

- thrush: *Candida albicans,* is a fungal infection that often follows the use of antibiotics to treat mastitis or other infections. The skin may become sore and itchy. Both mother and baby may be infected and should be referred to the GP for treatment.
- Reynaud's syndrome where some women's nipples become blanched due to lack of blood supply. There is no ready cure for this but heat treatment and feeding in a warm room may help.
- Cracked nipples which may follow from poor attachment. Mothers should be encouraged to continue breastfeeding, as with improved attachment nipple pain should lessen considerably after about the first 20 seconds of feeding. Nipples will then begin to heal. Occasionally, cracked nipples may bleed and the infant may posit or vomit bloodstained milk. Ingesting blood is harmless for the infant and there is no cause for alarm.

Engorgement

Engorgement occurs when the breast becomes full of milk and the blood and lymph flow slows and enters the breast tissue, causing oedema. Infrequent feeding or abrupt weaning off breastmilk may cause it. One or both breasts may be affected. It may be the areola or the body of the breast or both that are infected. Indications are:

- the breast is warm, painful, throbbing – this may extend up into the mother's armpit;
- skin may appear red, shiny, taut and oedematous;
- low-grade pyrexia may be present.

Possible actions to deal with engorgement include:

- massaging before feeds; kneading with fingertips using a circular motion, beginning at the chest wall and travelling around the breast in a spiral towards the nipple;
- applying warm water before a feed (shower/bowl of water/warm compress)
- combination of massage and heat (e.g. shower and massage together);
- expressing gently, aiming to soften the areola and enabling the baby to attach and feed;
- breastfeeding more often, finishing the first breast before moving on to the second;
- changing breastfeeding position;
- applying cold compresses after feeds to help reduce swelling and relieve pain
- using cabbage leaves – anecdotal evidence says women find these soothing when worn inside the bra next to the skin with a hole cut out for the nipple.

Analgesics such as paracetamol can be used to reduce symptoms. Aspirin should NOT be taken by breastfeeding mothers.

Blocked ducts

Blocked ducts may be caused by engorgement or poor positioning and attachment. The mother should be shown how to massage the affected area and express her breast. Hot flannels and a bath or shower may help. Cold, washed cabbage leaves around the breast are a traditional method still used but without evidence to support it.

Mastitis

Mastitis can be prevented by early diagnosis of, and successful treatment of blocked ducts. However, if it does occur the mother should continue to breastfeed, but it is essential that her positioning and attachment be improved. If it fails to respond or gets worse, the mother may need to take antibiotics in addition to correct management. Unless positioning and attachment are improved, mastitis may re-occur. Unresolved mastitis may lead to a breast abscess.

Breast abscess

A breast abscess may require a surgical aspiration or operation and drainage. However, breastfeeding should continue. If the abscess is close to the nipple, the mother may wish to express on the affected side, until it is a little more comfortable.

Inadequate milk supply

Inadequate milk supply is a common reason that mothers cite when they perceive that their milk is not satisfying their infant. This may be true in about 5 per cent of mothers but in most this perception may simply be due to persistent crying or fussing by infants. As infants do not only cry because they are hungry, they often cry because they are uncomfortable, cold, lonely or bored. A crying infant may just need comforting and someone to talk and interact with them. Some infants experience more discomfort than others (e.g. those who have colic or reflux). Comforting an infant who has colic, reflux or some other cause for discomfort other than hunger can be very stressful and time consuming for parents and carers.

Any of the following measures may help to increase milk supply:

- Different positioning (e.g. underarm or lying down) may help the infant to feed more efficiently.
- The infant needs to feed on both breasts at each feed and for as long as he or she wishes on each breast to ensure adequate intake.
- More frequent feeding may help some infants but it is important they are allowed to feed as long as they wish on both breasts.
- Mothers may need to adapt their lifestyle to allow more time for feeding. Help with their household tasks and looking after other children may encourage some mothers to be more relaxed about the time taken for breastfeeding.

Tongue-tie

On occasions an infant with a marked tongue-tie may experience difficulty with breastfeeding. This can be resolved with minor surgery.

Mixed breast and bottle feeding

Infants find bottle feeding easier than breastfeeding as they suck against more pressure when feeding from the breast than when feeding from a bottle teat. Giving expressed breast milk from a bottle may improve breast milk intake in infants who are having feeding problems.

Introducing formula milk in bottles is likely to decrease an infant's breast milk intake and subsequently the mother's supply of breast milk. If a breastfeeding mother has chosen to supplement with formula milk, one formula feed per day at a specific time will have less effect on her supply of breast milk than topping up with formula milk after every breastfeed.

Expressing breast milk

NICE recommends that all mothers are taught to hand express their breast milk (National Institute for Health and Care Excellence 2014). It may be necessary to express breast milk if:

- the infant is too small or sick to breastfeed;
- the mother needs help to attach her infant to a full breast;
- the mother's breasts feel full and uncomfortable;
- the mother needs to be away from her infant for long periods of time such as social engagements or returning to work;
- the mother requires surgery;
- the mother chooses to bottle feed her infant with her own expressed milk rather than breastfeeding.

There are 3 main methods of expressing breast milk:

- hand expression;
- using a hand pump;
- using an electric pump/battery pump.

Whichever method is chosen it is important that:

- the mother washes her hands thoroughly before she starts;
- all containers, bottles and pump pieces are washed in hot soapy water and sterilised before use.

Milk can be expressed from 1 breast for around

five minutes or until the supply slows down or appears to stop. Milk can then be expressed from the other breast. Then the mother can go back to the first breast and start again. Expressing from alternative breasts can continue until the milk stops or drips very slowly.

If there are problems beginning, the following may help the milk to flow:

- the mother should be comfortable and as relaxed as possible – sitting in a quiet room with a warm drink may help;
- if possible, skin-to-skin contact with the infant;
- having her infant close by or having a photograph of the infant to look at or being able to smell the infant's scent (e.g. on a baby blanket or garment);
- having a warm bath or shower prior to expressing, or applying warm flannels to her breast;
- light, gentle massage of the breast by the mother using her fingertips or by rolling her closed fist over her breast towards the nipple. She should work around the whole breast, including underneath. She should not slide her fingers along her breast as this can damage the skin. After massaging, light stimulation of the areola between her first finger and thumb encourages the release of hormones which stimulate the breast to produce and release the milk.

As mothers get used to expressing their milk, they will find that they do not need to prepare so carefully. Just like breastfeeding, it gets easier as time goes by.

Hand expressing is free and convenient and is particularly useful if a mother needs to relieve an uncomfortable breast. The best way to learn is to practise (perhaps in the bath) so that the mother can find what works for her. As a guide, the mother should be instructed to try the following steps:

1. Place your first finger under your breast, towards the edge of the areola, with your thumb on top of the breast opposite the first finger. These should then be in about the same position as the baby's mouth. You may be able to feel the knobbly sinuses underneath the areola.
2. Keeping your fingers and thumb in the same places on your skin, press them together for 2 seconds and release. A hard squeeze will be painful and not effective.
3. This press and release action should be repeated, keeping the thumb and the finger in the same place and taking care not to slide your finger and thumb up or down the breast.
4. Once you have acquired the technique, press and release every few seconds, building up a steady rhythm. The exact rate and rhythm needed to express milk efficiently varies from woman to woman.
5. The milk may take a minute or 2 to flow. When it does it will drip or spurt from the breast. Collect it in a sterile, wide-mouthed container – a measuring jug is ideal.
6. It is important to rotate your fingers around the breast to ensure that milk is expressed from all the lobes.
7. With practice it is possible to express from both breasts at the same time.

Using a breast pump

It is best to establish a good breastfeeding routine if possible before beginning to use a pump. There are 3 main types of pump available – hand, battery and electric. There are many varieties for personal preferences and circumstances. For mothers with infants in special care it may be necessary to hire a hospital-grade electric pump.

Simultaneous pumping may be recommended in some circumstances. This is expressing both breasts at the same time. It is thought that this significantly raises the prolactin, fat and volume levels and may be useful for long-term expressing.

Expressing milk for new-born infants

It is important to start expressing as soon as possible after birth for infants who cannot be put to the breast. Mothers who have infants in Neonatal Intensive Care Unit (NICU) should be encouraged to express at least 6–8 times in 24 hours, including at least once during the night. From 2–3 days after birth, milk production is related to milk removal and if milk remains in the breasts too long, there is a build-up of a protein called the 'feedback inhibitor of lactation', which may decrease the milk supply.

Storing expressed breast milk (EBM)

After expressing into a sterilised container, the container should be covered with a tight-fitting lid, labelled with the date and put into the fridge or freezer as quickly as possible (National Institute for Health and Care Excellence 2014). EBM stored in a fridge retains the properties more effectively than freezing.

In a fridge

EBM should be stored at the back of the fridge where it remains coldest. It should not be stored on the door of the fridge where it is more likely to be warmer. It can be stored for up to five days if the parents are confident that the fridge remains at 4°C or lower. This cannot necessarily be guaranteed in a domestic fridge that is frequently opened. Hence in a busy household it may be preferable to freeze the EBM if it is not going to be used within 48 hours.

In a freezer

EBM can be stored for up to 2 weeks in the freezer compartment of a fridge or for 6 months in a domestic freezer, at minus 18°C or lower.

In hospital

Storage times within hospital guidelines should be followed.

Thawing frozen breast milk

Frozen EBM should only be defrosted in the fridge and then used within 24 hours. It should not be re-frozen once it has begun to thaw. A microwave oven should not be used to warm or defrost EBM.

Continuing breastfeeding when returning to work

Mothers returning to work after giving birth can consider continuing breastfeeding by:

- expressing milk so that someone else can feed her infant while she is away;
- finding childcare close to her work and arranging to breastfeed during breaks in her work day;
- asking her employer for flexible hours around breastfeeding; employers now have a duty to consider such requests;
- asking her employer for support and logistics to express and store her milk while she is at work. The Workplace Regulations and Approved Code of Practice require employers to provide suitable facilities for pregnant and breastfeeding mothers to rest.

Information on the rights of mothers returning to work is available on the Maternity Action website (maternityaction.org.uk).

Infants reluctant to take a bottle

Infants who steadfastly refuse a bottle from their mother may be more likely to take it from someone else when the mother is not around. However, for infants who refuse any bottle, the following may work:

- trying a different teat;
- running the teat under warm water to raise it to body temperature;
- breast milk given in a cup or beaker or on a teaspoon;
- wrapping something that smells of the mother around the bottle or cup.

Introducing a cup or beaker

Infants can learn to drink from a cup from the time they are capable of sitting (around 5–6 months). Many infants are never bottle fed as they go directly from breastfeeding to taking EBM or formula milk from a cup.

Nutritional needs for breastfeeding mothers

Although requirements for some nutrients are increased during lactation, eating a balanced nutritious diet based on the five food groups as for during pregnancy (see Table 7.1 page 82) will usually ensure nutritional requirements are met, except for vitamin D – a daily supplement of 10 micrograms of vitamin D3 is recommended.

Pregnancy and breastfeeding are times when families are often well motivated to adapt their lifestyles and change to healthier eating habits.

The nutritional quality of breast milk is only affected by the mother's diet if she is undernourished. Strict dieting regimes with restricted food choices in order to lose weight while breastfeeding are not appropriate. Undernourished women and those on very restrictive diets may require some extra nutrient supplementation. Vegan mothers who are breastfeeding need to plan their diets well and will need additional supplements of calcium, iodine and vitamin B12 in addition to vitamin D.

Foods to limit

Oily fish and large fish should be limited as for pregnancy (see Chapter 7, page 90).

Alcohol is absorbed directly into the bloodstream and passes into breast milk. The highest level of alcohol in milk will occur between 30 and 90 minutes after ingesting alcohol. Breastfeeding mothers who choose to drink alcohol should not ingest alcohol for about 2 hours before breastfeeding and should keep alcohol intake to a minimum (e.g. 1 or 2 units once or twice a week). Regular or binge drinking should be avoided.

Caffeine in tea, coffee, chocolate and energy drinks does not need to be avoided but some mothers find large amounts of caffeine unsettle their baby.

Food hypersensitivity

Very occasionally, a food that the mother eats can cause an allergic response in the infant. Common triggers are dairy products, eggs and nuts. If a mother needs to exclude a whole food group (e.g. milk and dairy products) then she should be referred to a registered dietitian for advice to make sure her diet remains adequate in all nutrients, particularly calcium, riboflavin and iodine.

Formula milks for infants

The standard infant formulas are made from skimmed milk powder with added fats and nutrients to make the composition nutritionally adequate for infants. Formula milks have been modified as knowledge and technology progresses. However, their composition must always comply with strict criteria set by European Union regulations, which are updated from time to time as scientific research advances. Current regulations can be found at https://ec.europa.eu/food/safety/labelling_nutrition/special_groups_food/children_en.

The EU regulations allow the protein in formula milks to be from either cow or goat milk or soya. They also specify minimum and maximum levels of all nutrients in addition to maximum limits on food additives and contaminants. The maximum levels on pesticides levels are very strict making them similar to those required by organic regulations.

Some of the nutrients in typical infant formula milks are listed in Table 8.3. The list of nutrients is not complete but the table highlights key differences between breast milk and different infant formula milks.

Infant formulas are suitable as the main milk for infants throughout their first year of life. Follow On milks may be given from 6 months of age although changing from an infant formula to a follow on formula is not necessary.

Choosing an infant formula suitable from birth

Infant and follow on formulas based on cow or goat milk protein

The several types of infant and follow on formulas set out in Table 8.4:

- *Whey-dominant infant formula:* The protein has the same whey-to-casein ratio (60: 40) as mature breast milk.

Table 8.3 Nutritional components in breast milk and infant formula milks

Nutrients		Breast milk	Infant formulas – suitable from birth
Proteins	Whey and casein	Main proteins in breast milk	Present in whey-dominant formula in the ratio 60: 40
		Whey: casein ratio changes and is 60: 40 in mature breast milk	Present in casein-dominant formula in ratio 20: 80
	Alpha-lactalbumin	Main component of whey protein	Added to some formulas
	Beta-lactalbumin	Very small proportion of the whey protein	Main component of whey protein in other formula milks
	Lactoferrin	An iron-binding protein. It binds the iron, rendering it unavailable to pathogenic gut bacteria whose growth is thereby inhibited, reducing the risk of gastrointestinal infections	Currently not present but being trialled
	Immunoglobulins (anti-infective proteins)	Remain relatively constant throughout lactation regardless of the amount of breast milk provided by the mother. This happens because concentrations increase as total volume diminishes	Not present
	Cytokines (affect the interactions and communications between cells):Growth factors Interferon	Poly-peptides specific to each mother.	Not present
		Growth factors are especially high in the breast milk of mothers who give birth prematurely. Epidermal growth factor, for example, stimulates the proliferation of epidermal and epithelial tissues in the gut lining.	
		Interferon – antiviral factor	
	Lysozyme	Has antibacterial activity and is also responsible for the development of intestinal flora	Not present
	Taurine	An amino acid essential for the myelination of the central nervous system and brain. In new-borns, bile acids are almost exclusively conjugated with taurine, which helps excretion	Present
Fats	Total fat	Provides about 50 per cent of the energy content of breast milk	Present at same level
	Short chain and long chain omega 3 and omega 6 fatty acids	Important in brain and retina development and in myelination of the nervous system	Present – docosahexaenoic acid, linoleic acid and alpha linolenic acid are required by the legislation.
			Some formulas add eicosapentaenoic and arachidonic acids which are

(*Continued*)

Table 8.3 (Continued)

Nutrients		Breast milk	Infant formulas – suitable from birth
			not required by the regulations
	beta palmitate	Present	Present in some – not required by regulations
Carbohydrates	Lactose	The main digestible sugar in breast milk and is about 7 per cent by weight. It is digested to the monosaccharides galactose and glucose	Present at same level but not present in lactose free formulas
	Maltodextrin Glucose syrup	Not present	Used in lactose free formulas
	Prebiotics	Types of fibre that remain undigested in the gut. They promote the growth of bacteria (e.g. bifidobacteria) in the gut flora that have a positive effect on digestion and absorption. Human milk contains a much wider variety of prebiotic carbohydrates than other mammalian milks and maternal Human Milk Oligosaccharides (HMO's) vary between mothers causing different bacterially induced effects on each infant's metabolism and immunity.	Galacto-oligosaccharides, fructosaccharides and HMOs are added to some formulas - not required by the regulations
Iron		Low in breast milk but in a form that is highly absorbable -about 70 per cent is absorbed	Added in higher amounts as there is only about 10 per cent absorption from infant formula. The excess iron remaining in the gut promotes bacterial growth
Vitamin D		Naturally low as the main source of vitamin D is from skin synthesis when outside – only during the summer months, April-September in the UK	Added in higher amounts as a supplement – required by the regulations
Nucleotides		Essential precursors for DNA and RNA and important for the function of cell membranes and the normal development of the brain. They may act as co-factors for the growth of *Lactobacillus bifidus* bacterium which reduces the presence of pathogens, such as *Escherichia coli,* in the faecal flora	Added to some – not required by the regulations
Carnitine		Essential for the catabolism of long-chain fatty acids. It enables fatty	Present

(*Continued*)

Table 8.3 (Continued)

Nutrients	Breast milk	Infant formulas – suitable from birth
	acids and ketone bodies to be oxidised to provide alternative fuels to glucose. This helps prevent neonatal hypoglycaemia	
Milk fat globule membrane (MFGM)	The mainly lipid and protein structure that surrounds milk fat globules	Added to some formulas – not required by the regulations
Probiotics	Present – specific to each mother	Not present
Stem cells	Present – specific to each mother	Not present
Immune cells	Present – specific to each mother	Not present

- *Hungry infant milk:* These casein dominant milk based formulas have the same energy and nutrient content as the whey dominant formulas. The protein has the same whey-to-casein ratio (20: 80) as cow's milk. There is no evidence to support the claim that these formulas are suitable for hungrier babies but there is some evidence that they may take longer to empty from the stomach and infants may therefore feel satisfied for longer (Taitz and Scholey 1989, Billeaud et al. 1990).
- *Modified infant formulas* for infants with mild digestive problems such as colic and reflux are labelled Comfort, Anti-reflux or Lactose free.
- *Partially hydrolysed whey protein formula* – for infants at risk of food allergies, however scientific evidence is not yet clear on whether they reduce the risk of a cow's milk protein allergy.

Differences between and within brands

There are several different brands of infant formula in the United Kingdom as in addition to the four most popular brands some supermarkets have their own brands. The formula manufacturers research and develop their milk formulas in different ways and each brand promotes the benefits of their formulas to healthcare professionals based on different additions, not required by the regulations, shown in Table 8.3. However, these differences are minimal and healthcare professionals cannot promote 1 brand over another.

Within some brands there is a choice of formulas:

- Formulas which comply with the regulations without any extra additions. Priced more cheaply.
- Formulas which have some added components which are not required by the regulations but research suggests they may have small advantages. Priced more expensively.
- Organic formulas which are made from milks from cows raised on certified organic farms.

Soya-based infant formula

Soya-based infant formulas were previously recommended as an alternative to cow and goat milk-based infant formulas, but they are no longer recommended for infants in the United Kingdom under 6 months as they have a high content of phytoestrogens and may have an oestrogenic effect. The consequences of this are uncertain.

Phytoestrogens are naturally occurring chemicals similar to human oestrogen and are found in some foods of plant origin (e.g. soya beans). One study found that the production of testosterone was suppressed in neonatal marmoset monkeys that were partially fed soya formula. No study has definitely proven that soya formula can cause

Table 8.4 Infant and follow-on formulas available in the United Kingdom

Formulas		Labelled as	Brands
Infant Formulas	Cow's milk whey-dominant infant formula – whey-to-casein ratio is 60: 40 Several varieties depending on the additives Some have partially hydrolysed milk protein	1 First infant milk	Aptamil Cow & Gate Hipp Organic SMA Supermarket own brands
	Goat's milk whey-dominant infant formula – whey-to-casein ratio is 60: 40	1 Infant Milk Goat Milk based	Kabrita
	Goat's milk casein-dominant infant formula – whey-to-casein ratio is 20: 80	1 First Infant Milk Goat milk based	Nannycare
	Soya infant formula	Soya infant formula from birth	SMA Wysoy
	Cow's milk casein-dominant infant formula – whey-to-casein ratio is 20: 80	Hungry /Extra Hungry infant milk	Aptamil Cow & Gate Hipp Organic SMA Nutrition Supermarket own brands
	Modified infant formulas for minor digestive problems – based on cow's milk Protein is partially hydrolysed, fat is modified, some of the lactose is replaced with starch, added thickeners	Comfort milk	Aptamil Cow & Gate Hipp SMA Supermarket own brands
	Modified infant formulas using either carob bean gum or starch to thicken the formula	Anti -Reflux	Aptamil Cow & Gate Hipp SMA
	Partially hydrolysed whey protein	1 First Infant Milk	Aptamil Sensavia SMA HA formula
Follow On Formulas	Cow's milk Follow On milks Suitable from 6 months	2 Follow On milk	Aptamil Cow & Gate Hipp SMA Supermarket own brands
	Goat's milk Follow On formulas	2 Follow-on milk Goat milk based	Kabrita Nannycare
	Partially hydrolysed milk Follow On Formula	2 Follow On Milk	Aptamil Sensavia

Table 8.5 Ready-to-feed and powdered formulas compared

	Liquid ready-to-feed formula	Powdered formula
Sterile	Yes – until opened	No – because it cannot be manufactured and packaged without the chance of some bacterial contamination
Making up	Ready-to-feed	Must be made up with boiled water as per instructions on the packaging
Storage	Once opened it can be stored in a refrigerator kept at 5°C or below for up to 24 hours	Keep tin in cool dry cupboard
		Once made up it can be stored in a refrigerator kept at 5°C or below for up to 24 hours
		Ideally it should be made up just before feeding to the infant
Cost	More expensive	Less expensive

long-term damage to human infants, and a paediatrician, GP or dietitian may recommend them if there is a clinical need while the infant is still under 6 months of age. In 2004 the Chief Medical Officer advised that: 'Soya-based formulae should only be used in exceptional circumstances to ensure adequate nutrition. For example, they may be given to infants of vegan parents who are not breastfeeding or infants who find alternatives prescribed for allergy treatment unacceptable.'

Specialised infant formulas

There are a range of specialised infant formulas available for infants with certain medical conditions (see Table 10.1 pages 143). They should only be used on the advice of a doctor or dietitian. They are usually prescribed by a doctor or GP but can be ordered directly from a pharmacy by parents.

Making up and storing infant formula

To reduce the risk of bacterial contamination, up until an infant is 12 months old all bottles and teats must be washed in hot soapy water and then sterilised before formula milk is added to them.

Most formula milks are offered in 2 formats: dry powder and liquid ready-to-feed. They are compared in Table 8.5.

Only safe water should be used for making up powdered formula feeds:

Safe water sources in the UK	Unsafe water sources
Freshly drawn cold tap water	Water from the hot tap
Bottled water that complies with tap water regulations – it may be labelled as 'suitable for making up infant formula'. The sodium content should be less than that allowed in tap water which is 200 mg/L	Spring or mineral water that does not comply with tap water regulations
	Carbonated water
	Water that has been softened with a sodium exchange pump
	Well water

Water for feeds, whether freshly drawn tap water or bottled water, should be boiled, but only once, and allowed to cool, covered, for up to 30 minutes. This ensures it is still above 70°C when the formula powder is added to it. Directions for making up are on the packaging. Ideally each bottle should be made up just before feeding to the infant and discarded if not consumed within 2 hours. Storing prepared infant formula is no longer recommended but there may be times when feeds need to be prepared in advance. The prepared feeds must be cooled quickly and stored in a refrigerator kept at 5°C or below. The maximum storage time is 24 hours and any prepared feed not used after this time should be discarded.

To make up a feed outside the home, parents should take the powdered milk and a vacuum flask of water that has been boiled and poured into the vacuum flask within 30 minutes of boiling. The feed can then be made up in a sterilised bottle when needed.

Care should be taken not to over- or under-concentrate the feed:

- the scoop supplied with the milk powder should always be used;
- 1 level scoop of powder should be added for each 30 ml boiled water;
- care should be taken not to overpack the milk powder in the scoop as this will over-concentrate the feed.

Over-concentrated feeds can cause constipation, vomiting and excess weight gain. Under-concentrating feeds will not provide the infant with sufficient energy or nutrients for growth and development.

Warming refrigerated feeds

Refrigerated feeds can be warmed to room temperature by standing in a jug of hot water for a few minutes. Microwaving formula feeds is NOT recommended practice and should be discouraged because of:

- ongoing heating – the milk will continue to heat after removal from the microwave;
- 'hot spots' – hot fluid in the centre of the bottle may be undetected and scald the infant.

Making up formula feeds while travelling or on holiday outside the United Kingdom

The customer care line of each formula milk company can advise on a suitable formula milk available in the country to which a family is travelling. Taking at least 1 unopened can of powder with them will allow some time in which to find a supply abroad.

As in the United Kingdom, tap water and bottled water should be boiled for making up a formula feed using powdered formula. Bottled water should be still and unflavoured and the label checked to make sure that the sodium level is less than 200 mg/L.

Bottle feeding infants

Average fluid requirements for 24 hours are:

Age	ml/kg body weight/ 24 hours
0–2/3 days	minimal
3/4 days–6 months	About 150
7–12 months	About 120

New-borns may take very small volumes of milk. From about day 3 the volume of feeds demanded will gradually increase to around a total of about 150 ml per kg bodyweight every 24 hours. The total volume increases as infants gain weight. As with breastfed babies, younger infants feed more frequently than older infants. When fed responsively the vast majority of infants will regulate their own energy needs and take the volumes of milk they need to satisfy their energy needs. The example volumes suggested for age and weight on packaging do not apply to all infants as there is a wide range of weights at each age and some infants take small volumes more frequently and others larger volumes less frequently. Table 8.6 shows the variations indicating how important it is to feed each infant responsively.

To bottle feed responsively parents and carers should:

- learn the cues that their infant uses to show he or she is hungry;
- wait for the infant to open his or her mouth and accept the feed and never force the teat into the mouth;

Table 8.6 Variations of feed volumes at different ages

Age of infant	Weight range (Kg)	Range of Energy requirements (kcals/day)	Range of milk volumes (ml/day)	Range of demanded feeds per day
Birth to 2 days	2.4 – 4.5	Low	Low	3 – 6
Day 3–7	2.6 – 4.5	325 – 562	500 – 866	6 – 10
1–4 weeks	2.6 – 5.5	325 – 687	500 – 1057	6 – 8
1–2 months	3.5 – 6.5	420 – 780	647 – 1201	6 – 8
3 months	4.5 – 7.3	463 – 752	713 – 1158	5 – 8
4 months	4.9 – 7.5	431 – 660	663 – 1016	5 – 7
5–6 months	5.4 – 9.8	459 – 833	707 – 1282	4 – 6

- cuddle their infant and if appropriate use some skin-to-skin contact when feeding to ensure the same closeness as when breastfeeding;
- tilt the bottle so there is always milk in the teat;
- allow the infant to pause from time to time while feeding from a bottle, and to wind him or her at some stage during the feed to allow a break before offering more;
- allow their infant to stop feeding when he or she has had enough rather than encouraging him or her to finish each bottle, which may lead to excess weight gain which is a risk factor for childhood obesity;
- discard any leftover milk at the end of the feed.

There is no evidence to support dream feeding which is giving an infant a feed while they are sleeping – it is usually done with the aim of encouraging the infant to sleep through the night. Beginning to sleep through the night is related to the hormonally driven development of infants' circadian rhythm and is not related to their energy or nutritional intake. The earliest that any infant will begin sleeping through the night is 6–8 weeks (McGraw et al. 1999).

Precautions:

- Infants should never be left alone with a bottle.
- Adding solid foods to a bottle of milk is not recommended in the United Kingdom, however it is part of complementary feeding practices from 4–6 months in other countries.

Extra fluid

In exceptionally hot weather formula-fed infants may become thirsty in between their usual feeds as the water content of formula feeds does not vary as during breastfeeding. They can be offered drinks of cooled, boiled water. Flavoured or sweetened waters are not suitable.

Introducing a cup

From about 6 months of age a lidded cup with a spout can be introduced for water drinks. Once the infant is drinking competently from a cup, milk feeds can also be given in a cup. Breast fed babies who change to formula milks from around 9 months may move onto a cup without ever using bottles

Bottles of milk can be phased out from around the age of 12 months as toddlers may begin to associate bottles of milk with comfort and can become stubborn about giving them up.

Vitamin D supplementation for formula-fed infants

All formula milks are fortified with vitamin D but only at least 500 mls per day of infant or follow-on formula will provide the RNI for infants of 8.5–10 μg. However the European Food Safety Authority and the European Society for Paediatric Endocrinology recommend a supplement of 10 μg per day for all infants from birth to 12 months of age, independent of their mode of feeding, to prevent nutritional rickets (Braegger et al. 2013, Munns et al. 2016). The European tolerable upper intake level (UL) for infants of 25 µg/day is very unlikely to be reached.

Those families who are entitled to receive Healthy Start vouchers are entitled to free Healthy Start children's vitamin drops providing 10 µg of vitamin D per day (www.healthystart.nhs.uk). Some NHS Trusts also sell the vitamin drops but for families who cannot access these, a range of infant supplements are available in pharmacies and some large supermarkets.

Vitamin drops are best given from a spoon or syringe, not added to bottles, to ensure the full dose is taken.

References and further reading

Adgent MA, Umbach DM, Zemel BS, Kelly A, et al. (2018) A longitudinal study of estrogen-responsive tissues and hormone concentrations in infants fed soy formula. *The Journal of Clinical Endocrinology & Metabolism*, doi: 10.1210/jc.2017-02249.

Ballard O, Morrow AL (2013, Feb) Human Milk Composition: Nutrients and Bioactive Factors. *Pediatric Clinics of North America*. **60**(1): 49–74. doi: 10.1016/j.pcl.2012.10.002.

Braegger C, Campoy C, Colomb V, Decsi T, Domellof M, Fewtrell M, Hojsak I, Mihatsch W, Molgaard C, Shamir R, Turck D and van Goudoever J (2013) Vitamin D in the healthy European paediatric population. *Journal of Pediatric Gastroenterology and Nutrition* **56**: 692–701.

Billeaud C, Guillet J and Sandler B (1990) Gastric emptying in infants with or without gastro-oesophageal reflux according to the type of milk. *European Journal of Clinical Nutrition* **44**: 577–583.

Bramson L, Lee JW, Moore E et al. (2010 May) Effect of early skin-to-skin mother--infant contact during the first 3 hours following birth on exclusive breastfeeding during the maternity hospital stay. *Journal of Human Lactation* **26**(2): 130–137. doi: 10.1177/0890334409355779. Epub 2010 Jan 28.

Dollberg S, Lahav S, Mimouni FB (2001) A comparison of intakes of breast-fed and bottle-fed infants during the first two days of life. *Journal of the American College of Nutrition* **20**: 209–211.

Hester SN, Hustead DS, Mackey AD, et al. (2012) Is the macronutrient intake of formula-fed infants greater than breast-fed infants in early infancy? *Journal of Nutrition and Metabolism*. 891201. Available from: doi:10.1155/2012/891201.

Ip S, Chung M, Raman G, et al. (2009 Oct) A summary of the Agency for Healthcare Research and Quality's evidence report on breastfeeding in developed countries. *Breastfeeding Medicine* 4 Suppl 1: S17–S30. doi: 10.1089/bfm.2009.0050.

Julies P, Lynn RM, Pall K, Leoni M, Calder A, Mughal Z, Shaw N, McDonnell C, McDevitt H, Blair M (2020 Jan 16) Nutritional rickets under 16 years: UK surveillance results. *Archives of Disease in Childhood* pii: archdischild-2019-317934. doi: 10.1136/archdischild-2019-317934. [Epub ahead of print].

Kent JC (2007, Nov-Dec) How breastfeeding works. *Journal of Midwifery & Women's Health* **52**(6): 564–570.

Kent JC, Mitoulas LR, Cregan MD, et al. (2006) Volume and frequency of breastfeedings and fat content of breast milk throughout the day. *Pediatrics* **117**(3): e387–e395.

Li F, Wu SS, Berseth CL, Cheryl L, et al. (2019) Improved Neurodevelopmental Outcomes Associated with Bovine Milk Fat Globule Membrane and Lactoferrin in Infant Formula: A Randomized, Controlled Trial. *The Journal of Pediatrics*, doi: 10.1016/j.jpeds.2019.08.030.

McAndrew F, Thompson J, Fellows L, et al. (2012) *Infant Feeding Survey 2010*. Health and Social Care Information Centre. Available from: https://digital.nhs.uk/catalogue/PUB08694 Accessed 01February2018.

McGraw K, Hoffmann R, Harker C, et al. (1999 May 1) The development of circadian rhythms in a human infant. *Sleep* **22**(3): 303–310.

Munns CF, Shaw N, Kiely M, et al. (2016 Feb) Global Consensus Recommendations on Prevention and Management of Nutritional Rickets. *The Journal of Clinical Endocrinology and Metabolism* **101**(2): 394–415. doi: 10.1210/jc.2015-2175. Epub 2016 Jan 8.

National Institute for Health and Care Excellence (November 2014) *Public Health Guidance 11. Improving the nutrition of pregnant and breast-feeding mothers and children in low-income households*. London: NICE. (accessed April 2020).

National Institute for Health and Care Excellence (February 2015) *Clinical Guidance 63. Diabetes in pregnancy: management of diabetes and its complications from preconception to the postnatal period*. www.nice.org.uk/Guidance/CG63 (accessed April 2020).

Neifert MR (2001) Prevention of breastfeeding tragedies. *Pediatric Clinics of North America* **48**: 273–297.

Neville MC, Morton J (2001) Physiology and endocrine changes underlying human lactogenesis II. *Journal of Nutrition* **131**(11): 3005S–30058S.

Quigley MA, Kelly YJ and Sacker A (2007) Breastfeeding and hospitalisation for diarrheal and respiratory infection in the UK Millennium Cohort Study. *Pediatrics* **119**: 837–842.

Scientific Advisory Committee on Nutrition (2018) *Feeding in the first year of Life*. London: The Stationery Office.

Taitz LS and Scholey E (1989) Are babies more satisfied by casein-based formulae? *Archives of Disease in Childhood* **64**: 619–662.

World Health organization 2020 *Infant and Young Child Feeding: Key Facts*. Available at: www.who.int/en/news-room/fact-sheets/detail/infant-and-young-child-feeding Accessed 01April2020.

World Health Organization (2003) *Global Strategy for Infant and Young Child Feeding*. Geneva: WHO.

World Health Organization (2002) *Infant and Young Child Nutrition*. 55th World Health Assembly. Geneva, Switzerland: World Health Organization.

Victora CG, Bahl R, Barros AJ, França GV, Horton S, Krasevec J, Murch S, Sankar MJ, Walker N, Rollins NC; Lancet Breastfeeding Series Group (2016 Jan 30) Breastfeeding in the 21st century: epidemiology, mechanisms, and lifelong effect. *Lancet* 387(10017): 475–490. doi: 10.1016/S0140-6736(15)01024-7.

Resources

Maternityaction.org.uk

EU Regulations on Infant and Follow-on Formulas (2015): https://eur-lex.europa.eu/legal-content/EN/TXT/?uri=CELEX:32016R0127

9

Complementary feeding

Summary

- Infants develop at different rates and parents can be supported to decide when their infant is ready to begin having complementary foods (CFs) alongside their milk feeds.
- Most term infants are ready to begin between 4 and 6 months.
- Breast milk is the ideal main milk drink during complementary feeding but most infants in the United Kingdom are already on formula milks by this age.
- Offering spoon feeding and finger foods from the beginning encourages the development of all feeding skills including self-feeding skills.
- A responsive and positive feeding environment allowing infants to decide how much they eat and drink enhances progression. Milk feeds should decrease as more food is eaten.
- Infants progress through the food textures at different rates depending on their oromotor development.
- Progression onto more complex textures and a wide variety of tastes of family foods by 12 months decreases the likelihood of feeding problems in toddlers.

Terminology

Both the terms 'complementary feeding' and 'introduction of complementary foods' are used internationally for the introduction of solid foods alongside an infant's milk feeds.

In the United Kingdom, the term 'weaning' is also used for the introduction of complementary foods (CFs) alongside milk feeds, whereas the World Health Organization (WHO) uses 'weaning' for the process of reducing and stopping breastfeeding or breast milk intake – either to replace breastmilk with formula milk or during complementary feeding.

Why begin complementary feeding?

The purpose of introducing CFs is to:

- provide extra energy (calories) and nutrients when breast milk or infant formula alone no longer supplies them in sufficient amounts to sustain normal growth and optimal health and development;
- provide infants the opportunity to develop their oromotor skills to manage different food textures in their mouths;
- provide infants the opportunity to learn to like and accept new tastes and textures, based on family foods, at a time when they are receptive to learning to like them.

Ideally, breast milk should continue as the main milk drink throughout complementary feeding.

When to begin

There is an ideal age range, not a specific age, because infants all develop at different rates. Healthcare professionals can support parents to decide when their infant is ready to begin complementary feeding.

Physiology and skills necessary of infants for safe introduction of CFs are:

Physiology and skills necessary in infants	Age observed
Gross motor skills for spoon feeding smooth foods: able to hold the head in midline when supine and to control the head well when sitting, with or without support	Between 3 and 4 months (EFSA 2019)
Diminished rooting and the extrusion reflexes	Assumed to be between 3 and 4 months (EFSA 2019)
Oromotor skills	3 and 6 months (Carruth and Skinner 2002)
Motor skills for self-feeding finger foods	At 4 months in some infants, but more commonly between 5 and 7 months (EFSA 2019)
Gastrointestinal and renal functions	are not limiting factors once the necessary neuromotor skills are present and an infant shows interest in non-milk foods and feeding (EFSA 2019).

Over the last few decades scientific opinion and recommendations on the ideal age to begin complementary feeding have changed and conflicting advice is sometimes given to parents in the United Kingdom. The key population recommendations from various agencies are summarised in Table 9.1.

Delaying clamping of the umbilical cord until the cord stops pulsating is now recommended as, during the few minutes of delay, extra iron and fluid are transferred to the infant (National Institute for Health and Care Excellence 2017, SACN 2018).

Mothers tend to choose to begin CFs earlier for larger and male infants than smaller and female infants (Wright et al. 2004) and this is probably because they perceive that infants growing more quickly are ready for more than just milk at an earlier age.

Within Europe, national recommendations vary from country to country, with most recommending beginning CFs between 4 and 6 months of age or around 6 months as exclusive breastfeeding for six months may not be appropiate for all infants and their stage of readiness should also be considered (Pérez-Escamilla, Buccini, Segura-Pérez and Piwoz 2019). Between 4 and 6 months infants learn to accept new tastes and foods relatively quickly (Carruth et al. 2004).

The developmental signs that suggest that an infant is ready to accept solid foods are:

- able to sit with or without support and with good head and neck control;
- putting toys and other objects in the mouth;
- watching others with interest when they are eating;
- seeming hungry between milk feeds by chewing fists or demanding feeds more often even though larger feeds have been offered.

Night-time waking and crying are not necessarily signs of hunger at this age. Sleeping patterns change around this time and some infants are more easily aroused and may begin to wake during the night. Some parents hope that beginning CFs will help their infant sleep through the night, but little evidence supports this theory. The EAT (Enquiring About Tolerance) Study found that parents who had been randomised to begin complementary feeding from 3 to 4 months reported that at 6 months their infants slept for slightly longer 10–25 mins/night and woke less frequently than the parents who had been randomised to begin CFs at 6 months of age. Serious sleep problems were less common in the group who began complementary feeding at 3–4 months (Perkin et al. 2018). EFSA considered these findings to be of little biological relevance (EFSA 2019).

Table 9.1 Summary of scientific opinions on complementary feeding

Year	Organisation	Scientific opinions
1994	UK Department of Health	'The majority of infants should not be given solid foods before the age of 4 months and a mixed diet should be offered by the age of 6 months' (Department of Health 1994)
2001	World Health Organisation	1. Exclusive breastfeeding until 6 months of age to reduce the incidence of gastroenteritis, which causes death in developing countries 2. Begin complementary feeding at 6 months of age 3. Each country must interpret these recommendations for the needs of their own population and each infant should be considered individually because exclusive breastfeeding to 6 months could lead to iron deficiency in susceptible infants, and growth faltering and other micronutrient deficiencies in others.
2003	World Health Organization recommendations for Europe	Introduce complementary foods between 4 and 6 months
2017	European Society for Paediatric Gastroenterology, Hepatology and Nutrition (ESPGHAN)	'Exclusive breast feeding should be promoted for at least 4 months (17 weeks) and continuing through to approximately 6 months (26 weeks) is a desirable goal Complementary foods should not be introduced before 4 months but should not be delayed beyond 6 months.
2018	UK Scientific Advisory Committee on Nutrition (SACN)	From around 6 months of age, a diverse complementary diet is needed to meet the increasing iron requirements of older infants. Allergenic foods such as peanut, hen's egg, gluten or fish can be introduced from around 6 months of age and need not be differentiated from other CFs.
2019	European Food Safety Authority (EFSA)	There is an appropriate age range, not a single age, for the introduction of CFs for infants living in Europe. Each infant's characteristics and development will determine their ideal age. There are no adverse or beneficial health effects to introducing safely prepared and nutritionally and age appropriate CFs at any age before 6 months except for infants at risk of iron* depletion who may need high iron CFs before 6 months. Gluten and potentially allergenic foods (egg, cereals, fish and peanut) can be introduced at the same time as other CFs. For nutritional reasons, the majority of infants need CFs from around 6 months of age.

Notes

*Infants at risk of iron deficiency are exclusively breastfed infants:

- born to mothers with low iron status, or;
- with early umbilical cord clamping (< 1 min after birth), or;
- born small-for-gestational age or;
- with high growth velocity – larger male infants are those who grow most quickly.

Nutrient and energy density of complementary foods

Nutrient dense, particularly iron-rich foods, need to be offered from the beginning of complementary feeding when infants are taking more than 1–2 teaspoons. The best food sources of iron are meat, oily fish, pulses, eggs and nut butters. Meat and oily fish provide the haem form of iron, which is easily absorbed. Pulses, eggs and nut butters contain the non-haem form of iron, and absorption is less efficient, but can be improved by combining them with a high vitamin C food.

Once infants are eating more than 1 or 2 teaspoons, savoury courses for infants should ideally contain by volume:

- ⅓ high iron foods: meat/fish/eggs/nut butter/pulses (lentils, hummus, starchy beans);
- ⅓ starchy foods: potato/rice/pasta/couscous/bread;
- ⅓ vegetables.

This will meet the WHO recommendation that CFs are energy and nutrient dense providing about 80–120 kcal (335–500 kJ)/100 g food (Dewey et al. 2001).

Fruit and/or unsweetened yoghurt/custard/milk pudding can be given as a third meal early in complementary feeding or later as a second course to replace the milk feed at 1 and then 2 meals.

Milk feeding 6–12 months

Breast milk or formula milk continue to be an important part of an infant's nutritional intake, however, these milk feeds should decrease as the quantity of CFs increases:

- The amount of breast milk demanded and taken will naturally decrease as the vast majority of infants are able to regulate their own milk intake if allowed to continue feeding on demand. Bottle-fed infants need to be allowed to decrease their milk intake in the same way.
- Early morning milk feeds can be discontinued from around 9 months to encourage more food to be eaten at breakfast. A milk feed can then be offered after breakfast.
- An unsweetened yogurt, custard or milk pudding can be substituted for the milk feed following the meal, once 2 courses are being offered at the meal.

Parents feeding formula milk should be advised to offer less milk after meals and not to encourage finishing the whole bottle but to let the infant stop when he or she indicates they have had enough. Over 9 to 12 months, formula milk intake can decrease down to about 500–600 ml milk per day. Follow-on formula can be given in place of infant formula after 6 months but this is not necessary.

Expected intakes of meals and milk feeds at each complementary feeding stage are listed in Table 9.2. The food groups are listed in Tables 9.3 and 9.5.

Suitable drinking cups

Water can be offered from a lidded cup from about 6 months. Non-valved lidded cups are the ideal as they allow infants to learn to sip. Cups with valved lids only allow infants to suck and should be discouraged. Once an infant becomes adept at drinking from a cup, milk drinks can be offered in a cup. It is ideal to phase out all drinks from bottles around an infant's first birthday. This is to help prevent tooth decay known as 'bottle caries' in the toddler years which can occur in toddlers who use bottle feeding for comfort.

Table 9.2 Expected milk and food intake at each stage

Stage	Age guide	Milk feeds	Meals	Variety of foods
1	4–6 months	5–4	1–2	From 1 or 2 food groups Vitamin D supplement
2	6–9 months	4–3	3	3 different meals with foods from all 4 food groups 1 or 2 courses per meal Offer water in a lidded cup with each meal Vitamin D supplement
3	9–12 months	3–2 No early morning milk feed	3	3 different meals from 4 food groups 2 courses per meal – 1 savoury and 1 of fruit and/or milk pudding Offer water in a cup with each meal Vitamin D supplement

Table 9.3 Appropriate items from each food group

Food groups	Appropriate foods to introduce
1: Bread, rice, potatoes, pasta and other starchy foods	Potato, toast crusts, rice, couscous, pasta, quinoa, porridge and other breakfast cereals
2: Fruit and vegetables	Soft ripe fruits, cooked harder fruits, cooked vegetables
3: Milk, cheese and yogurt	Yogurt, cheese, unsweetened custard and milk puddings
4: Meat, fish, eggs, nut butters and pulses	Well-cooked and soft textured meat, fish, eggs, pulses (peas, beans and lentils) and nut butters or pastes of finely ground nuts

Vitamin D supplement

The supplement of 8.5–10 μg/day begun at birth to prevent vitamin D deficiency should continue. Infant formula is supplemented with vitamin D and infants drinking 500 ml or more formula per day, will obtain their vitamin D requirement in their formula but there is no disadvantage in continuing the full supplement throughout the first year. Infants in the United Kingdom most at risk of low vitamin D are those of Asian, Black or Middle Eastern origin whose mothers did not take a vitamin D supplement during pregnancy.

Foods to avoid until 12 months of age

- Added salt;
- Added free sugars – table sugar, all syrups, jam and honey – unpasteurised honey carries a risk of botulism;
- Sweet drinks including fruit juices, smoothies and sweetened herbal teas.

Acquiring feeding skills in a positive feeding environment with responsive feeding

Accepting and managing complementary foods is a learning process and infants only learn to develop their feeding skills and accept and enjoy new tastes and textures when they are given the opportunity to try them (Carruth et al. 2004).

Feeding infants in a positive and responsive environment allows infants to develop new oromotor skills, to eat to their appetite and enjoy mealtimes. Components of a responsive feeding environment include:

- infant sitting with support for both back and feet;
- infant and carer facing each other;
- pleasant and positive interaction between infant and carer;
- allowing infant to set the pace and with the carer following his or her cues;
- having food where the infant can see it and allowing the infant to touch and play with food;
- offering finger foods from early in complementary feeding;
- no distractions such as TV or toys so that the infant can concentrate on eating;
- use bibs/cloths/plastic sheets/newspaper to ‘contain’ mess so that it can be cleaned up at the end of the meal.

The amount of CFs given should always be as much as the infant is happy to eat. Practicing new oromotor skills is tiring for infants and they may wish to stop before eating very much. Many parents find it disappointing and frustrating when their infant eats less than they expect and they may need a lot of reassurance to allow their infant to decide when he or she has had enough food or enough milk to drink. Infants who are coerced or forced to eat more than they need may develop a negative association with food or may gain weight rapidly and cross centiles upwards on their growth chart. Excess weight gain in infancy is a risk factor for future obesity (Reilly et al. 2005) (see Chapter 18, page 235).

Following infant cues

Hunger cues change with age:

Approximate age	Hunger cues
4–6 months	Cries or fusses Smiles, gazes at caregiver, or coos during feeding to indicate wanting more Moves head toward spoon or tries to swipe food towards mouth
5–11 months	Reaches for food Points to food Gets excited when food is presented
10–12 months	Expresses desire for specific food with words or sounds

The vast majority of infants can regulate their energy needs if allowed to. When happy to eat more food, infants will:

- open their mouth to accept a spoon of food;
- pick up food and put it in their mouth themselves.

Satiety cues

When they have had enough food through tiredness or satiation of hunger, infants will:

- keep their mouths shut when food is offered;
- turn their head away from food offered;
- put their hand in front of their mouth;
- push away a spoon, bowl or plate;
- hold foods in their mouth and refuse to swallow.

Older infants may

- spit out food repeatedly;
- cry, shout or scream;
- try to climb out of their high chair;
- gag, retch or vomit.

By offering both spoon feeding and soft finger foods from the beginning complementary feeding infants will develop both types of feeding skills. As infants' feeding skills become more adept, they will gradually eat larger amounts. Younger infants need more help with feeding as they may not be able to feed themselves adequate quantities of food fast enough to satisfy their hunger.

Infants who are allowed to become involved in learning to self-feed will feel more engaged in the feeding process and are more likely to develop a positive relationship with food and be less likely to want to end the meal because they have become bored. Finger foods give this opportunity, but touching and playing with soft or liquid foods in their bowl or plate is also important. Some parents find the mess involved hard to accept and may need to be encouraged to allow this important part of an infant's learning experience.

In recent years, offering only finger foods to infants has been promoted as baby led weaning, but there is no evidence to support the energy and nutritional adequacy of this method for all infants (Wright et al. 2011).

Learning to like new tastes

When offered a new taste, infants may show surprise and be reluctant to take more at that meal. However, if new tastes are offered repeatedly infants will usually learn to like that taste as they become more familiar with it. Parents often give up offering new foods if they perceive that their infant does not like that food. However, this narrows down the range of foods the infant has the opportunity to learn to like. By persevering in offering small tastes of a new food every day or every few days, the infant will have the opportunity to learn to like that food (Birch 1998, Maier et al. 2007).

Learning to cope with new textures

When infants are learning to manage new textures they may gag or cough back food that they cannot yet manage or that needs more chewing. This is part of the learning process and parents should be advised not to panic; the infant might just need more experience to cope easily with that texture. If an infant gags or coughs frequently,

Table 9.4 **Skills to learn and food textures to introduce at different developmental stages**

Stage	Age	Skills to learn	New food textures to introduce
1	4–6 months	Taking food from a spoon Moving food from the front of the mouth to the back for swallowing Managing thicker purees and mashed food Picking up and bringing soft finger foods to the mouth to suck	Smooth well mashed or pureed foods Soft finger foods
2	6–9 months	Moving lumps around the mouth Chewing lumps Self-feeding using hands and fingers Sipping from a cup	Thicker mashed foods Mashed food with soft lumps Soft finger foods Water in a lidded beaker or cup
3	9–12 months	Chewing minced and chopped food Self-feeding attempts with a spoon	Hard finger foods Minced and chopped family foods

families may need further assessment from a speech and language therapist.

Even without teeth infants can learn to chew as the gums are very hard with the unerupted teeth already present in them. A study found that when infants are kept on smooth foods for too long and not offered lumps and finger foods by 10 months they are more likely to be fussy eaters at the age of 3 years compared to those who progressed onto lumpy textures and finger foods appropriately (Northstone et al. 2001).

Progressing through the feeding stages

The food textures to introduce at each stage are summarised in Table 9.4.

Stage 1: Beginning CFs

CFs may be introduced at any time during the day that is convenient for the carer and infant. For the first few tastes it is best to give some of the milk feed first, then offer first tastes of foods before offering the rest of the milk feed. Before a milk feed, infants might be too hungry and thirsty and not prepared to try anything new, while at the end of their feed they may be too satisfied to bother with anything else in their mouth. As the infant becomes accustomed to CFs, he or she can be offered CFs before the milk feed.

Once an infant is managing to take and swallow food at 1 meal, a second and then a third meal can be introduced. Offering different foods at the three meals provides a wider range of nutrients.

Texture of foods

A smooth well-mashed or pureed food is best for the first few tastes, offering it from a shallow teaspoon. Parents can then make thicker purees or mashed food once their infant becomes used to taking food from a spoon. Offering some soft finger foods at the same time allows the infant to touch and play with foods and they may be brought to the mouth. If only finger foods are offered infants are unlikely to be able to eat enough to significantly increase the energy (calories) and nutrients from food.

Foods to offer

Any appropriate nutritious family foods from the list below can be introduced as the first CFs, but most parents begin with cereal, potato, root vegetables or fruit, often mixed with a little of their infant's usual milk:

- all cooked vegetables;
- all soft or cooked fruits;

- all cereal foods;
- well-cooked lean meat, poultry, fish and eggs;
- dhal, lentils, hummus, chick peas and other pulses, nut butters;
- plain yogurt or fromage frais.

Herbs and mild spices can be used to flavour food but salt should not be added.

Quantities of freshly prepared foods can be frozen in small quantities in ice cube trays and then the frozen cubes transferred to sealed bags for convenience.

Infants at high risk of developing food allergies

Food allergies are on the increase and infants with moderate to severe eczema are most at risk. For these infants the highly allergenic foods should be introduced 1 at a time so that any reaction to 1 of these foods can be noted. There is no benefit in delaying introducing these foods to a later age: research suggests that early introduction may prevent food allergies developing for all infants (See Chapter 17 p220). The highly allergenic foods are:

- cow's milk;
- egg;
- nuts – as nut butters or finely ground nuts;
- fish and seafood;
- wheat
- soya;
- sesame seeds e.g. tahini in hummus;
- lupin;
- celery;
- mustard.

Menu planners

First meals

	Day 1	Day 2	Day 3
Before a morning feed	Baby cereal with milk	Porridge with milk	Baby cereal with milk
Before a midday feed	Well-mashed or pureed potato and carrot	Well-mashed or pureed sweet potato and cauliflower	Well-mashed or pureed pasta and broccoli
Before an evening feed	Well-mashed or pureed cooked apple	Well-mashed or pureed peach	Well-mashed or pureed avocado

More nutritious first meals as the infant begins to eat more than 1–2 teaspoons

	Day 1	Day 2 – vegetarian	Day 3
Breakfast	Baby porridge with well mashed or puréed pear and milk	Wholegrain wheat breakfast cereal with well-mashed or pureed banana and milk	Baby cereal with well-mashed or pureed cooked apple and milk
Midday meal	Puréed lamb with well mashed potato and spinach	Well-mashed or well mashed or pureed lentils with pasta, carrot and coriander	Well-mashed of puréed white fish with sweet potato, broccoli and courgette
Evening meal	Well-mashed or pureed mango mixed with plain yogurt	Well-mashed or pureed apple and pear and unsweetened fromage frais	Well-mashed or pureed peach and apricot with unsweetened custard

Stage 2: 6–9 months

Texture

Thicker mash with soft lumps is introduced at this stage foods alongside soft finger foods. Meat may still need to be pureed at first but can be mashed if it is very soft.

Infants who begin CFs at or just before 6 months of age should be moved onto mashed food as quickly as possible to ensure nutritional adequacy and for them to learn to cope with new textures. Finger foods offered with all meals will keep infants engaged in the meal and give them the opportunity to develop self-feeding skills.

Some infants are more sensitive to texture changes and benefit with slow gradual changes. Those who spit out lumps need more practice managing them rather than being moved back to smooth purees.

Examples of soft finger foods

Soft ripe fruit pieces	banana, mango, melon, pear, peach, papaya, kiwi, avocado
Cooked vegetables - steamed, roasted or boiled	carrot sticks, green beans, courgette sticks, potato and sweet potato pieces, parsnip sticks, pepper sticks, beetroot pieces, cauliflower and broccoli florets
Cooked pasta pieces	
Crusts of bread or toast	
Soft cheese cubes	

During this age infants learn to move their tongue from side to side and can therefore manage to move soft lumps to between their hard gums to be munched or chewed.

Foods to offer

By offering different foods at the three different mealtimes, a variety of foods and nutrients from all the four food groups can be included (Table 9.4). For example:

- breakfast: cereal and fruit with milk;
- midday meal: meat/fish/dhal with potatoes/rice/quinoa and vegetables. From around 7–8 months a second course of fruit and an unsweetened yogurt or milk based pudding can be offered to replace the milk feed;
- evening meal: egg/grated cheese/nut butter with pasta, couscous or bread and a vegetable. Follow with a second course of fruit.

Meals can finish with the usual milk feed or an unsweetened milk pudding.

By the age of 6 months, an infant's iron stores are unlikely to be adequate to meet the infant's iron requirements. Breast milk is low in iron and so the iron-rich foods from food group 4 as well as iron-fortified breakfast cereals and green leafy vegetables should be offered. Potatoes, tomatoes and fruits rich in vitamin C will increase the absorption of non-haem iron from eggs and plant-based foods.

Drinks with meals

Once infants are eating thickly mashed food they will need to be offered some water with all meals to satisfy their thirst. Carers will need to help control the flow from a lidded cup without a valve until the infant is competent to do this alone.

Menu planner for 6–7 months

	Day 1	Day 2	Day 3 – vegetarian
Breakfast	Breakfast wheat biscuit (e.g. Weetabix) with mashed pear and milk	Porridge with mashed banana and milk	Baby muesli with mashed strawberries and milk
	Finger food: ripe pear slices	Finger food: sticks of ripe banana	Finger food: strawberries
Midday meal	Chicken with mashed potato and broccoli	Poached white fish with sweet potato and vegetables	Courgette, cauliflower and chickpea curry with rice
	Finger food: cooked broccoli florets	Finger food: steamed vegetable sticks	Finger food: cooked courgette sticks and cauliflower florets
Evening meal	Mashed mango and yogurt	Mashed cooked apple and pear	Mashed peach and apricot
	Finger food: mango slices	Finger food: ripe pear slices	Finger food: ripe peach slices

Menu planner for 7–9 months

	Day 1	Day 2	Day 3 – vegetarian
Breakfast	Breakfast wheat biscuit (e.g. Weetabix) with mashed peach and milk	Porridge cooked with sultanas and milk	Scrambled egg with toast
	Finger food: peeled ripe peach slices	Finger food: banana slices	Finger food: toast fingers and ripe fruit pieces
Midday meal	Baked mackerel with roasted sweet potato and vegetables	Lamb stew with potato and carrots	Vegetable curry with dhal and rice
	Finger food: roasted potato and vegetable pieces	Finger food: cooked vegetable sticks	Finger food: cooked vegetable sticks
	Rice pudding with cooked plums and slices of peeled ripe plum as finger food	Egg custard and slices of peeled ripe pear	Yogurt with soft melon pieces as finger food
Evening meal	Scrambled egg with toast	Poached fish with mashed potato	Pasta with red pepper and lentil sauce
	Finger food: toast fingers	Finger food: potato chips	Finger food: cooked pasta and vegetable pieces
	Mashed kiwi fruit with fruit slices	Mashed peaches and slices of ripe peach	Mashed banana and banana slices

Stage 3: 9–12 months

Foods to offer

A variety of foods from all the four food groups over the three meals and 2 courses at the 2 main meals will provide a wider range of nutrients and tastes. These should comprise:

- a savoury first course with starchy food, vegetables and 1 of meat, fish, eggs, pulses or nut butters;
- a fruit and/or milk-based second course.

The average numbers of servings to be included from each food group per day are listed in Table 9.5.

Family foods should be the main foods offered at this stage to ensure infants learn to like the taste of their family foods. When infants join in family meals they continue to develop their own feeding skills by watching and copying other family members' eating habits.

The family foods offered should have been prepared without the addition of salt or free sugars and should not be based on convenience foods that are high in salt.

Texture

Minced and chopped foods can be introduced along with harder finger foods such as raw ripe fruit and raw vegetable sticks. Family foods such as sandwiches are also suitable.

Examples of harder finger foods
Pieces of raw fruit e.g. apples, pears
Fruits with the pips or stones removed e.g. cherries, halved grapes,[a] and segments of oranges, satsumas and clementines
Raw vegetables (e.g. sticks of cucumber, carrot, peppers, courgette)
Breadsticks and crackers
Pitta bread strips with hummus
Rice cakes
Sandwiches with soft fillings
Slices of hard boiled egg
Pieces of soft cooked meats
Sausage pieces [a] that are not round

[a] Soft round foods are a choking hazard and should be cut in half.

Table 9.5 Average number of servings from each food group at 9–12 months

Food groups	Daily servings
1: Bread, rice, potatoes, pasta and other starchy foods	3–4 servings (i.e. at each meal)
2: Fruit and vegetables	3–4 servings (i.e. fruit at breakfast and a vegetable and fruit at the 2 main meals)
3: Milk, cheese and yogurt	1–2 servings
4: Meat, fish, eggs, well-ground nuts and pulses	1–2 servings or 2–3 for vegetarians

Menu planner for 9–12 months

		Day 1	Day 2	Day 3 – vegetarian
Breakfast		Porridge with mashed fruit	Baby muesli with milk	Boiled egg with toast
	Finger foods	Banana slices	Blueberries	Kiwi fruit slices
		Milk feed	Milk feed	Milk feed
Midday meal	1st course	Beef casserole with potato and green beans	Fried fish fillet with mashed sweet potato and peas	Vegetable curry with rice and dahl
	Finger foods	Green beans	Steamed sweet potato sticks	Cooked vegetable sticks
	2nd course	Banana with custard	Rice pudding with apple and cinnamon	Yogurt and mashed peach
	Finger foods	Banana slices	Apple slices	Ripe peach slices
	Drink	Water	Water	Water
Evening meal	1st course	Scrambled egg with toast	Peanut butter sandwiches	Macaroni cheese
	Finger foods	Toast fingers and button mushroom pieces	Carrot and cucumber sticks	Cooked macaroni pieces and cherry tomatoes
	2nd course	Yogurt and mashed raspberries	Strawberries and fromage frais	Fruit compote
	Finger foods	Raspberries and grapes	Fresh strawberries	Clementine segments
	Drinks	Water and milk feed to finish	Water and milk feed to finish	Water and milk feed to finish

Activity 1

Develop menus specifying the milk feeds, food textures and finger foods for infants aged 5½ months, 6 ½ months, 8 months and 11 months.

Vegetarian diets in infancy

Vegetarian foods from food group 4 should be offered 2–3 times per day alongside a high carbohydrate food from food group 1 and a food high in vitamin C. To ensure an adequate iron intake a food high in iron is offered at each meal. For example:

- breakfast: iron-fortified breakfast cereal or oats with fruit;
- the 2 main meals: eggs/finely ground nuts or nut butters or pulses such as hummus, chickpeas, lentils or other beans.

Vegan diets are not recommended unless under strict medical and dietetic supervision with carefully planned supplements. Even then, growth will not be optimal (see page 24)

Activity 2

Make a menu plan for a week for an infant 7–12 months on a vegetarian diet.

Dental care

Dentists recommend tooth brushing should begin in infancy from the time the first tooth erupts:

- Teeth should be brushed twice daily with fluoridated tooth paste once in the morning and last thing at night.
- Use a smear of paste containing at least 1000 ppm of fluoride.

Commercial baby foods

Commercial baby foods, such as pouches, cans, jars and dried food, are regulated by EFSA. They may be convenient in some circumstances, but their exclusive use provides much less variety of taste and texture. Learning to like family foods is a key aim of complementary feeding but the family foods when used for infants need to be nutritious and balanced as described above. Some families may need support to improve their cooking skills and knowledge of healthy eating.

The European regulations for commercial foods sold for infants and young children up to the age of three years are being updated in 2020 and currently have a generous allowance of free sugars. Organic baby foods have become much more popular in recent years but they are low in iron content as organic regulations prevent fortification with iron. In addition most manufacturers only add the minimum amounts of meat or fish required by the regulations governing the nutritional content, which is 8–10 per cent.

Food safety

Preventing choking

Infants must never be left unattended with foods or drinks as they can easily choke. Tragic cases of choking are very rare in infants and more likely during the toddler years. Having infants seated and in a calm atmosphere at all times when eating is a safeguard against this. Cutting finger foods into short lengths rather than round pieces will also reduce the risk. Soft round foods such as cherry tomatoes, grapes and sausages should be cut in half.

Hygiene

- Bottles and teats for formula milks should always be sterilised.
- Plates, bowls, drinking cups and cutlery do not need to be sterilised but should be scrupulously clean.
- Freshly cooked food can be stored for up to 24 hours in the fridge.
- Frozen food should be thawed in the fridge and used within 24 hours. Thawed frozen food should not be refrozen.
- Cooked food for infants should be reheated

until piping hot right through and then cooled before feeding. Food should not be reheated more than once.

- Eggs, meat, fish and shellfish should all be well cooked right through. The exception is eggs with the British Lion Mark which can be offered partially cooked, e.g. soft boiled egg.

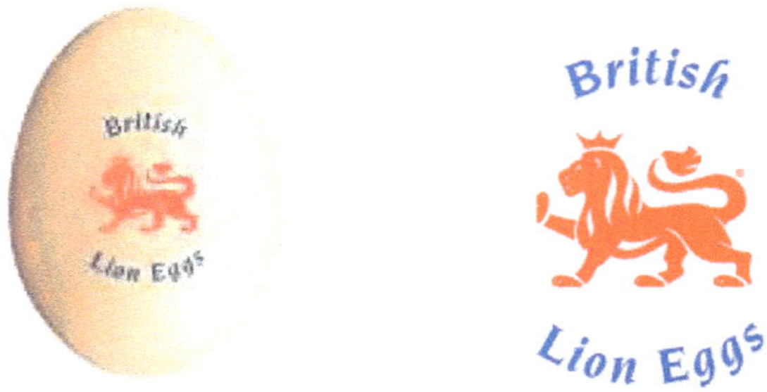

Figure 9.1 British Lion Mark

Foods to limit and avoid

Foods that should be limited and/or avoided are listed in Table 9.6.

Activity 2

Make up some meals for each of the three stages of complementary feeding, taking care to mix them to the correct texture. Buy some commercial baby foods and compare the flavour, texture and nutrient levels to those you have prepared from fresh ingredients.

Table 9.6 Foods to limit and avoid

Foods	Reason
Foods to limit	
Foods with added sugar	They provide excess calories with fewer nutrientsInfants are born with a preference for sweet foods and complementary feeding is a time for learning to like the other savoury other tastesIn homemade puddings and cooked fruit a small amount may be added if necessary to reduce the tart flavour of very sharp fruits
Foods with added salt such as adult ready meals and commercial sauces, soups and packet snacks	An excess of salt could cause dehydration if an infant becomes ill. However, nutritious foods that are preserved with salt, such as bread and cheese, do not need to be limited as infants need a certain amount of sodium to grow. See Chapter 2, page xx
Liver	Should be limited to 1 small serving per week because of the very high levels of vitamin A
Foods to avoid	
Unpasteurised Honey	It carries a small risk of botulism
Under-cooked meat, fish and shellfishUnpasteurised soft cheeses	Likely to cause gastroenteritis
Under-cooked or foods containing raw eggs unless they contain carry the British Lion Mark	Only partially cooked eggs with a British Lion Mark are safe (Figure 9.1)
Large fish such as marlin, swordfish and shark	May contain mercury
Whole nuts	A choking hazard and nuts can cause severe reactions if inhaled

References and further reading

Birch LL (1998) Development of food acceptance patterns in the first years of life. *Proceedings of the Nutrition Society* **57**(4): 617–624.

Carruth BR and Skinner JD (2002) Feeding behaviours and other motor development in healthy children (2–24 months). *Journal of the American College of Nutrition* **21**(2): 88–96.

Carruth BR, Ziegler PJ, Gordon A, et al. (2004 Jan) Developmental milestones and self-feeding behaviours in infants and toddlers. *Journal of the American Dietetic Association* **104**: 51–56.

Department of Health (1994) *Weaning and the Weaning Diet. Report on Health and Social Subjects No. 45*. London: HMSO.

Dewey K (2001) *Guiding Principles of Complementary Feeding for the Breastfed Child*. Division of Health Promotion and Protection Food and Nutrition Program, Pan American Health Organization; World Health Orgaization. www.who.int/nutrition/publications/guiding_principles_compfeeding_breastfed.pdf Accessed 01April2018.

European Food Safety Authority NDA Panel (EFSA Panel on Nutrition, Novel Foods and Food Allergens) (2019 Sept) Appropriate age range for introduction of complementary feeding into an infant's diet. *EFSA Journal* 17(9): 5780.

Castenmiller J, de Henauw S, Hirsch-Ernst K-I, Kearney J, Knutsen HK, Maciuk A, Mangelsdorf I, McArdle HJ, Naska A, Pelaez C, Pentieva K, Siani A, Thies F, Tsabouri S, Vinceti M, Bresson J-L, Fewtrell M, Kersting M, Przyrembel H, Dumas C, Titz A and Turck D (2019). Scientific Opinion on the appropriate age range for introduction of complementary feeding into an infant's diet. *EFSA Journal* 2019;**17**(9): 5780, 241 pp. EFSA Journal 2019;17(9): 5780 https://doi.org/10.2903/j.efsa.2019.5780 https://www.efsa.europa.eu/en/news/age-start-complementary-feeding-infants.

Fewtrell M, Bronsky J, Campoy C, Domellöf M, Embleton N, Fidler Mis N, Hojsak I, Hulst JM, Indrio F, Lapillonne A, Molgaard C (2017) Complementary Feeding: Position Paper by the European Society for Paediatric Gastroenterology, Hepatology, and Nutrition (ESPGHAN) Committee on Nutrition *Journal of Pediatric Gastroenterology and Nutrition* **64**(1): 119–132 doi: 10.1097/MPG.0000000000001454.

Maier A, Chabanet C, Schaal B, et al. (2007) Food-related sensory experience from birth through weaning: Contrasted patterns in two nearby European regions. *Appetite* **49**(2): 429–440.

Mughal MZ, Salama H, Greenway T, et al. (1999) Florid rickets associated with prolonged breast-feeding without vitamin D supplementation. *British Medical Journal* **318**: 39–40.

National Institute for Health and Care Excellence (November 2014) *Public Health Guidance 11. Improving the nutrition of pregnant and breast-feeding mothers and children in low-income households*. London: NICE (accessed April 2020).

National Institute for Health and Care Excellence (2017) Clinical Guideline 190: Intrapartum care. Care of healthy women and their babies during childbirth. Currently being updated. Available from: www.nice.org.uk/guidance/cg190 (accessed April2020).

Northstone K, Emmett P, Nethersole F andthe ALSPAC study team (2001) The effect of age of introduction to lumpy solids on foods eaten and reported feeding difficulties at 6 and 15 months. *Journal of Human Nutrition and Diet* **14**: 43–54.

Obbagy JE, English LK, Wong YP, Butte NF, Dewey KG, Fleischer DM, Fox MK, Greer FR, Krebs NF, Scanlon KS and Stoody EE (2019) Complementary feeding and food allergy, atopic dermatitis/eczema, asthma, and allergic rhinitis: a systematic review. *American Journal of Clinical Nutrition*, **109** (Suppl 1): 890s–934s.

Obbagy JE, English LK, Psota TL, Wong YP, Butte NF, Dewey KG, Fox MK, Greer FR, Krebs NF, Scanlon KS and Stoody EE (2019) Complementary feeding and micronutrient status: a systematic review. *American Journal of Clinical Nutrition* **109** (Suppl 1): 852s–871s.

Pérez-Escamilla R, Buccini GS, Segura-Pérez S, Piwoz E (2019) Perspective: Should Exclusive Breastfeeding Still Be Recommended for 6 Months? Advances in Nutrition **10**(6): 931–943. doi: 10.1093/advances/nmz039.

Perkin MR, Bahnson HT, Logan K, et al. (2018 Aug 6) Association of Early Introduction of Solids With Infant Sleep: A Secondary Analysis of a Randomized

Clinical Trial. JAMA Pediatrics **172**(8): e180739. doi: 10.1001/jamapediatrics.2018.0739. Epub 2018 Aug 6.

Quigley MA, Kelly YJ and Sacker A (2009) Infant feeding, solid foods and hospitalisation in the first 8 months after birth. *Archives of Disease in Childhood* **94**: 148–150.

Reilly JJ, Armstrong J, Dorosty AR, et al. (2005) Early life risk factors for obesity in childhood: cohort study. *British Medical Journal* **330**: 1357–1359.

Scientific Advisory Committee on Nutrition. (2018) Feeding in the First Year of Life. London: The Stationery Office.

Shaw V (2020) *Clinical Paediatric Dietetics*, 5th edn. Oxford: Wiley Blackwell.

WHO Regional Office for Europe (World Health Organization Regional Office for Europe) (2003). Feeding and nutrition of infants and young children. Guidelines for the WHO European region, with emphasis on the former Soviet countries. 288 pp.

WHO (2001) *World Health Organization 54th World Health Assembly 2001. Global strategy for infant and young child feeding. The optimal duration of exclusive breastfeeding.* A54/INF.DOC./4. Geneva: WHO.

Wright, CM, Cameron, K, Tsiaka, M, Parkinson, KN-(2001) Is baby-led weaning feasible? When do babies first reach out for and eat finger foods? Maternal and Child Nutrition **7**: 27–33.

Wright CM, Parkinson KN and Drewett RF (2004) Why are babies weaned early? Data from a prospective population based cohort study. *Archives of Disease in Childhood* **89**: 813–816.

Resources

European Regulations on Food intended for infants and young children: https://eur-lex.europa.eu/legal-content/EN/TXT/PDF/?uri=CELEX:32006L0125&from=EN.

These regulations are currently being updated.

10

Common feeding problems in infancy

Summary

- Early feeding difficulties may be related to slow development of feeding skills or neurodevelopmental delay.
- Better attachment and positioning may help with breastfeeding problems.
- The most common feeding problems in infants are colic, posseting and vomiting, gastro-oesophageal reflux disease, diarrhoea and gastroenteritis, constipation, food hypersensitivity and faltering growth.
- There are several specialist infant formulas that can be prescribed for formula-fed infants with specific conditions.

Many parents have concerns and anxieties about feeding infants. In breastfed infants, poor feeding may be a consequence of poor attachment, as discussed in Chapter 8. It may be a consequence of slow feeding skills development in both breast and bottles fed babies. Most feeding problems resolve with time but those that may need support from healthcare professionals and possibly intervention include:

- oromotor delay;
- colic;
- gastro-oesophageal reflux;
- persistent diarrhoea and gastroenteritis;
- constipation;
- food hypersensitivity;
- faltering growth.

Slow development of feeding skills and oromotor delay

Difficulty in feeding and food refusal is commonly seen during infancy. From birth, some infants are slow to develop feeding skills and coordinate their suck, swallow and breathing. Without adequate fluid intake they can dehydrate quickly and may need medical intervention. They may lose more than 10 per cent of their birthweight and may take longer to regain their birthweight. Breastfeeding mothers find this distressing and are often persuaded to change to bottle feeding, which is an easier mode of feeding as bottle feeding infants suck against less pressure than breastfeeding infants.

For some infants, poor feeding may be the first indication of oromotor delay or neurodevelopmental delay. Wright found about a fifth of mothers reported poor appetite and oromotor delay in their 6-week-old infants (Wright et al. 2006).

Taking longer to manage solid food and moving more slowly from smooth to lumpy textures may be an indication of delayed oromotor development.

Unsettled infants/colic

Some young infants have a period during the day when they are unsettled and cry with unexplained abdominal discomfort but appear not to be hungry. It occurs both in exclusively breast fed and formula fed infants and commonly in the late afternoon and evening. It usually resolves by the age of about 5 months. In 2016 the Rome Foundation updated their Rome IV criteria on gastrointestinal disorders and defined infantile colic as (Benninga et al. 2016):

- an infant who is less than five months of age when symptoms start and stop;
- has recurrent and prolonged periods of infant crying, fussing or irritability reported by caregivers that occur without any obvious cause and cannot be prevented or resolved by caregivers;
- and with no evidence of infant failure to thrive, fever or illness.

The previous definition involved an infant crying for more than 3 hours/ day on more than 3 days per week.

Causes of colic are still unknown and it can be extremely distressing for parents and carers. Comforting and soothing the baby with a massage or a warm bath sometimes helps. Anecdotal evidence suggests some infants improve when lactase drops are added to their milk feed to break down most of the lactose in the milk into the 2 monosaccharides glucose and galactose. However current NICE guidance (National Institute of Care and Clinical Excellence 2017) do not endorse any pharmacological treatment.

Healthcare professionals can investigate gastrointestinal discomfort by:

- asking about the infant's feeding routine and bowel movements;
- observing a feed and correct positioning and attachment in breastfed infants;
- checking that formula feeds are being made up correctly and not over- or under-concentrated;
- checking the teat hole size is suitable in bottle fed infants;
- checking that infants are being winded correctly during and after the feed.

Posseting and gastro-oesophageal reflux

Posseting or regurgitation is seen in most young infants. It occurs when the immature valve mechanism where the oesophagus and stomach meet (gastro-oesophageal sphincter) allows the stomach contents to regurgitate back up into the mouth without any harmful effects. Infants with mild posseting will gain weight and thrive normally.

More severe reflux/regurgitation, resulting in distress to the infant is called gastro-oesophageal reflux disease (GORD). In this case the acidic stomach contents come up into the oesophagus but not always into the mouth causing discomfort or pain for the infant but the carer will not necessarily be aware that it is happening. Screaming episodes during or after milk feeds may be caused by GORD.

Both conditions usually resolve with time as the infant grows and the length of the oesophagus increases and the gastro-oesophageal sphincter becomes more efficient. GORD may continue throughout infancy and beyond in some children. Symptoms often improve when complementary feeding begins, or when the infant starts to walk and is in a more upright position.

Management in primary healthcare is usually sufficient and should include explanation and reassurance to the parent. Positional management of holding infants upright for some time after feeding may help. Changing breastfed infants to infant formula will not help. NICE Guidelines suggest the following pathways:

Breastfed infants:

1. a breastfeeding assessment to check latching and feeding position;
2. Alginate therapy e.g. Infant Gaviscon, for a trial period of 1–2 weeks. Continue if symptoms resolve and monitor by stopping at intervals to check if the infant has recovered.

Formula-fed infants:

1. review the feeding history and check volumes and whether powdered feeds are being made

up correctly. If volumes are excessive for the infant's weight, reduce feed volumes;
2. offer a trial of smaller, more frequent feeds while maintaining an appropriate total daily amount of milk unless the feeds are already small and frequent;
3. offer a trial of thickened formula and if unsuccessful, trial alginate therapy for 1–2 weeks.

If the problems persist, despite having taken the above measures, or if the infant has faltering growth, referral to a paediatrician is recommended.

GORD that does not respond to treatment may be caused by, or a result of, dietary protein allergy (Hait & McDonald 2019). A trial diet, free of the suspected protein, for 2–4 weeks can be initiated to see if symptoms resolve. Cow's milk protein allergy is the most common in early infancy and for a diet free of this protein:

- the mother of a breastfed infant would need to exclude milk and foods containing milk from her diet;
- formula-fed infants can be changed to an extensively hydrolysed milk formula;
- infants who have begun complementary feeding need milk-free complementary foods.

Diarrhoea and gastroenteritis

Diarrhoea or loose stools occur frequently in infants. It can be seen in those experiencing pain during teething and resolves as the pain subsides.

Acute gastroenteritis is an infectious disease of the alimentary tract, producing damage to the mucosa, either structural or functional and of variable extent and severity. The main aim in managing gastroenteritis in infants is the correction of dehydration and maintenance of hydration and electrolyte balance. Infants under 6 months are particularly vulnerable to gastroenteritis and dehydration and may require hospital admission.

Gastroenteritis is uncommon in infants who are exclusively breastfed. In the rare event that it occurs, it is important that breastfeeding is continued, as discontinuation of breastfeeding is a major risk factor for the development of dehydration. Severe cases may require oral rehydration fluids to be given.

Infant formula feeds may be stopped for a short time (6–24 hours) and an oral rehydration solution (e.g. Dioralyte or Rehydrat) given to replace lost fluids (i.e. after vomiting or diarrhoea) and to provide the infant's fluid requirement. Formula feeds should then be re-commenced at full strength and not diluted.

If infants have begun complementary feeding, it may also be necessary to discontinue foods for a similarly short period of time.

Continued diarrhoea after acute gastroenteritis may be associated with a temporary intolerance to lactose in a small minority of infants. Breastfeeding should continue, but formula-fed infants can be changed to a lactose-free formula. Advice on excluding foods containing milk and lactose will be needed for infants who have begun complementary feeding. Reintroduction of a lactose formula must be gradual as the infant's production of the enzyme lactase will build up slowly. Lactose containng formula should be mixed with the lactose free formula in increasing amounts over about 7 days.

Constipation

In the first 3–4 months infants normally pass frequent, loose, bright yellow stools, at least 2–3 times in 24 hours. From 3 to 4 months, stools will become less frequent. It is not unusual for an infant to go several days without a bowel movement, and providing the infant is well and happy this is of no significant concern. After the introduction of complementary food, stools may change in frequency and colour.

Constipation can be simply defined as 'difficult passage of hard stools'; it may present as:

- abdominal pain;
- soiling from 'overflow' diarrhoea;
- passage of very large stools;

- stool withholding behaviour to avoid the pain on passing a stool;
- rectal bleeding which may indicate anal fissure.

Most constipation in infants and young children is idiopathic in origin – that is there is no underlying cause, including dietary factors, that can be identified. It is rare in exclusively breastfed infants and may begin when:

- infant formula is introduced or;
- complementary feeding begins.

Management of constipation

Most infants will grow out of constipation by 4–5 years of age if it is well-managed and the development of behavioural problems is avoided by preventing pain with laxatives. . With constipation an infant may have abdominal discomfort and changing the diet or feeding regimes may not be possible until the constipation is managed. National Institute of Care and Clinical Excellence (2017) recommends that management should be:

1. Introduce osmotic laxatives to treat the constipation.
2. Then assess and adjust dietary factors if necessary and possible.
3. Monitor laxative use and reduce as appropriate.

Parents are often reluctant to introduce laxatives and need some reassurance that the osmotic laxatives do not stimulate or affect the colon wall but work by retaining more water in the stool to ensure a softer stool which is easier and less painful to pass.

Dietary factors which can cause or exacerbate constipation:

During breastfeeding

- inadequate milk intake due to poor attachment or positioning. If this can be improved it may resolve the problem but additional fluids other than breast milk are not recommended;
- cow's milk protein intolerance – this is more likely in infants that have asthma or eczema. If so, it should resolve if the breastfeeding mother removes milk and dairy products from her own diet. She will need to begin a calcium supplement to ensure her own nutritional adequacy.

During infant formula feeding

- the calcium salts in the formula harden the stools in susceptible infants – this often develops when infants change from breastfeeding to formula feeding or from a whey-dominant formula to a casein-dominant 'hungry' formula;
- inadequate fluid intake through over-concentrating of the infant formula or underfeeding
- cow's milk protein allergy.

When complementary feeding begins

- inadequate fluid or fibre.

Dietary management of constipation

In formula-fed infants

- Fluid intake: Ask parents to keep a feed diary for 2–3 days. Check the volume of feed given/kg actual body weight/24 hours against recommended intake (see Chapter 8, page 109).
- Check that the infant formula is being made up according to the manufacturer's instructions and not being over-concentrated or under-concentrated.
- Change from a casein-dominant 'Hungry'milk formula to a whey-dominant formula.
- Change to a comfort formula for minor digestive problems may help as the fats in these formula are different to standard formulas (Moro et al. 2002, Schmelzle et al. 2003).
- Trial for 2-weeks an extensively hydrolysed protein or amino acid-based formula which will indicate if the cause is cow's milk protein intolerance.
- Additional drinks of cooled boiled water can be offered in between milk feeds and particularly in hot weather.

During complementary feeding

- check if drinks of water are being offered with meals and milk feeds are appropriate;
- check if fibre containing meals including fruit, vegetables, pulses, nut butters and cereals are being offered. More wholegrain cereals can be offered such as porridge or whole grain breakfast cereals (e.g. Weetabix or Shreddies). However, bran should not be given to infants.

Food hypersensitivity (food allergy and food intolerance)

About 2–5 per cent of infants are sensitive to certain foods, but many more parents suspect that a food is causing problems for their infant (Venter et al. 2006). Infants with moderate or severe eczema are most at risk.

The foods that most commonly cause problems are milk, eggs, soya, fish, wheat and peanuts. Many infants grow out of food hypersensitivity by 12 months so it is important that the condition is monitored carefully to ensure exclusion diets are not continued for longer than necessary.

Symptoms

Symptoms of immediate-onset allergy may occur up to 1 hour after food ingestion and include skin manifestations (urticaria, itching, rash), vomiting, angioedema and respiratory symptoms including wheezing or exacerbation of asthma. Anaphylaxis is rare in infants. Delayed-onset reactions are harder to diagnose and may not manifest until hours or days after the ingestion of the offending food. Possible symptoms include eczema, chronic diarrhoea, abdominal pain and faltering growth.

Diagnosis

The gold standard test is the placebo-controlled double-blind food challenge. In clinical practice, however, open challenges are usually performed where parents and practitioners know what is in the food. Food challenges are an integral part of diagnosis in order to:

- detect a specific food which causes symptoms -a positive result confirms the need to exclude that food from the diet; or
- prove that a specific food is not responsible – an absence of symptoms confirms that a restricted diet is not needed.

Once diagnosed, a food causing symptoms can be excluded.

In breastfed infants the mother may need to exclude foods from her diet and take a calcium supplement to ensure nutritional adequacy.

For cow's milk protein allergy formula-fed infants can be changed to an extensively hydrolysed formula. As these are less palatable, older infants who reject them could be given soya based infant. However, cow's milk protein and soya protein allergy may be present together.

Advice is needed to ensure an infant's milk and complementary food intake continues to provide all the necessary nutrients for optimising growth and development. A supplement may be needed in some cases.

Faltering growth

Infants who are not eating and drinking adequate energy for their needs will not grow as expected. The Avon Longitudinal Study of Parents and Children (Emond et al. 2007) showed the following feeding problems to be associated with poor growth:

- sucking problems and slow feeding in the first few weeks;
- difficulties in beginning complementary feeding at around 6 months.

Oromotor dysfunction may be the cause of both these feeding problems.

Other indications of inadequate milk intake in young infants are:

- apathetic or weakly crying infant;
- poor muscle tone and skin turgor;
- concentrated urine, a few times/day;
- infrequent, scanty stools;
- fewer than 8 short breastfeeds/day.

The NICE definition of faltering growth is outlined in Chapter 4, p. 56–57. However, interpreting growth charts requires taking into consideration:

- infants lose weight in the first few days of life but should have regained it by 2 weeks of age.
- over the first 6 - 8 weeks of life infants with a weight above the 50th centile may cross centile lines downwards and small infants with a birthweight below the 50th centile may cross centile lines upwards, moving closer to the 50th centile line.
- breastfed and formula-fed infants have slightly different growth patterns during the first year of life. Breastfed infants grow more quickly in the first 3–4 months and then grow more slowly from about 5 months when compared to formula-fed infants. Infants should all be plotted on the UK WHO growth charts based on breastfed infants.

The management of faltering growth is different for breast- and formula-fed infants.

Management of faltering growth in breastfed infants

A person skilled in breastfeeding management should assess mother and infant feeding.

- The infant should feed at least eight times in 24 hours (including at night).
- Infants should be fed until they come off the breast spontaneously. If sleepy, a nappy change may help to rouse them and the infant can then be fed on the second breast.
- The mother and infant should be in skin-to-skin contact as often as possible.
- The mother should be encouraged to express milk from her breasts after the infant has finished feeding as, after completely emptying the breast, more milk will be produced for the next feed.
- Different positioning for feeding (e.g. underarm, or especially with mother lying down) may help the infant to feed more efficiently.
- If the mother's milk supply has diminished, she may benefit from taking domperidone 10 mg three times a day in consultation with a lactation specialist.
- If the infant is sleepy or reluctant to feed it may be necessary for the mother to express her milk for some time and feed her infant with her expressed breast milk by syringe, cup or bottle until the infant is passing frequent yellow stools and is more alert. The infant can then be re-introduced to the breast.
- A healthcare professional should check that the mother is eating a balanced diet and drinking adequate fluid.
- The interaction between the mother and infant should be considered.
- The mother should be asked about any emotional stress or anxieties as this can reduce her milk production.
- The social circumstances of the family should be assessed and support arranged where necessary.

Management of faltering growth in formula-fed infants

The healthcare professional should first take a diet history and/or ask parents to keep a feed and food diary and check:

- frequency and volume of feeds taken;
- that the appropriate formula is being used and that it is being made up correctly with good hygienic practices;
- the size of the teat on the bottle is appropriate;
- the infant is not constipated;
- that suitable complementary foods are being offered.

For preterm infants, check that the parents are continuing to use a preterm formula as directed by the paediatrician or dietitian.

If there are no obvious dietary causes of faltering growth or the above measures do not result in improvement in weight gain, the infant should be referred to a paediatrician.

Some infants with certain diseases or syndromes have particularly high energy requirements and those unable to take sufficient volumes of standard infant formula should be referred to a paediatric dietitian.

Table 10.1 UK specialised infant formulas – suitable from birth or, where stated, from 6 months of age

Type of formula	Examples	Relevant compositional details	Used for infants with
High-energy	Infatrini (Nutricia)	100 kcal/100 ml	Faltering growth
	Similac High Energy (Abbott)	100 kcal/100 ml	
	SMA High Energy	91 kcal/100 ml	
High Energy extensively hydrolysed	Infatrini Peptisorb (Nutricia)	100 kcal/100 mls Extensively hydrolysed whey protein	Faltering growth with cow's milk or whole protein allergy
Thickening feeds for GORD	Aptamil Anti-Reflux	Contains carob bean gum which thickens the formula in the bottle	Gastro-oesophageal reflux disease
	Cow & Gate Anti-Reflux		
	HIPP organic Anti-reflux		
	Enfamil AR (Mead Johnson)	Rice starch which thickens in the stomach on contact with gastric acid	
	SMA Staydown Infant Milk	Corn starch thickens in the stomach on contact with gastric acid	
Lactose-free	Aptamil Lactose Free	Lactose is replaced with glucose	Lactose intolerance
	Enfamil O-Lac (Mead Johnson)		
	SMA LF		
Soya formulas	SMA Wysoy	Soy proteinLactose and sucrose free	For infants over 6 months who need to avoid cow's milk protein
Extensively hydrolysed formulas	Aptamil Pepti 1Aptamil Pepti 2 -suitable from 6 months	Extensively hydrolysed whey protein Reduced lactose	Cow's milk protein allergy without suspected lactose intolerance
	Aptamil Pepti-Junior	Extensively hydrolysed whey protein; 50% of fat is MCT; trace lactose	Whole protein and/or disaccharide intolerance, multiple malabsorption, short bowel syndrome
	Nutramigen 1 Nutramigen 2 - suitable from 6 months (Mead Johnson)	Extensively hydrolysed casein protein	Whole protein or disaccharide intolerance
	Pregestimil Lipil (Mead Johnson)	Extensively hydrolysed casein; 50- 55% of fat is MCT	Whole protein and/or disaccharide intolerance, fat or multiple malabsorption, short bowel syndrome
	Alimentum (Abbott)		
	SMA Althera	Hydrolysed whey protein	Cows milk allergy and/or multiple protein allergies

(Continued)

Table 10.1 (Continued)

Type of formula	Examples	Relevant compositional details	Used for infants with
	Pepdite (Nutricia)	Protein is hydrolysed pork collagen and soya; 3% of fat is MCT	Whole protein and/or disaccharide intolerance, multiple malabsorption, short bowel syndrome
Partially Hydrolysed	Aptamil Sensavia Range	Partially hydrolysed whey protein	
	SMA HA Infant Milk	Partially hydrolysed whey protein	SMA claims this reduces risk of developing eczema and cow's milk protein allergy but it is not suitable for diagnosed cow's milk protein allergy
Amino acid formulas	Neocate LCPNeocate Syneo (Nutricia)	Protein is a mixture of free amino acids with no peptide chains; Some MCT fat	Infants who have not responded to an extensively hydrolysed formula
	Nutramigen Puramino (Mead Johnson)		Whole protein/hydrolysate intolerance, multiple malabsorption, short bowel syndrome
	SMA Alfamino		
Carbohydrate disorders	Galactomin 17 (Nutricia)	Carbohydrate is glucose	For lactose intolerance, galactosaemia and glucokinase deficiency
	Galactomin 19 (Nutricia)	Carbohydrate is fructose	For glucose-galactose intolerance
Modified fat	Lipistart (Nestle)	81% fat is MCT	Fat malabsorption, pancreatic insufficiency, short bowel syndrome, multiple malabsorption, short bowel syndrome, whole protein intolerance requiring MCT
	Monogen (Nutricia)	84% fat is MCT	
	MCT Pepdite (Nutricia)	75% of fat is MCT Protein is hydrolysed pork collagen and soya	
High-fat, low-carbohydrate	Ketocal Infant (Nutricia)	73% fat	Infants on a ketogenic diet for treatment of epilepsy
Formula for renal disease	Kindergen (Kindergen)	Higher in energy (101 kcals/100 ml), fat, carbohydrate and sodium but lower in potassium than standard infant formulas	For chronic renal failure and where peritoneal rapid overnight dialysis (PROD) or continuous cycling peritoneal dialysis (CCPD) is required
Very low-calcium formula	Locasol (Nutricia)	Very low in calcium and vitamin D	For infants with hypercalcinaemia

GORD, gastro-oesophageal reflux disease; MCT, medium-chain triglycerides; LCP, long-chain polyunsaturated fatty acids

A 'high-energy' infant formula may be recommended (see Table 10.1). These should only be used with dietetic and/or medical recommendation and ongoing assessment.

Vitamin D deficiency

Infants born to mothers with low vitamin D levels before and during pregnancy may be born with low vitamin D levels themselves. This can lead to low plasma calcium and they may present with:

- stridor or seizures;
- tetany;
- cardiomyopathy;
- reduced muscle tone – floppy infant
- delayed closure of anterior fontanelle – prominent forehead;
- rickets - may be seen in late infancy but is usually seen in toddlers.

Specialist infant formulas

Specialist infant formulas (Table 10.1) are prescribable for certain medical conditions as specified in Borderline Substances section in the British National Formulary for Children. Only a qualified doctor can prescribe them, although doctors often do so on the advice of a paediatric dietitian. The formulas are available over the counter if a parent asks a pharmacist to order them. However, they are much more expensive than standard formulas.

References and further reading

Benninga MA, Faure C, Hyman PE, St James Roberts I, Schechter NL, Nurko S. (2016) Childhood functional gastrointestinal disorders: neonate/toddler. *Gastroenterology* **150**: 1443–1455. e2

Emond A, Drewett R, Blair P and Emmett P (2007) Postnatal factors associated with failure to thrive in term infants in the Avon Longitudinal Study of Parents and Children. *Archives of Disease in Childhood* **92**: 115–119.

Guarino A, Albano F, Ashkenazi S, et al. (2008) ESPGHAN/ESPID Evidence-based guidelines for the management of acute gastroenteritis in children in Europe. Expert Working Group. European Society for Paediatric Gastroenterology, Hepatology, and Nutrition/European Society for Paediatric Infectious Diseases. *Journal of Pediatric Gastroenterology and Nutrition* **46** (suppl 2): S81–S122.

Hait EJ, McDonald DR. (2019) Impact of Gastroesophageal Reflux Disease on Mucosal Immunity and Atopic Disorders. *Clin Rev Allergy Immunol* **57**(2): 213–225. doi:10.1007/s12016-018-8701-4

Moro G, Minoli L, Mosca M, et al. (2002) Dosage-related bifidogenic effects of galacto- and fructooligosaccharides in formula-fed term infant. Journal of Paediatric Gastroenterology and Nutrition 34: 291–295.

National Institute of Care and Clinical Excellence. (2017) Clinical Knowledge Summary: Colic – Infantile.

National Institute of Care and Clinical Excellence. (July 2017) *Constipation in children and young people: diagnosis and management Clinical guideline* [CG99]. https://www.nice.org.uk/guidance/cg99/chapter/1-Guidance#clinical-management

National Institute of Care and Clinical Excellence. (October 2019) *Gastro-oesophageal reflux disease in children and young people: diagnosis and management NICE guideline* [NG1]. Next planned review by December 2020.

Perry R, Leach V, Penfold C, Davies P. (2019) An overview of systematic reviews of complementary and alternative therapies for infantile colic. *Systematic Reviews* **8** (1) DOI: 10.1186/s13643-019-1191-5

Rybak A, Pesce M, Thapar N, Borrelli O. (2017) Gastro-Esophageal Reflux in Children. *Int J Mol Sci* **18**(8): 1671. Published 2017 Aug 1. doi:10.3390/ijms18081671

Schmelzle H, Wirth S, Skopnik H, et al. (2003) Randomised double-blind study of the nutritional efficacy and bifidogenicity of a new infant formula containing partially hydrolysed protein, a high ß-palmitic acid level and non-digestible oligosaccharides. *Journal of Paediatric Gastroenterology and Nutrition* **36**: 343–351.

Vandenplas Y, Abkari A, Bellaiche M, et al. (2015) Prevalence and health outcomes of functional gastrointestinal symptoms in infants from birth to 12 months of age. *J Pediatr Gastroenterol Nutr* **61**(5): 531–537.

Vandenplas Y, Gutierrez-Castrellon P, Velasco-Benitez C, et al. (2013) Practical algorithms for managing common gastrointestinal symptoms in infants. *Nutrition* **29**: 184–194.

Venter C, Pereira B, Grundy J, et al. (2006) Incidence of parentally reported and clinically diagnosed food hypersensitivity in the first year of life. *Journal of Allergy and Clinical Immunology* **117**: 1118–1124.

Wright CM, Parkinson KN and Drewett RF (2006) How does maternal and child feeding behavior relate to weight gain and failure to thrive? Data from a prospective birth cohort. *Pediatrics* **117**(4): 1262–1269.

Zeevenhooven J, Koppen IJN, Benninga, MA. (2017 Mar) The New Rome IV Criteria for Functional Gastrointestinal Disorders in Infants and Toddlers. *Pediatr Gastroenterol Hepatol Nutr* **20**(1): 1–13. doi: 10.5223/pghn.2017.20.1.1

Resources

British National Formulary for Children: https://bnfc.nice.org.uk/borderline-substance-taxonomy/specialised-formulas-infant-and-child.html

The Children's Bowel & Bladder Charity (ERIC; www.eric.org.uk) has a range of leaflets on constipation and soiling, such as the Constipation toilet tool, and runs a helpline (telephone 0845 370 8008).

Cry-sis charity for families with excessively crying or sleepless children www.cry-sis.org.uk and runs a national telephone helpline (0845 122 8669).

11

Preterm infants

Summary

- Preterm infants are those born before 37 weeks gestation.
- The nutritional needs of preterm infants are higher per kg body weight than those of term infants and vary depending on the infant's gestation and size.
- Infants born very preterm and/or very small are likely to require neonatal parenteral nutrition while establishing enteral feeds.
- Maternal breast milk, either enterally via a feeding tube or orally, provides health benefits.
- Mothers may need skilled support to express breast milk for their preterm infant.
- Preterm infants may need protein supplements or breast milk fortifiers added to maternal breast milk to aid growth and ensure adequate nutritional status.
- If breast milk is unavailable there are preterm formulas and nutrient-enriched post discharge formula milks which have been designed to meet the specific nutritional needs of preterm infants.
- Development of oral feeding is individual and dependent on many factors, including gestation and size at birth and the medical condition and history of the baby.
- Complementary feeding can begin at the same age as term infants – 4–6 months post term age – but preterm infants and those small for gestational age are at higher risk of iron deficiency and may benefit from high iron complementary feeding before 6 months post-term age.

Classification of preterm and small-for-gestational-age infants

About 1 in 13 infants in the United Kingdom are born before 37 weeks gestation and are classified as preterm. They, and those born with a low birth-weight (LBW), below 2500 g (2.5 kg), have special nutritional needs which vary according to the infant's maturity and any medical complications that are present at birth or develop subsequently. The terms used to classify preterm and low-birthweight infants are defined in Table 11.1. About 80 per cent of preterm infants are born 32–36 weeks i.e. late and moderately preterm (LMPT).

Growth charts for classification and assessment

In the United Kingdom, the Neonatal and Infant Close Monitoring Chart are used. However, other charts have been developed and there is some debate around which charts are the most suitable as they differ in the way they were developed and the techniques and assumptions that underpin them. They include:

- INTERGROWTH-21st Fetal charts
- International Fetal and Newborn Growth Consortium for the 21st Century Preterm Postnatal Growth Standards

Table 11.1 Classification of preterm and low-birthweight infants

Preterm	Born before 37 weeks gestation
Late Preterm	Born 34–<37 weeks gestation
Moderately preterm	Born 32–<34 weeks gestation
Very preterm	Born 28–32 weeks gestation
Extremely preterm	Born less than 28 weeks gestation
Low birthweight (LBW)	Birthweight: 1500–2500 g
Very low birthweight (VLBW)	Birthweight: 1000–1500 g
Extremely low birthweight (ELBW)	Birthweight: <1000 g
Small for gestational age (SGA)	Birthweight below the 9th centile for gestational age. Can result from a number of causes such as infection and genetic reasons
Intrauterine growth restriction (IUGR)	Born with a low weight but may show normal head and length growth depending on how long there has been a placental deficiency. Often at high risk of feeding problems as there may have been redirection of blood flow from the gut to brain and other organs

- World Health Organization (WHO) fetal charts
- Gestation Related Optimal Weight (GROW) charts

Nutritional requirements

Growth failure is almost universal among preterm infants but the goal is to meet the growth rate of a healthy fetus of the same gestational age as growth velocities affect neurodevelopment and anthropometric outcomes (Hickey et al. 2020).

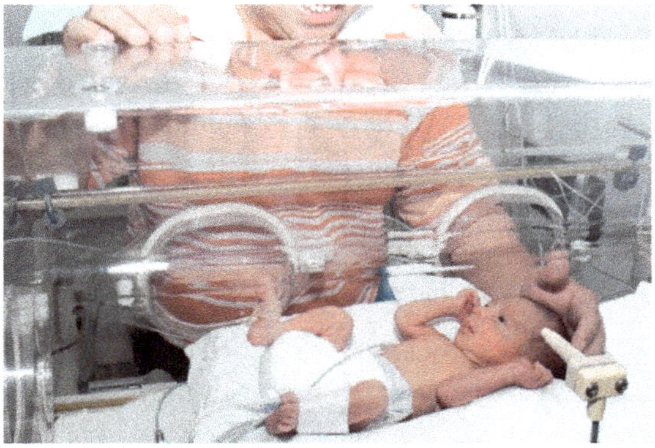

Figure 11.1 Preterm infant in an incubator

The energy and nutrient requirements are calculated based on their body weight in kilograms and the need to support energy expenditure and growth. As preterm infants have not accumulated the body stores of nutrients that term infants accumulate during the third trimester of pregnancy, they have higher nutrient needs per kilogram of body weight than term infants.

As preterm infants' risk of iron deficiency may impair neurodevelopment, ESPGHAN recommends for LMPT infants:

- 1 to 2 mg iron//kg/day up to 6 months age for those weighing less than 2.5 kg at birth
- 2 to 3 mg iron//kg/day at least up to 6 months for those weighing less than 2 kg at birth

LMPT infants are also at high risk of hypoglycemia and proactive nutritional support is required to address this.

Nutritional requirements of preterm infants up to 1.8 kg compared to those of term infants are shown in Table 11.2. Ranges of advisable micronutrient intakes for preterm infants published by ESPGHAN in 2010, are generally used in the United Kingdom (ESPGHAN Committee on Nutrition 2010). Guidelines on parenteral nutrition for preterm infants were published in 2018 from a collaboration of 3 organisations:

Table 11.2 Comparison of average daily nutritional requirements of term infants with preterm infants feeding enterally

	Term infants	Enteral nutrition for infants 1 to 1.8 kg (ESPGHAN Committee on Nutrition 2010)	Enteral nutrition for infants <1 kg (ESPGHAN Committee on Nutrition 2010)
Fluids (ml/kg)	150	135–200	135–200
Energy (kcal/kg)	96	110–135	110–135
Protein (g protein/ kg)	2.1	3.5–4.0	4–4.5
Sodium (mg/kg)	35	69–115	69–115
Potassium (mg/kg)	133	66–132	66–132

ESPGHAN, European Society for Clinical Nutrition and Metabolism and the Chinese Society for Parenteral and Enteral Nutrition (ESPGHAN/ESPEN/CSPEN 2018).

Feeding routes for preterm infants in the neonatal unit

The feeding route or routes used for preterm infants will depend on gestation, size and condition at birth (Table 11.3). Where possible, all infants will receive enteral nutrition as soon as clinically indicated.

Parenteral nutrition

Parenteral nutrition has been used in neonatal units for many decades to feed infants born too early to tolerate an adequate amount of enteral feeds. It is now common practice on neonatal units. NICE recommend parenteral nutrition for the following groups of infants (NICE 2020):

- infants born before 31 weeks gestation
- infants born after 31 weeks gestation who do not make sufficient progress with enteral nutrition in the first 72 hours following birth
- infants with a congenital gut disorder or a critical illness

Maintenance parenteral nutrition is usually by standardised solutions to meet vitamin and mineral requirements and providing:

Energy	75–120 (kcal/kg/day)
Amino acids	3–4 (g/kg/day)
Glucose	9–16 (g/kg/day)
Lipids	3–4 (g/kg/day)

Parenteral nutritional requirements may be lower than those for enteral and oral nutrition because absorption of nutrients across the gut wall is not complete.

Parenteral nutrition is decreased as enteral nutrition is tolerated and NICE recommends stopping parenteral nutrition when enteral nutrition has reached:

- 140 to 150 ml/kg/day for infants born before 28 weeks gestation
- 120 to 140 ml/kg/day for infants born at or after 28 weeks gestation

Trophic feeds or minimal enteral feeding

Trophic feeds or minimal enteral feeding is recommended, even for the smallest sickest infants on parenteral nutrition. Very small amounts of feed of <24 ml feed/kg/day are given. Meanwhile parenteral nutrition provides all the nutrition for the infants.

The benefits of trophic feeding include:

- gut priming

Table 11.3 Feeding routes for preterm infants

	Route	Feeds used	When to use
Parenteral nutrition	Administered directly into the bloodstream usually via peripherally sited central venous access	A sterile complete feed delivered as an aqueous solution with a standardised composition of dextrose, amino acids, electrolytes, vitamins and minerals. Alongside this, a lipid solution containing fat-soluble vitamins is also infused	For infants who are born at <1000 g, and some <1500 g Some intrauterine growth restriction infants
Enteral nutrition	Milk feed via a nasogastric (NG) tube (from nose to stomach) or an orogastric tube (mouth to stomach)	In order of preference: 1. Expressed breast milk (EBM) 2. Donor expressed breast milk (DEBM) 3. Breast milk fortifiers may be added to either EBM or DEBM 4. Preterm formula	Begin as soon as clinically indicated as trophic feeding (minimal enteral feeding) and increase as tolerated
Breastfeeding	Oral feeding direct from the mother's breast	Breast milk	Can begin when infant starts to coordinate suck, swallow and breathing for short periods
Bottle feeding	Oral feeding using sterilised bottles and teats	Expressed breast milk Preterm formula Nutrient-enriched post-discharge formula	Can begin when infant starts to coordinate suck, swallow and breathing for short periods

- a reduced dependence on parenteral nutrition as there is a more rapid tolerance to enteral feeds
- lower peak bilirubin and alkaline phosphatase levels
- enhanced gut motility
- increased lactase activity
- less hyperglycaemia
- reduced rate of sepsis.

Maternal colostrum and breast milk are the first choices for trophic feeding but where they are unavailable and the infant is thought to be at risk of developing necrotising enterocolitis, donor breast milk may be used if available. If neither source of breast milk is available, a preterm formula milk (discussed below) can be used.

Increasing enteral feeds will commence once clinicians are confident that the infant is tolerating trophic feeds. Advancing feeds is on an individual basis depending on each infant's tolerance.

Enteral nutrition

Enteral nutrition is used for infants with:

- immature suck/swallow
- mechanical ventilation with an endotracheal tube in place preventing oral feeding
- limited oral intake that is less than adequate and requires top-up of feeds via a nasogastric or orogastric tube (see Figure 11.2).

ESPGHAN recommend enteral feeding for infants with a birth weight less than 1800g and in 2010 they published guidelines for the enteral nutrient supply for preterm infants.

The route of the tube will depend on how the baby is receiving ventilation or oxygen support.

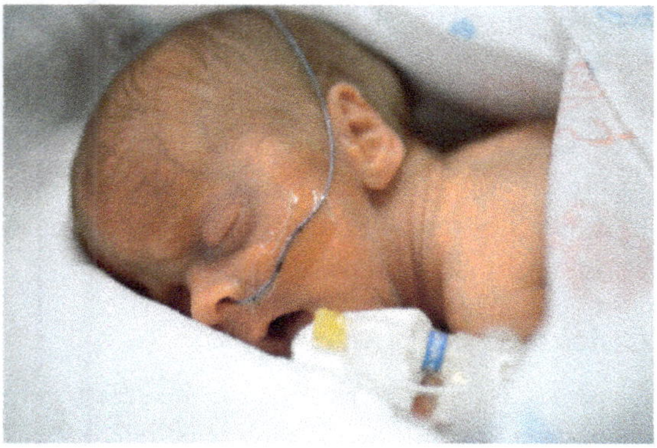

Figure 11.2 A preterm infant with a nasogastric tube

Breast milk

The health benefits of breast milk for term infants also apply to preterm infants and are described in Chapter 8. Additional specific benefits for preterm infants include:

- reduced incidence of necrotising enterocolitis
- reduced incidence of sepsis
- improved neurodevelopmental outcomes
- associated with later improved bone mineralisation.

These benefits are dose-dependent so the more breast milk an infant receives the greater the benefit to them. Breast milk is also better tolerated than formula milk so can reduce the duration of parenteral nutrition.

Expressing breast milk for preterm infants

Until their infant is old enough or well enough to feed directly from the breast, mothers must express their breast milk. Mothers often say that it is the one thing they can do for their preterm infant in an intensive medical environment where skilled staff do most of the care for their infant. It also helps bonding and attachment between mother and infant.

Mothers of even the most preterm infants can provide all or some of the milk needed by their baby. When infants are born extremely prematurely, breast development will be at an earlier stage than those of the mothers of term infants. Compensatory breast growth can be achieved by efficient early and frequent milk removal by expressing. When mothers have given birth before 28 weeks gestation, expressing their milk about 10–12 times in 24 hours for the first 2 weeks supports catch-up growth of the breast and effective initiation of lactation.

Ideally, mothers should initiate expressing within 6 hours after delivery. Initially, hand expression will provide the first few drops of colostrum. After 2–3 days, as maternal milk increases in volume, mothers can move to electric pumping to express their breast milk. A trained member of staff should ensure that mothers have the correctly fitting equipment and should show them how to use the pump.

Levels of anxiety, depression and psychological distress correlate negatively with early lactation success. Maintaining lactation through expression can be a long and tough process, so these mothers need good, consistent advice and support from the outset. The following tips may help them through the process:

- Prepare the breast through gentle massage before beginning to express.
- Hand expression can be useful before pump expressing or breastfeeding to initiate milk flow.
- Express regularly: a minimum 8–10 times per day.
- Don't leave the gap between expression longer than six hours.
- Express once at night – preferably between 2 and 4 am.
- Ensure the breast is fully emptied before stopping expressing.
- Make sure mothers are fully confident about using the breast pump.
- Check the funnel size as they come in different sizes and can cause trauma if not fitting correctly.
- Where possible double pump from both breasts at the same time.

- Engage in regular skin-to-skin contact (e.g. kangaroo care).
- Sensory stimulation encourages oxytocin hormone levels and the let-down reflex. This may be by expressing beside the infant's cot or expressing with a picture of the infant and/or toys/muslin cloths with the infant's smell.

Evidence suggests that mothers should be encouraged to express 750–1000 ml of breast milk in 24 hours by 2 weeks post delivery in order to enable them to maintain long-term lactation. Once lactation has been established, some mothers may be able to express less frequently to achieve this volume. The volume produced at each expression depends on the glandular tissue content of the breasts, which varies from mother to mother. Some mothers can therefore produce larger volumes than others at each expression.

Nutrient content of preterm breast milk

Preterm breast milk, like term breast milk, starts out as colostrum rich in protein and immunoglobins specifically designed to help protect the preterm infant from infection. After 2–3 days the milk goes through a transitional phase for about 15 days and then becomes mature milk.

The composition varies during the course of an expression/feed and also depends on:

- time since birth
- the time of the day
- expressing technique
- how much the milk is handled after expressing.

Energy

As the transitional and mature milks increase in fat and energy throughout the feed, mothers are encouraged to 'empty' both breasts each time they express to include the high-fat, high-energy content at the end of the expression.

Protein

The maternal protein is of a higher bioavailability compared to formula milk and so is better absorbed by preterm infants. The protein content is higher at 1.8 g/100 ml in the transitional milk from the mothers whose infants were born before 31 weeks gestation. It then falls to about 1.3 g/100 ml in mature milk – similar to that of mature milk in mothers of term infants. The higher content in transitional milk promotes better growth.

Calcium and phosphorus

These are also better absorbed from breast milk than from formula milk. However, phosphorus can become a limiting nutrient for bone development and is therefore always given to the infant as a supplement.

Vitamins and iron

The vitamin and iron content of breast milk is lower than preterm requirements so preterm infants feeding only on breast milk need a vitamin supplement once on full enteral feeds and an iron supplement from around 4 weeks of life. Local policies for supplementation vary.

Most infants less than 1500 g grow satisfactorily on maternal breast milk and vitamin supplements for the first weeks of life, however, some may need additional phosphorus and sodium. Beyond this, many will require additional protein as the breast milk levels decrease over time.

Supplements for breast milk

Protein supplements contain hydrolysed whey and casein and can be added to either breastmilk or preterm formula to increase protein intakes.

Breast milk fortifiers contain protein as hydrolysed whey and casein, along with a wide range of nutrients. Currently the SMA product contains iron but the Cow & Gate product does not. In the United Kingdom, only powdered supplements are used and are added to expressed breast milk if the infant is not gaining sufficient weight on breast milk alone.

There is no consensus on either routinely fortifying breast milk or only fortifying on a case by case basis. Fortification is probably not required in early breast milk while the protein level is high.

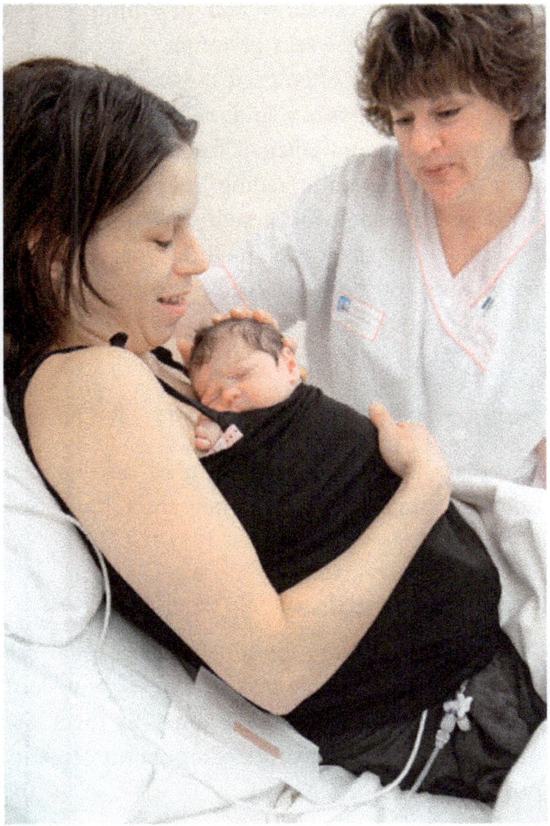

Figure 11.3 A baby being held in kangaroo care

There are no current recommendations on when breast milk fortifiers should be added to expressed breast milk. Ideally they should be added to the breast milk just prior to feeding if possible.

Breast milk fortifiers are usually discontinued before discharge from the neonatal unit.

Oral feeding

Feeding development in the preterm infant is individual and dependent on many factors, including gestation and size at birth, the medical condition and history of the baby.

Breastfeeding

With appropriate support preterm infants may be able to start breastfeeding attempts from around 32 weeks gestation as an extension of 'kangaroo care', but they are unlikely to achieve full nutritive breastfeeding until around 36 weeks gestation.

Kangaroo care (Figure 11.3) involves the infant being secured against the mother or father's skin – often on the mother's chest between her breasts. This maintains the infant's body heat and the benefits for the infant include reduced morbidity and mortality. Benefits are also seen in low birth weight infants cared for at home (Mazumder et al. 2019).

As breastfeeding development is reliant on the mother and infant dyad, every effort should be made to enable mothers to be with their infant as much as possible. An overview of breastfeeding progression is summarised in Table 11.4. but progression may be slower depending on an infant's medical condition.

Patience, practice and persistence are needed in the transition from tube feeding to breastfeeding. Ongoing practical and emotional support from staff trained in breastfeeding care is needed as they can observe and support breastfeeding attempts and help mothers to:

Table 11.4 Breastfeeding progression in preterm infants

Gestational age	Breastfeeding skills of preterm infants
Less than 30 weeks	Smell, open mouth, protrude tongue, dribble saliva, lick milk from the nipple, take some breast tissue into the mouth and make a few weak sucks
30–32 weeks	Attach to the breast and may make some weak to strong sucks with long pauses in between
32 weeks and over	Root, organise sucking bursts with long pauses, take part of a feed from the breast and as he or she becomes older may take 1 to all complete feeds from the breast
36 weeks and over	Breastfeed in a well-coordinated way

From Lang 2002.

- understand normal feeding behaviours of preterm infants
- understand the development to effective attachment and positioning on the breast and sucking behaviours
- assess success and progress of their infant's breastfeeding.

Physiological benefits for preterm infants of breastfeeding compared to bottle feeding include:

- improved temperature control
- improved oxygen saturations
- improved suck swallow breathe coordination.
- better cognitive and behavioural outcomes if still breastfeeding at discharge

There is some evidence that breastfeeding facilitates earlier discharge from neonatal units than bottle feeding (Altman *et al.* 2009). Bottle feeding may interfere with the development of breastfeeding if introduced before breastfeeding is fully established.

Establishing breastfeeding in late preterm infants is frequently more problematic than in term infants and as a consequence they are less likely to be breastfed and less likely to breastfeed for a long duration.

Bottle feeding

If a mother chooses not to breastfeed, preterm infants can start attempting bottle feeding once the infant is old enough and well enough to coordinate suck, swallow and breathing; this is usually around 34 weeks gestation.

Preterm infants often need slow milk flow teats, supportive positioning and careful monitoring to achieve safe and efficient feeding, especially if their breathing and feeding are less well co-ordinated. Parents will therefore need support to feed safely and effectively. As they progress, bottle fed infants can be fed according to their hunger cues as for term infants.

Formula milks for preterm infants

There are 2 types of formula used on neonatal units for preterm infants. They are summarised in Table 11.5.

Preterm formulas

Preterm formulas are for supervised hospital use only and only available in a sterile, ready-to-feed format. They have been designed to meet the nutritional requirements of preterm infants providing:

- adequate energy and protein levels with a protein-to-energy ratio to optimise growth
- phosphate and calcium levels at the optimum ratio for bone mineralisation
- required vitamin, mineral and iron content.

Preterm formulas are also given to infants who weigh less than 2 kg at birth.

Table 11.5 Types of formula milk available for preterm infants

Type of formula milk	Examples	Relevant compositional details	Used for:
Preterm formula	Nutriprem 1 (Cow & Gate)	Higher in energy and nutrients than term formulas and nutrient-enriched post-discharge formulas	Preterm or low-birthweight infants in hospital
Hydrolysed Preterm formula	Hydrolysed Nutriprem (Cow & Gate) SMA Gold Prem 1	Hydrolysed protein	Preterm or low birthweight infants in hospital, who are not tolerating standard preterm formula.
Nutrient-enriched post-discharge formulas	Nutriprem 2 (Cow & Gate) SMA Gold Prem 2	Higher in some nutrients than term formula	Discharged preterm and low-birthweight infants

Nutrient-enriched post-discharge formula

Nutrient-enriched post-discharge formula may be given to preterm infants still in hospital who have been on a preterm formula and have reached 2–2.5 kg. They contain less energy and protein than preterm formulas but are higher in energy, protein, vitamins and minerals, especially calcium and phosphorus and iron, than standard formulas for term infants. They are used to support the higher nutritional requirements for catch-up growth in preterm infants once they have been discharged home.

They are available both as:

- sterile ready-to-feed and
- non-sterile powder that must be reconstituted with boiled water.

Discharge home from the neonatal unit

Individual discharge plans depending on local resources should be developed. Some preterm infants may go home with some nutritional deficits but most will demand feed orally and should be allowed to 'catch up' any growth deficit in their own time. Their nutritional intake and growth should be regularly assessed and monitored.

Breastfeeding infants require additional vitamin and iron supplements, as directed by the consultant paediatrician or dietitian. ESPGHAN Committee on Nutrition 2019 recommend a daily vitamin D supplement of at least 10 µg/day (400 IU/day).

Formula-fed infants do not usually require extra supplements as the nutrient-enriched post-discharge formula is fortified with all nutrients. It is usually prescribed until 6 months post term age or until adequate catch-up growth has been achieved. However, the evidence for benefit beyond 3 months after their expected date of delivery is limited (Young, Embleton and McGuire 2016).

Some neonatal units recommend that the sterile ready-to-feed formula should be used until 4 weeks post term age to reduce the risk of food-borne infections. Infants can then be switched onto the cheaper powdered formula. Preparation and storage recommendations for these formula milks are the same as for standard formulas for term infants (see Chapter 8).

Beginning complementary feeding

The medical team for each preterm infant is best placed to advise when to begin complementary feeding and, beginning around the same biological age as for term infants, i.e. four to six months post term age. As preterm infants are at higher risk of being iron depleted by six months they may benefit from high iron foods before six months post term age (European Food Safety Authority NDA Panel EFSA Panel on Nutrition, Novel Foods and Food Allergens et al. 2019). They may begin complementary feeding as early as 3–4 months post term age.

Preterm infants may need more support to sit upright and control their head as some experience developmental delay. Parents need to be advised to make sure the head and neck are well supported during feeding, as seen in Figure 11.4 where a rolled towel is placed behind and round the sides of the neck to keep the head in a stable position.

Complementary feeding should then progress as for term babies, introducing new textures to give infants the opportunity to learn to manage them in their mouth. Unfortunately, preterm babies are more likely to have feeding problems than term babies (Johnson et al. 2016).

Activity 1

What advice for complementary feeding would you give the mother of a fully breastfed preterm infant born at 30 weeks gestation?

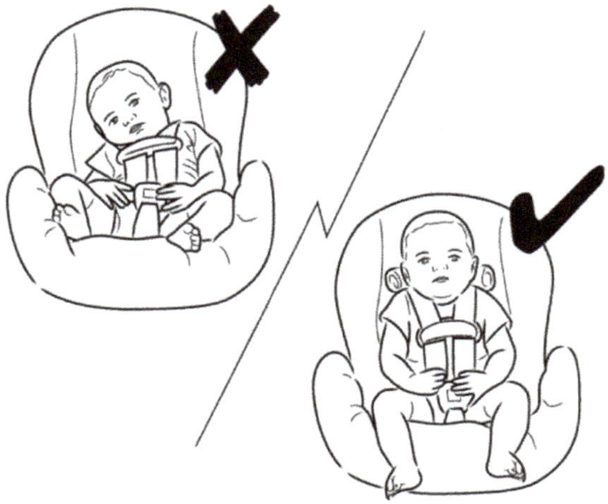

Figure 11.4 Safe positioning for complementary feeding for pre-term infants

Acknowledgements

Kate Arnold, Specialist Neonatal/Paediatric Gastroenterology Dietitian, Chelsea and Westminster Hospital, London.

References and further reading

Agostoni C, Buonocore G, Carnielli VP, et al. (2010) Enteral nutrient supply for preterm infants: commentary from the European Society of Paediatric Gastroenterology, Hepatology and Nutrition Committee on Nutrition. Journal of Pediatric Gastroenterology and Nutrition **50**(1): 85–91.

Altman M, Vanpée M, Cnattingius S and Norman M (2009) Moderately preterm infants and determinants of length of hospital stay. *Archives of Disease in Childhood; Fetal Neonatal Edition* **94**(6): F414–F418.

Aylward GP (2014 Jul-Aug) Neurodevelopmental outcomes of infants born prematurely. The Journal of Developmental and Behavioral Pediatrics **35**(6):394–407. Available from: doi: 10.1097/01.DBP.0000452240.39511.d4.

Blesa M, Sullivan G, Anblagan D, Telford EJ, Quigley AJ, Sparrow SA, Serag A, Semple SI, Bastin ME, Boardman JP (2019) Early breast milk exposure modifies brain connectivity in preterm infants. *NeuroImage* **184**: 431 doi: 10.1016/j.neuroimage.2018.09.045.

Brennan AM, Murphy BP, Kiely ME (2016 May) Optimising preterm nutrition: present and future. Proceedings of the Nutrition Society **75**(2):154–161. doi: 10.1017/S0029665116000136. Epub 2016 Apr 1.

Brennan AM, Kiely ME, Fenton S, Murphy BP (2018 Feb 2) Standardized Parenteral Nutrition for the Transition Phase in Preterm Infants: A Bag That Fits. *Nutrients* **10**(2). pii: E170. doi: 10.3390/nu10020170.

Cheong JLY, Wark JD, Cheung MM, et al. (2019) Impact of extreme prematurity or extreme low birth weight on young adult health and well-being: the Victorian Infant Collaborative Study (VICS) 1991-1992 Longitudinal Cohort study protocol. *BMJ Open* **9**(5):e030345. Published 2019 May 9. doi:10.1136/bmjopen-2019-030345.

Conde-Agudelo A, Díaz-Rossello JL (2016 Aug 23) Kangaroo mother care to reduce morbidity and mortality in low birthweight infants. *Cochrane Database Systematic Reviews* **2016**(8): CD002771. doi: 10.1002/14651858.CD002771.pub4. PMID: 27552521; PMCID: PMC6464509.

European Food Safety Authority NDA Panel (EFSA Panel on Nutrition, Novel Foods and Food Allergens)Castenmiller J, de Henauw S, Hirsch-Ernst K-I, Kearney J, Knutsen HK, Maciuk A,

Mangelsdorf I, McArdle HJ, Naska A, Pelaez C, Pentieva K, Siani A, Thies F, Tsabouri S, Vinceti M, Bresson J-L, Fewtrell M, Kersting M, Przyrembel H, Dumas C, Titz A and Turck D (2019) 2019. Scientific Opinion on the appropriate age range for introduction of complementary feeding into an infant's diet. EFSA Journal **17**(9):5780, 241 pp. *EFSA Journal* 2019;17(9):5780 https://doi.org/10.2903/j.efsa.2019.5780 https://www.efsa.europa.eu/en/news/age-start-complementary-feeding-infants.

European Food Safety Authority NDA Panel (EFSA Panel on Nutrition, Novel Foods and Food Allergens) (2013) Scientific Opinion on nutrient requirements and dietary intakes of infants and young children in the European Union. *EFSA Journal* 2013 **11**(10): 3408, 103 pp. doi:10.2903/j.efsa.2013.3408.

ESPGHAN Committee on Nutrition (2019 Aug) Feeding the late and moderately preterm infant: A position paper of the ESPGHAN Committee on Nutrition. Journal of Pediatric Gastroenterology and Nutrition **69**(2):259–270. doi: 10.1097/MPG.0000000000002397. http://www.espghan.org/fileadmin/user_upload/Society_Papers/Feeding_the_late_and_moderately_preterm_infant.pdf.

ESPGHAN Committee on Nutrition (2010) Enteral nutrition supply for preterm infants: Commentary from the European Society for Paediatric Gastroenterology, Hepatology, and Nutrition Committee on Nutrition. *Journal of Paediatric Gastroenterology and Nutrition* **50**: 1–9.

ESPGHAN/ESPEN/CSPEN (2018 Dec) Guidelines on pediatric parenteral nutrition. *Clinical Nutrition* **37**(6 Pt B):2303–2305. doi: 10.1016/j.clnu.2018.05.029. Epub 2018.

Healy DB, Brennan AM, O'Donovan R, Daly V, Doolan A, Dempsey EM (2016 Jun) Structured promotion of breastmilk expression is associated with shortened hospitalisation for very preterm infants. *Acta Paediatri ca* **105**(6):e252–e256. doi: 10.1111/apa.13399.

Hickey L, Burnett A, Spittle AJ, *et al.* Extreme prematurity, growth and neurodevelopment at 8 years: a cohort study. *Archives of Disease in Childhood* Published Online First: 03 August 2020. doi: 10.1136/archdischild-2019-318139.

Klingenberg C, Embleton ND, Jacobs SE, O'Connell LAF and Kuschel CA (2011) Enteral feeding practices in very preterm infants: an international survey. *Archives of Disease in Childhood; Fetal Neonatal Edition* **97**: F56–F61.

Koletzko B, Poindexter B, Uauy R (eds): (2014) Nutritional Care of Preterm Infants: Scientific Basis and Practical Guidelines. *World Rev Nutr Diet.* Basel, Karger **110**: 297–299. doi: 10.1159/000360195.

Johnson S, Matthews R, Draper ES, Field DJ, Manktelow BN, Marlow N, Smith LK, Boyle EM (2016 Feb) Eating difficulties in children born late and moderately preterm at 2 y of age: a prospective population-based cohort study. The American Journal of Clinical Nutrition **103**(2): 406–414. doi: 10.3945/ajcn.115.121061. Epub 2015 Dec 30.

Lang S (2002) The position and attachment of the baby at the breast. In: *Breastfeeding Special Care Babies*. Oxford: Elsevier, p. 31.

Mazumder S, Taneja S, Dube B et al. (2019) Effect of community-initiated kangaroo mother care on survival of infants with low birthweight: a randomised controlled trial. *The Lancet* **394** (10210): 1724 DOI: 10.1016/S0140-6736(19)32223-8.

Pritchard NL, Hiscock RJ, Lockie E, Permezel M, McGauren MFG, Kennedy AL, Green B, Walker SP, Lindquist AC (2019 Oct) Identification of the optimal **growth charts** for use in a **preterm** population: An Australian state-wide retrospective cohort study. *PLoS Med* **16**(10): e1002923. Published online 2019 Oct 4. doi: 10.1371/journal.pmed.1002923.

Pereira-da-Silva L, Virella D, Fusch C (2019 Sep) Nutritional Assessment in **Preterm** Infants: A Practical Approach in the NICU. *Nutrients* **11**(9): 1999. Published online 2019 Aug 23. doi: 10.3390/nu11091999.

Quigley M, Embleton ND, McGuire W (2018 Jun 20) Formula versus donor breast milk for feeding preterm or low birth weight infants. *Cochrane Database Syst Rev* **6**(6):CD002971. doi: 10.1002/14651858.CD002971.pub4. Update in: *Cochrane Database Syst Rev.* 2019 Jul 19;7:CD002971. PMID: 29926476; PMCID: PMC6513381.

Tudehope D, Vento M, Bhutta Z, Pachi P (2013 Mar) Nutritional requirements and feeding recommendations for small for gestational age infants. The Journal of Pediatrics **162**(3 Suppl): S81–S89.

Villar J, Giuliani F, Barros F, Roggero P, Coronado Zarco IA, Rego MAS, Ochieng R, Gianni ML, Rao S, Lambert A, et al. (2018 Feb) Monitoring the Postnatal Growth of Preterm Infants: A Paradigm Change. *Pediatrics* **141**(2). Epub 2018 Jan 4.

Young L, Embleton N, McGuire W (2016 Dec 13) Nutrient-enriched formula versus standard term formula for preterm infants following hospital discharge. *Cochrane Database Systematic Reviews* **12**(12) **3**: CD004696.

Resources

BLISS – For Babies born premature or sick (www.bliss.org.uk)

British Association of Perinatal Medicine (www.bapm.org)

Neonatal Dietitians Interest Group (https://www.bda.uk.com/specialist-groups-and-branches/paediatric-specialist-group/neonatal-dietitians-sub-group.html)

Section 5

Preschool children: 1–4 years

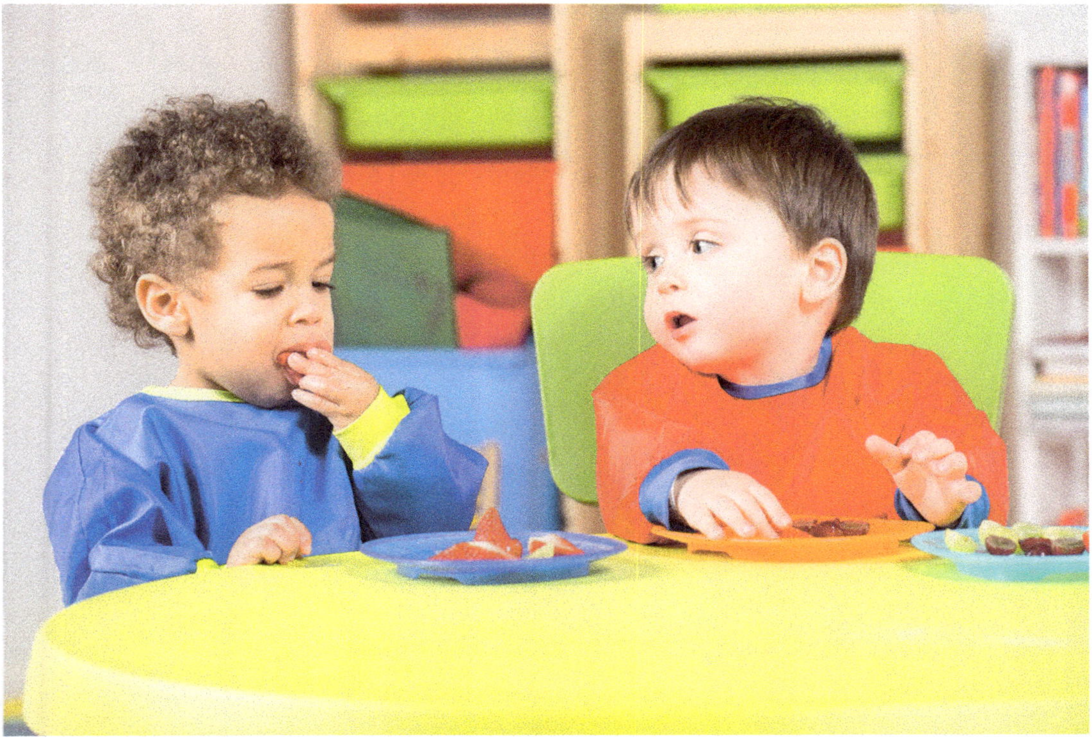

12

Preschool children: 1–4 years

Summary

- 1–4 year olds need a balanced diet based on a combination of foods from the food groups along with a supplement of vitamin D.
- A daily meal and snack routine of 3 meals and 2–3 planned nutritious snacks will provide adequate energy and nutrients and prevent toddlers becoming over hungry or too tired to eat.
- Toddlers' appetites vary from day to day and over the day and by feeding responsively parents will ensure they eat to their appetite and finish eating when they have had enough.
- Nutritious snacks are necessary as under-fives are unlikely to eat an adequate amount of nutrients in just 3 meals.
- Iron is the most critical nutrient in this age group.
- Sweet drinks, confectionery and high fat packet snacks should be limited to 1 item per week.
- Teeth of under-fives are vulnerable to dental decay and limiting foods containing free sugars to four occasions per day (e.g. 3 meals and 1 snack) will reduce the risk of dental caries.

This age group should be offered nutritious family foods and included in as many family meals as possible. Younger toddlers usually need their food cut up for them for some time and some continue to need help with feeding as they may not be able to feed themselves fast enough to satisfy their hunger. However, self-feeding should continue to be encouraged until they can manage by themselves. Finger foods make self-feeding easier for this age group.

Achieving nutrient and energy requirements

Preschool children have high nutrient requirements relative to their size as they are still undergoing quite rapid growth and development and, if allowed, are usually very physically active. They need about 70 kcal per kg body weight per day, whereas adults only need about a half of this – that is about 30–35 kcal for every kilogram body weight.

Larger amounts of most nutrients per kilogram body weight are also needed compared to adults. To achieve this, nutritious foods are needed at all meals and snacks to ensure a good nutrient intake. Iron is the most critical nutrient at this age and 10 per cent of 1–3 year olds have intakes below the LRNI for iron (Food Standards Agency and Public Health England 2018).

The vast majority of under-fives will self-regulate their energy intake to meet their activity, growth and developmental needs through responsive feeding of nutritious foods. A routine of 2 or 3 planned nutritious snacks in addition to 3 meals each day will help to give them all the energy and nutrients they need in food portion sizes that they can manage comfortably.

Combining the food groups

A balanced nutritious diet for 1–4 year olds is based on the food groups as discussed in Chapter 2.

Food group 1: Bread, rice, potatoes, pasta and other starchy foods

This group provides a good source of energy. It is also a good source of fibre, but under-fives can be offered a mixture of both wholegrain and refined bread and cereals (e.g. white and wholemeal bread and white and brown rice). Too much fibre in younger children can be very filling and fibre binds with certain minerals, thereby reducing their absorption. Wholegrains can be slowly increased for those with constipation, or decreased if they cause a tendency towards diarrhoea.

Food group 2: Fruit and vegetables

This is the food group some young children have most trouble eating, particularly vegetables with a bitter taste. Offering them at every meal is important, even though they may be refused, to teach under-fives that fruit and vegetables are a normal part of each meal. Seeing others, particularly their parents, eating and enjoying them is a powerful encouragement for under-fives to taste and then, with time, learn to like them. Small portions should be offered and more can be given when children request it.

Food group 3: Milk, cheese and yogurt

This food group involves the biggest change from feeding during infancy. These very low iron foods need to be limited to an average of 3 portions a day to ensure they do not replace iron-containing foods of the food groups 1, 2 and 4. Three portions per day will provide adequate calcium for children from 1 year of age onwards.

A portion for children 1–4 years old is:

- 1 cup of milk (120 ml);
- cheese in a sandwich or sauce, or on pasta or pizza;
- a small pot of yogurt (about 125 g).

Bottles of milk should have been discontinued around a child's first birthday. Children who drink excess milk for comfort will be filling up on this at the expense of eating more iron-rich foods and will be at risk of iron-deficiency anaemia. If no yogurt or cheese is eaten, then 3 cups of milk a day, about 350 ml in total, is adequate.

Whole/full fat cow's milk is higher in vitamin A than low-fat milks and is given until a child is at least 2 years old. Semi-skimmed milk can be introduced from this age providing the toddler eats a wide variety of foods. However, whole milk can continue to be given and will provide more vitamin A than semi-skimmed milk. Skimmed milk is not suitable for children under 5 years of age as it contains very little vitamin A.

Follow-on or growing up milks may be used for milk drinks in place of cow's milk to provide extra nutrients for toddlers who eat poorly. They provide the same range of nutrients as cow's milk but in addition they are fortified with iron. However they are more expensive than cow's milk.

Food group 4: Meat, fish, eggs, nuts and pulses

This food group is the richest source of iron and under-fives have high iron requirements. A significant number become anaemic from not having enough food from this group (see Chapter 13).

Chicken is a popular texture in this group and darker meat from the thigh and leg provide more iron.

Toddlers often reject hard, chewy red meats and prefer softer cuts and minced meat in burgers, meatballs, meat loaf and sausages. When good-quality products with a high lean meat content are used, adequate iron will be provided. Liver, if offered, should be limited to 1 small serving per week because of the very high levels of vitamin A.

Fish in fishcake and fish pies are popular alternatives to fried fish products such as fish fingers. The Food Standards Agency advises that:

- Oily fish should be limited for girls to 2 servings per week as these fish can contain dioxins and polychlorinated biphenyls. Girls can retain an excess of these chemicals into their childbearing years. Boys may have up to four servings per week.

- Swordfish, marlin and shark should not be given to under-fives because of their possibly high mercury content.

Pulses include baked beans, kidney beans, other starchy beans, chickpeas, hummus, lentils and dhal.

Ground and chopped nuts and nut butters can be offered but whole nuts should be avoided as they can cause choking or severe lung inflammation if inhaled.

Food group 5: Oils, butter and fat spreads

These can be used sparingly in food preparation. Using rapeseed oil in cooking provides a better source of short chain omega 3 fats than other oils. Olive and soya oils provide some omega 3 but peanut, corn, sunflower and safflower have virtually no omega 3 content. Butter is a less processed food than fat spreads.

Extra food groups 6, 7 & 8 includng foods high in free sugars

These energy-dense foods add flavour and enjoyment but need to be limited and not given in place of foods from the other more nutritious food groups. A nutritious pudding with added sugar can be given as the second course at 1 main meal each day. A nutritious pudding is one that contains 1 or more of the following: milk, eggs, flour, fruit, dried fruit and ground or chopped nuts. Over the day all food and drinks sweetened with sugar should be limited to four times to reduce the risk of dental decay – that could be the 3 meals and 1 snack per day (Moynihan and Petersen 2004).

Vitamin and mineral supplementation

A daily supplement of 10 µg (400IU) vitamin D3 per day is recommended for all under fives. Suitable supplements are available over the counter in pharmacies and parents should be advised to buy only brands sold in pharmacies as they have good quality control. Other brands are not regulated and may or may not contain the nutrient amount listed on the label. The Healthy Start children's vitamin drops are the least expensive but they are not widely available. They provide vitamins A & C in addition to vitamin D. Healthy Start beneficiaries are entitled to them free and access is via their NHS Trust.

Under-fives who may need a supplement with a wider range of vitamins and minerals, especially iron, include:

- persistent poor eaters;
- children who eat a very limited number of foods;
- those on restricted diets by choice;
- vegans;
- children on restricted diets because of food allergy or intolerance.

A dietitian can advise on a supplement for these children after assessing which nutrients are insufficient in their diet.

Portion sizes for children 1–4 years

There are no specific portion sizes of food for under-fives as there is a wide variation in the quantities eaten by this age group. It varies from 1 meal to another, 1 day to another and depends on how active the child is and whether they like the food or not. The portion size ranges listed in Table 12.1 give parents and carers an idea of the quantities to offer. If preschool children are eating amounts within these ranges then parents can be reassured that they are eating an adequately nutritious diet.

Drinks

Children need to be offered 6–8 drinks, each of 100–120 ml per day to provide adequate fluid. They may need more drinks in very hot weather or after extra physical activity as young children can dehydrate quite quickly.

Water and milk are the safest drinks to offer between meals as they do not cause tooth erosion nor increase the risk of dental decay. Up to 3 drinks per day can be milk (see above).

Table 12.1 Portion size ranges recommended for children aged 1–4 years (More & Emmett 2015)

Food groups	Portion size
1: Bread, rice potatoes, pasta and other starchy foods 5 portions per day, 4 for vegetarians	½–1 slice wholegrain or white bread, muffin, roll or chapatti 3–6 heaped tbsp dry breakfast cereals 5–8 tbsp of hot cereals like porridge made up with milk 2–5 tbsp of rice or pasta ½–1½ egg-sized potatoes or 1–4 tbsp of mashed potato ½–2 crispbreads or 1–3 crackers
2: Fruit and vegetables 3 portions or fruit and 3 portions of vegetables per day	¼–½ apple, orange, pear, banana 3–10 small berries or grapes 2–4 tbsp freshly cooked, stewed or mashed fruit 1–2 tbsp raw or cooked vegetables
3: Milk, cheese and yogurt 3 portions per day	100–120 ml whole cow's milk as a drink 1 small pot (125 ml) yogurt or fromage frais 2–4 tbsp grated cheese Cheese in a sandwich or on a piece of pizza 4–6 tbsp custard or a milk pudding
4: Meat, fish, eggs, nuts and pulses 2 portions per day or 3 for vegetarians	2–4 tbsp ground, chopped or cubed lean meat, fish or poultry ½–1 whole egg 2–4 tbsp whole or mashed pulses (peas, baked beans, lentils, hummus, dhal) ½–1 tbsp peanut butter or 1–2 tbsp ground nuts
5: Oils, butter and fat spreads 2 portions per day	1 tsp butter, mayonnaise or oil 2 tsp double cream
Extra Food groups	
6: Cakes, biscuits & puddings 1 portion per day	½–1 digestive biscuit or 1–2 small biscuits 1 small slice cake
7: Sauces, and sweet/savoury spreads 2 portions per day	1–2 tbsp tomato or curry sauce 2–3 tsp tomato ketchup ½–1½ tbsp gravy 1 tsp jam, honey or sugar
8: Sweet drinks, confectionery and high fat packet snacks (crisps) 1 portion of either sweet drinks, confectionery or crisps per week	120 mls high sugar drinks including fruit juices, smoothies, squash and cordials 3–4 crisps or 2–4 sweets 1 small fun-sized chocolate bar

The measures used are 1 tbsp = one 15 ml tablespoon and 1 tsp = one 5 ml teaspoon. These are the spoons found within a set of spoons for standard recipe measures.

Pure fruit juices provide small amounts of nutrients from fruit but they contain large amounts of the fruit sugar, fructose and they are acidic. Both this free sugar and acid can cause dental decay and therefore they are not recommended at all. If offered, they should be well diluted to reduce the acid and sugar content and the risk of dental decay and only given with a meal.

Fizzy drinks and squashes containing added free sugars are not necessary in a young child's diet as they add energy without providing nutrients and can contribute to dental caries and obesity.

'No added sugar' drinks may contain natural sugars and/or acids and can therefore still contribute to tooth decay. These include 'baby' juices, natural fruit juices, fruit smoothies, fruit juice drinks and sugar-free squashes and fizzy drinks.

Tea and coffee are not recommended for young children because the tannins and polyphenols in them bind with iron, reducing the availability of iron to the body. They also contain caffeine.

Meal and snack routines

With their small stomachs but high energy and nutrient needs, it is preferable to offer under-fives nutritious food about 5 or 6 times a day – that is 3 meals and 2–3 nutritious planned snacks. Energy and nutrient requirements in this age group are very unlikely to be met with just 3 meals if small meals are eaten. Ideally, a daily routine is planned with meals and snacks at regular times evenly spaced throughout the day around any daytime sleeps. The family routine may need to be adjusted to have family mealtimes fitting into this routine as preschool children eating at more family meals is associated with (Verhage et al 2018):

- more nutrient-dense food intake and a more balanced diet;
- more food enjoyment;
- less fussy and emotional eating.

A daily meal and snack routine:

- prevents toddlers becoming over hungry or thirsty by going too long between eating occasions;
- avoids attempts to feed toddlers when they are ready to sleep and too tired to eat;
- prevents grazing on less nutritious food throughout the day;
- prevents toddlers not being hungry at mealtimes because they have just eaten snacks or had large drinks just before the meal.

If a child has not eaten well at a meal a parent can be reassured that it will only be about 2 or 3 hours before a nutritious snack will be offered. If a child does not eat well at a meal, parents often give snacks or an extra milk drink just to make sure the toddler has at least eaten something. However, toddlers often prefer the snack foods or milk given at these times and may refuse to eat meals in order to have the snack or drink that they prefer.

At meal and snack times:

- children should be sitting comfortably with their feet on the floor or supported on a foot rest as supported feet make it easier for them to cough back food if they have tried to swallow pieces that are too large;
- offer finger foods often – to make self-feeding easier;
- if used, give cutlery and utensils that are appropriate to the child's age and feeding skills;
- toddlers up to about 3 years may still need help to eat;
- offer small portions as more can be offered if the first portion is finished quickly;
- accept mess as a normal part of the feeding process;
- avoid distractions like screens, toys and games so that toddlers can concentrate on eating and drinking.

Ideally, 2 courses are offered at each main meal – a savoury course followed by fruit or a small nutritious pudding. This provides a wider range of nutrients to be eaten and makes the mealtime more of an occasion and less boring. Offering the second course as a bribe or reward for eating the first course raises the value of the second course and lowers the value of the first course in the child's eyes.

A positive eating environment that helps under-fives to enjoy mealtimes, stay engaged and eat well includes:

- making mealtimes happy, social occasions with parents or carers eating with the children;
- making eye contact and interacting with the children in a positive way
- making positive comments about the food being offered;
- allowing plenty of time for the meal to ensure children are not rushed, but ensuring it is not prolonged beyond about 30 minutes except for those that eat very slowly;
- allowing children to decide when they have eaten enough. When parents accept that decision and do not try to coerce them to eat more, mealtime battles are not set up and children can become more confident in their perception of satiety.

Young children indicate they have had enough to eat by:

- saying 'no' when offered or encouraged to eat more food;
- keeping their mouth shut when food is offered;
- turning their head away from food being offered;
- putting their hand in front of their mouth;
- pushing away a spoon bowl or plate containing food;
- holding food in the mouth without swallowing it;
- vomiting or spitting out food;
- crying, shouting or screaming when food is offered;
- trying to get out of the chair or away from the table.

When a family meal is a positive experience it becomes an opportunity for under-fives to learn good social skills and behaviours associated with eating and drinking e.g. chatting to other children and adults, developing good table manners, offering and sharing food, learning to respect others.

Meal plans

The following menus use seasonal food and incorporate a mixture of finger foods and foods requiring a spoon and fork. Over each day the appropriate number of portions from each food group are offered or can be made up with snacks.

Meal plan for spring

		Day 1	Day 2	Day 3
Breakfast		Porridge with dried fruit and milk	Poached egg with toast fingers Kiwi fruit slices	Toasted hot cross bun with butter Slices of pear
	Drink	Water	Water	Hot chocolate to drink
Midday meal	1st course	Chicken nuggets with new potatoes and purple sprouting broccoli	Salmon fish fingers with pasta pieces Spinach and radish salad	Roast lamb Potato wedges Broccoli florets
	2nd course	Mini muffin with orange segments	Rhubarb crumble with custard	Yogurt and stoned cherries
	Drink	Milk	Water	Water
Evening meal	1st course	Hummus and baby spinach sandwich	Baked beans on toast with carrot sticks	Cheese omelette with asparagus spears
	2nd course	Banana and yogurt	Apple slices and yogurt	Kiwi fruit with a biscuit
	Drink	Water	Water	Water

Meal plan for summer

		Day 1	Day 2	Day 3
Breakfast		Muesli with milk and blueberries	Pancake with strawberries	Breakfast wheat biscuit with milk and peach slices
	Drink	Water	Milk	Water
Midday meal	1st course	Tuna pasta Green beans Carrot sticks	Mini lamb burger New potatoes Coleslaw	Cold chicken pieces Rice salad Fresh peas
	2nd course	Gooseberry fool	Biscuit with fresh berries	Strawberries and yogurt
	Drink	Water	Water	Water
Evening meal	1st course	Herb omelette with toast fingers and cherry tomatoes	Hummus dip with breadsticks and red pepper slices	Ham sandwich with cucumber and courgette sticks
	2nd course	Melon pieces and yogurt	Nectarine slices	Drop scones with raspberries
	Drink	Water	Milk	Milk

Meal plan for autumn

		Day 1	Day 2	Day 3
Breakfast		Muesli with milk and blackberries	Boiled egg with toast fingers Grapes	Porridge with milk Sliced pears
	Drink	Water	Water	Water
Midday meal	1st course	Chicken nuggets Potato wedges Stir-fried vegetables	Fish and potato cakes Roast butternut squash and parsnips	Mini meatballs Pasta Cauliflower florets
	2nd course	Fromage frais and pear slices	Cooked plums and yogurt	Apple and blackberry crumble with custard
	Drink	Water	Water	Water
Evening meal	1st course	Pasta and red pepper sauce with grated cheese	Mini pizza topped with ham, tomato diced peppers and cheese Carrot sticks	Mushroom omelette Toast fingers Cherry tomatoes
	2nd course	Chocolate cake and grapes	Mini muffin and plums	Fruit salad
	Drink	Water	Water	Water

Meal plan for winter

		Day 1	Day 2	Day 3
Breakfast		Boiled egg with toast fingers Tangerine segments	Porridge with dried apricots and yogurt	Breakfast wheat biscuit with milk Ripe pear slices
	Drink	Water	Water	Water
Midday meal	1st course	Chicken and vegetable curry Rice	Fish and potato pie Stir-fried leeks	Slow cooked beef stew Potato and swede mash Stir fried sliced brussels sprouts
	2nd course	Fromage frais and pear slices	Apple crumble and custard	Warm fruit salad with yogurt
	Drink	Water	Water	Water
Evening meal	1st course	Pesto pasta with grated cheese Cauliflower florets	Toast fingers with chicken liver paté Celery sticks	Butternut squash and lentil soup with a bread roll
	2nd course	Chocolate biscuit Apple slices	Banana	Drop scones Orange segments
	Drink	Water	Water	Water

Nutritious snacks

Any single or combination of finger foods from food groups 1–4 make nutritious snacks. If a child eats well at mealtimes, snacks may be simple such as crackers and/ fruit and vegetables sticks. If they have not eaten well a more substantial snack including foods from groups 3 or 4 may be offered.

Food Group	Snack foods
1. Bread, rice, potatoes, pasta and other starchy foods	crackers, crispbread, rice cakes, pretzels, oatcakes bread sticks chapatti pieces slices of bread or toast cut into pieces fresh or toasted pieces of pitta bread sandwiches dry breakfast cereals
2. Fruit and Vegetables	fruit cut into slices, sticks, kebabs grapes cut in half with pips removed raw vegetables cut into sticks or slices e.g. celery, carrot, courgette, peppers, cherry tomatoes cut in half
3. Milk, cheese and yogurt	cubed cheese pizza pieces creamed cheese spread on bread/toast Yogurt Glass milk
4. Meat, fish, eggs, nuts and pulses	small pieces of cold cooked meat mini sausages or frankfurters slices of boiled egg plain omelette cut into squares mini falafels mini bhajis

Nutrients at risk

Key nutrients that are often low in the diets of under-fives are:

- iron – usually due to an excess of milk, an unbalanced diet or selective eating;
- fibre;
- vitamin D in those who are not given a supplement.

The consequences of low intakes of these nutrients are discussed in more detail in Chapter 13.

Vitamin A plays a key role in several systems: the immune system, vision, maintenance of skin, hair and membranes. Major sources of vitamin A in the diets of under-fives are whole milk and carotene in fruits and vegetables.

Vitamin C is usually adequate in the diets of UK toddlers but low-income families have the lowest intakes and for this reason vitamin C is included in the Healthy Start vitamin supplements that are available to low-income families qualifying for this scheme (see www.healthystart.nhs.uk).

Vegetarian and vegan diets

A vegetarian diet for preschool children needs careful planning to make sure that 3 servings of high iron foods are offered each day to ensure adequate iron intake. Within each meal a high-vitamin C food will help the absorption of non-haem iron from vegetarian foods.

Meal plans for a vegetarian diet with high-iron and high-vitamin C foods

	Day 1	Day 2	Day 3
Breakfast	Boiled egg with toast fingers Orange segments	Baked beans on toast Banana slices	Toddler muesli with added ground almonds and strawberries
Midday meal	Chickpea and potato curry Courgette and cauliflower Yogurt and strawberries	Dhal and rice Broccoli and carrot Mango slices and fromage frais	Pasta with lentils in bolognaise sauce Green beans Custard and fresh peaches
Evening meal	Tofu stir fry with noodles, cherry tomatoes and spinach Pancake with raspberries	Cheese omelette with toast fingers Pepper slices and courgette sticks Banana slices and a muffin	Pitta bread with hummus Carrot and cucumber sticks Slices of kiwi fruit with a biscuit

Activity

Identify the high-iron and high-vitamin C foods within each of the aforementioned meals.

Vegan diets

Vegan diets are not recommended for young children because they do not provide milk or meat protein and consequently do not ensure optimal growth. They may not provide all the energy and nutrients required in adequate amounts, particularly if the child is a faddy eater or has a small appetite. Some children may not be able to eat enough vegan food, which can be bulky and is higher in fibre, to obtain all the energy and nutrients they need for growth and development.

Parents who insist of giving their child a vegan diet should always be referred to a dietitian for dietary assessment to ensure that the child is given an appropriate supplement as a vegan diet will not provide adequate calcium, iodine, iron, zinc or vitamin B12. Depending on eating preferences other nutrients may be insufficient.

Dental health

Under-fives are particularly vulnerable to dental decay which is the breakdown and wearing away of tooth enamel. Tooth brushing twice per day with fluoridated toothpaste is required as well as limiting high sugar foods to only four times per day. Further dental care principles are discussed in Chapter 13 as if any first teeth have to be extracted, the likelihood of overcrowding when the adult teeth come through increases.

Food safety

Under-fives are still susceptible to food poisoning and can become very ill quickly so great care should be taken with food hygiene:

- meat, fish and shellfish should all be well cooked.
- eggs with the British Lion Mark can be eaten raw or partially cooked but those without this food safety guarantee should be well cooked.

Choking

Children under 3 years are more at risk from choking than older children, however, children above this age can also be at risk. As children get older, they put fewer non-edible items into their mouths but food risks are present at any age and can be minimised by ensuring:

- children's meal and snack times are supervised;
- young children are seated and in a calm atmosphere when eating and do not run around or play while eating;
- foods are cut into small lengths rather than round pieces;
- stones and pips are removed;
- soft round foods such as meatballs, grapes and cherries are cut into halves or quarters.

The foods frequently implicated in choking incidents are:

- sweets;
- popcorn;
- grapes and cherries;
- hard fruit;
- hard vegetables – especially peas, celery, carrots;
- hot dogs/sausages;
- burgers;
- chunks of cheese;
- meatballs;
- whole nuts and seeds.

Faddy eating, selective eating and food refusal

Young children do not eat well when they are:

- tired;
- over hungry – they will just feel unhappy without realising that if they eat, they will feel better;
- distracted by TV, games, new environment;
- not feeling well – teething, sore throat, getting a cold;
- anxious, worried, scared, rushed, sad.

In addition to these factors, toddlers go through a phase of becoming quite choosy about what they will and will not eat. It may be most noticeable around 18 months of age, but it can begin any time in the second year. Toddlers may:

- eat less than expected;
- refuse to taste new foods that are offered;
- refuse to eat certain foods including some they have previously eaten well;
- refuse to eat a food that looks slightly different to the food they are familiar with e.g. if a piece of apple has a mark on the skin, a yogurt is a different colour or in a different carton, or a cracker or biscuit is broken, not whole.

Food neophobia

Becoming wary of trying new foods is a normal stage in their development and is called food neophobia because 'neophobia' means fear of new. It is more evident in some toddlers while hardly noticeable in others. Parents begin to notice it around the time toddlers become independently mobile and are becoming more adept at investigating their environment. The fear of new foods is probably a survival mechanism to prevent mobile young toddlers from harming themselves through eating anything and everything: if they were to taste any interesting looking berry on a bush they could poison themselves.

Once the neophobic stage begins toddlers may refuse to even try a taste of a new food they are not visually familiar with. They will take much longer to learn to like and eat new foods than during infancy.

Most toddlers will move through this stage in their own time if parents and carers follow some or all of the suggestions below:

- Offer a variety of foods and repeatedly introduce new foods from an early age to allow young children time to learn to accept different tastes and textures. It is the number of times they taste a food not the amount eaten that will determine how long it takes for them to learn to like a new food.
- Eat together as a family and make mealtimes happy, relaxed, social occasions. Parents should offer their toddler nutritious foods but allow the toddler to decide which foods and how much he or she will eat. Without any

pressure exerted to eat certain foods or quantities, toddlers will come to enjoy mealtimes and different foods.

- Parents are good role models for their toddlers who learn by copying what others do. When parents eat the foods they would like their toddlers to eat and make positive comments about foods, their toddlers will be more likely to try eating those foods. Siblings, other children and carers are also good role models for toddlers. Some toddlers may need to watch others eating a food that is new to them several times before they become confident to try it themselves.
- Make foods easy to eat by offering finger foods so that toddlers can feed themselves and have more control over how much they eat.
- Praise toddlers when they eat well or try new foods as toddlers respond to praise and tend to repeat behaviours they are praised for.
- Allow enough time to finish eating and drinking but do not extend the mealtime to try to coerce a toddler to eat more than they want to. Average ideal times are around 10 minutes for a snack and 20–30 minutes for a 2-course meal.
- Reward toddlers with attention but not with food or drinks. Foods used as rewards or treats become more desirable than other foods and this encourages taste preferences for sweet, high-energy foods that are generally used as rewards.

Some young children are much more likely to take longer to move out of this phase and strategies to help them are discussed in the next chapter.

References and further reading

Birch LL (1998) Development of food acceptance patterns in the first years of life. *Proceedings of the Nutrition Society* **57**(4): 617–624.

Birch LL and Marlin DW (1982) I don't like it; I never tried it: effects of exposure on two-year-old children's food preferences. *Appetite* **3**(4): 353–360.

Cooke L (2004) The development and modification of children's eating habits. *Nutrition Bulletin* **29**: 31–35.

Cooke LJ, Chambers LC, Añez EV, Wardle J (2011) Facilitating or undermining? The effect of reward on food acceptance. A narrative review. *Appetite* **57**(2): 493-497. doi:10.1016/j.appet.2011.06.016

Food Standards Agency and Public Health England (2018) *Results of the National Diet and Nutrition Survey (NDNS) rolling programme for 2014 to 2015 and 2015 to 2016*. www.gov.uk/government/statistics/ndns-results-from-years-7-and-8-combined Accessed 01November2018.

More JA, Emmett PM (2015 Apr) Evidenced-based, practical food portion sizes for preschool children and how they fit into a well balanced, nutritionally adequate diet. *Journal of Human Nutrition and Dietetics* **28**(2):135–154. doi: 10.1111/jhn.12228. Epub 2014 Mar 24.

Moynihan P, Petersen PE (2004) Diet, nutrition and the prevention of dental diseases. *Public Health Nutrition* **7**: 201–226.

Mura Paroche M, Caton SJ, Vereijken CMJL, Weenen H, Houston-Price C (2017) How Infants and Young Children Learn About Food: A Systematic Review. *Frontiers in Psychology* **8**: 1046. Published 2017 Jul 25. doi:10.3389/fpsyg.2017.01046

Nekitsing C, Hetherington MM, Blundell-Birtill P (2018) Developing Healthy Food Preferences in Preschool Children Through Taste Exposure, Sensory Learning, and Nutrition Education. *Current Obesity Reports* **7**(1): 60-67. doi:10.1007/s13679-018-0297-8

Remington A, Añez E, Croker H, Wardle J and Cooke L (2012) Increasing food acceptance in the home setting: a randomized controlled trial of parent-administered taste exposure with incentives. *American Journal of Clinical Nutrition* **95**(1): 72–77.

Russell CG and Worsley A (2008) A population-based study of preschoolers' food neophobia and its associations with food preferences. *Journal of Nutrition Education and Behavior* **40**(1): 11–19.

Taylor CM, Emmett PM (2019) Picky eating in children: causes and consequences. *Proc Nutr Soc* **78**(2):161-169. doi:10.1017/S0029665118002586

Verhage CL, Gillebaart M, van der Veek SMC, Vereijken CMJL (2018) The relation between family meals and health of infants and toddlers: A review. *Appetite* **127**: 97-109. doi:10.1016/j.appet.2018.04.010

Fox MK, Devaney B, Reidy K et al. (2006) Relationship between portion size and energy intake among infants and toddlers: evidence of self-regulation. *Journal of the American Dietetic Association* **106**(Suppl. 1): S77–S83. 72.

Rolls BJ, Engell D & Birch LL (2000) Serving portion size influences 5-year-old but not 3-year-old children's food intakes. *Journal of the American Dietetic Association* **100**: 232–234.

Resources

Public Health England (2017) Delivering Better Oral Health: An evidence-based toolkit for prevention. https://www.gov.uk/government/publications/delivering-better-oral-health-an-evidence-based-toolkit-for-prevention

Healthy Child self learning programme: Module 8 Growth and nutrition (www.e-lfh.org.uk/healthychild)

Infant and Toddler Forum (www.infantandtoddlerforum.org)

13

Common nutritional problems in preschool children

Summary

- The common nutritional problems seen in under-fives are dental caries, iron-deficiency anaemia, obesity, constipation, diarrhoea, gastro-oesophageal reflux disease, selective eating. Faltering growth and rickets are also seen but are not common.
- Following the healthy eating guidelines for children aged 1–4 will prevent most of these conditions except selective eating and constipation.
- Many parents need support to improve healthy eating, management of mealtimes and challenging eating behaviours in their young children.
- If their feeding problems affect health and growth, some children may need a referral to a specialist feeding clinic.

Dental decay

Dental caries are common in under-fives mainly due to:

- the frequent consumption of sugary foods and sugary acidic drinks
- poor dental healthcare in the home

Twenty three per cent of 5 years old have some experience of dental decay with an average of 3–4 teeth affected. (Public Health England, 2017). The risk is higher in children:

- from lower socio-economic groups;
- whose teeth brushing began at a later age;
- whose teeth were brushed less frequently than twice a day;
- who always brushed their own teeth compared to those who had an adult helping them;
- who used a bottle, dinky feeder or dummy;
- who more frequently consumed free sugars, confectionery and carbonated drinks;
- who had a drink containing free sugars in bed at night.

Prevention

- Brush teeth for two minutes, twice a day with fluoridated toothpaste containing 1000 ppm of fluoride: a smear for children up to 3 years and a pea sized amount for children over 3 years.
- Brush once in the morning and once last thing at night before bed.
- After brushing children should spit out excess toothpaste but not rinse, as rinsing washes away the fluoride. Swallowing toothpaste should also be avoided.
- Parents or carers must supervise tooth brushing as young children lack the dexterity to brush properly.

- Limit sweet and acidic food and drinks to just 4 feeding episodes each day.
- Avoid sweet acidic drinks including fruit juices and smoothies especially at night - water is the best drink to offer.
- Avoid grazing on food throughout the day and follow a routine of 3 meals and 2–3 planned nutritious snacks.

Saliva has a protective effect on teeth but saliva production reduces during sleep. Hence sweet or acidic drinks given at bedtime are very harmful. Most harmful are sweet and acidic drinks given in a bottle which is left with the child to suck as they fall asleep and during the night. This is also a choking risk.

Iron-deficiency anaemia

About 5 per cent of preschool children in the UK are iron deficient and anaemia is more common in this age group than other age groups except adolescent females. Blood tests are required for diagnosis and the World Health Organization definition is a haemoglobin of <11.0 g/dL. Low plasma ferritin levels indicate very low stores of iron.

A poor diet is by far the most common cause of iron-deficiency anaemia in children 1–4 years old. The dietary risk factors are:

- beginning complementary feeding after 6 months or inappropriate complementary foods during infancy;
- changing to cow's milk as the main drink before 12 months of age;
- consuming excessive amounts of cow's milk - frequently from a bottle - an excess is more than 400 mL per day (Thorisdottir et al., 2013);
- eating an unbalanced diet with excess milk, confectionery, or low-nutrient snack foods and eating too few high-iron foods.

Iron deficiency may cause:

- tiredness, irritability;
- poor appetite;
- reduced exercise tolerance;
- increased risk of infection;
- pallor;
- spoon-shaped nails (koilonychia);
- sores at the corner of the mouth (angular stomatitis);
- a sore tongue (glossitis);
- developmental delay;
- poor educational achievement;
- breath holding;
- swallowing difficulty with food sticking (pharyngeal web);
- pica (e.g. licking newspapers, eating soil, carpet underlay, wood, etc.).

To correct iron deficiency an iron supplement may be prescribed, but for the long term a diet as discussed above with the appropriate number of servings of foods from food groups 1 and 4 will prevent iron deficiency.

Maintaining iron stores and preventing deficiency in children 1–4 years old can be promoted by:

- advising against the change to cow's milk as the main milk drink before 12 months of age and then restricting it to 360 mL/day or less if the toddler is eating yogurt and cheese;
- encouraging consumption of iron-rich foods e.g. red meat, oily fish, eggs, iron-fortified breakfast cereals, beans and pulses, nuts, dark green vegetables and dried fruit. Liver is a good source but should be limited to once per week as it has a high vitamin A;
- giving vitamin C-rich fruit and vegetables with vegetarian meals as this promotes iron absorption, for example, citrus fruit, tomatoes, peppers, kiwi fruit, strawberries and potatoes;
- advising against giving tea as a drink with meals and snacks as it contains tannin, which decreases the absorption of iron from food.

Parents who have trouble reducing an excess cow's milk intake in their young child could consider changing from cow's milk to an iron-fortified formula such as a follow-on formula or a growing-up milk. However, the ultimate aim should be to cut down milk consumption so that more iron-rich foods will be eaten.

Obesity

Obesity in children 1–4 years old is becoming increasingly prevalent. The prevention, consequences and treatment are discussed in detail in Chapter 18.

Constipation

A simple definition of constipation is 'the difficult passage of hard stools' and it is often a complex problem. Usually there is no one underlying cause that can be identified. Infrequent passing of stools is not always indicative as normal stool habit in children 1–4 years old is considered to be within the range of passing a stool three times per day to one stool every three days. The average is passing one stool a day.

Factors exacerbating constipation include:

- insufficient intake of dietary fibre and/or fluid;
- cow's milk protein allergy – probably more common in children with atopic disorders (e.g. eczema and asthma);
- emotional disturbances;
- childhood infection;
- a change in routine
- an intentional or subconscious withholding of a stool after a traumatic event.

It may have begun in infancy but may begin in some children at around 2 years of age when potty training begins.

Symptoms include:

- abdominal pain;
- bleeding from the bottom (anal fissure);
- passage of very large stools that are difficult to flush away;
- stool-withholding behaviour which can be misinterpreted as 'straining' to open bowels;
- soiling (from 'overflow' diarrhoea) – usually a result of chronic faecal retention in children over 3 years old.

Chronic faecal retention desensitizes the rectum wall, which exacerbates the problem as large stool volumes are then required to signal the need for a bowel movement.

Constipation may cause poor eating if a child experiences discomfort when constipated. Fibre and fluid intake will then decrease, possibly exacerbating the constipation.

Treatment

National Institute of Care and Clinical Excellence (2017) recommends that treatment should begin with emptying the large bowel and then maintaining regular passage of soft stools with laxatives so that the fear of painful defecation subsides. Parents need to be reassured that laxatives are both necessary and safe. Stress in the family over a child's constipation, and poor compliance with treatment can both delay recovery. Families need frequent support and encouragement; in difficult cases involvement of the clinical psychology or child and adolescent mental health team may be essential. Coercive potty training is to be avoided.

Once the constipation is being treated young children may begin to eat more and dietary changes can be considered. In time and on an individual basis, slow weaning from laxative treatment can begin as most young children will eventually grow out of constipation.

Dietary changes to suggest

Encourage the child to eat more foods with higher fibre content, such as:

- wholegrain breakfast cereals and wholemeal bread;
- fruit and vegetables;
- beans, pulses and lentils (e.g. baked beans);
- ground and chopped nuts.

Offer 6–8 drinks per day of about 100–120 mls each. More fluid may be required in hot weather and after physical activity.

Unprocessed bran should not be given to young children as it can cause bloating and interferes with the absorption of micronutrients, such as iron, calcium and zinc.

Diarrhoea

Toddler diarrhoea may occur in children who are otherwise healthy and growing well. The condition is thought to be due to a degree of immaturity of gut function and often improves spontaneously at around 3 or 4 years of age. Frequent loose stools containing recognizable food matter (peas, carrots, sweetcorn) may be passed up to eight times a day.

Dietary causes include:

- the consumption of large quantities of some squashes and fruit juices (e.g. clear apple juice) because they contain large quantities of non-absorbable monosaccharides and oligosaccharides (Hoekstra, 1998);
- cow's milk protein allergy – a trial elimination diet for 2–4 weeks will prove whether this is the cause or not (see Chapter 17, page 213).

Dietary advice should be to continue with food consumption including milk but avoiding all sweet drinks including fruit juice.

Continued diarrhoea (>7 days) after acute gastroenteritis may be associated with a temporary intolerance to lactose (Guarino et al., 2014). The exclusion of dairy products and other lactose containing foods for a few weeks can be considered. Lactose-free milks can be used as a direct substitute for cow's milk.

Gastro-oesophageal reflux disease

Most children grow out of gastro-oesophageal reflux disease (GORD) around their first birthday, however, for a small minority it may continue and may be diagnosed after the age of 1 year rather than during infancy. It may be:

- a symptom of cow's milk protein allergy;
- a cause of faltering growth.

Investigations to aid diagnosis include:

- X-ray of a barium swallow to rule out something wrong with the way the gut has formed (e.g. hiatus hernia; narrowing in the bowel; malrotation/twisting of the small intestine -usually giving rise to green bile in the vomit);
- 24-hour pH (acid) monitoring with a probe inserted through the nose with acid-sensitive tip in the lower oesophagus, giving a continuous 24-hour record of when acid stomach contents spill back into lower oesophagus;
- endoscopy examination under anaesthetic of the oesophagus and stomach, with tissue samples taken to look at under the microscope for inflammation, including allergy.

Dietary treatments include giving 5–6 small meals each day rather than 3 larger meals and small snacks. Continuous nasogastric tube feeding may be tried in children with this disease who have faltering growth as a result of eating insufficient energy and nutrients.

Drug treatments which suppress acid secretion in the stomach can be used in children aged 1–4 (National Institute of Care and Clinical Excellence, 2017): proton pump inhibitors (PPIs) or H_2 receptor antagonists (H_2RAs) e.g. Ranitidine and Omeprazole.

Anti-reflux fundoplication surgery is reserved for very severe complications resistant to medical management. It is major surgery that carries inherent risks and is performed much less frequently now than in previous decades.

Selective eating and avoidant restrictive food intake disorder (ARFID)

As discussed in the previous chapter, most toddlers pass through this normal developmental stage of food neophobia and eventually widen the range of foods they eat if their parents manage mealtimes well.

Older toddlers from 2 years may refuse foods for other reasons:

- They may begin to associate things that look similar and may associate a food with something that is disgusting to them. Noodles may resemble 'worms' or sausages may look like 'dog poo'. They will be unable to bring themselves to eat a food that reminds them of something disgusting.

- A liked food may be contaminated with a disliked food or a food they are wary of. If a disliked food is touching or even just on the same plate as food usually eaten all the food, including the liked foods, may be rejected.

Toddlers who are much slower to grow out of this phase of food neophobia and eat very selectively causing more parental anxiety include:

- those who during infancy had little experience of different food textures and family foods or were mainly fed on commercial baby foods. They may not have been allowed to touch and play with food or to develop their self-feeding skills. Some parents prefer to do all the spoon feeding themselves and do not offer finger foods. Sometimes this is to minimise mess but it may be because they prefer to retain full control;
- those who were not offered food with lumps by 9 months of age;
- those with slow oromotor development which is indicated by speech delay and/or very slow by progression through the food textures during complementary feeding including preferring smooth foods and choking or gagging frequently making feeding uncomfortable or frightening;
- those with oral hypersensitivity who are reluctant to have their teeth cleaned and have other sensory issues such sound, touch, smells or bright lights. They may dislike getting their hands and face dirty or have been very reluctant to walk with bare feet on grass or sand when they first encountered it. These toddlers may prefer plain, dry foods of just one texture, and they may avoid mushy textures such as fruits and vegetables;
- very stubborn children who are less likely to copy their parents, siblings and others and so do not copy the eating habits of those around them;
- those with one or both parents who ate selectively during early childhood;
- those who had negative experiences at mealtimes from force feeding or pain with reflux
- those who were tube-fed throughout most of infancy for medical reasons;
- preterm infants or others who had the negative oral sensations of tubes inserted in their mouth and medications via syringe.

Underlying medical problems, such as constipation, anaemia, gastro-oesophageal reflux and delayed gastric emptying, can all cause toddlers to limit the quantity or type of food they will eat. Medical treatments to resolve these conditions need to be implemented before helping parents with other interventions to change mealtime behaviours.

Parents can become very anxious when young children do not eat as well as expected. They fear that their child may become malnourished and not grow and develop normally and may have unrealistic expectations of quantities of food their child needs and growth rates which are lower in 1–4-year olds than in infants. Mismanaging mealtimes can include the following:

- becoming very anxious at mealtimes and making them stressful and a negative experience for their child;
- coercing children to eat more and/or extending mealtimes when the child has indicated they have had enough to eat;
- giving frequent drinks of milk or juice: many young children prefer drinking to eating and readily fill themselves up with drinks (Houlihane and Rolls, 1995);
- allowing frequent snacking: some children end up eating most of their food between meals and the snack foods tend to be high in energy and low in nutrients. There is often little or no incentive for the child to eat an appropriate meal if they are allowed to fill up on confectionery, biscuits and crisps. Less frequent snacking and more appropriate snacks such as fruit or small sandwiches can be offered;

- giving snacks when a meal is refused: children may prefer snack foods and refuse meals in order to be given snacks instead.

Management of selective eating behaviour

A consistent approach is essential and all those involved in the care of the child, including relatives and child minders, need to cooperate with any management plan that is agreed. Table 13.1 details strategies for parents to consider adopting:

Growth and dietary intake can be assessed in children with selective eating by:

- measuring weight and height accurately on calibrated scales and plotting on growth charts;
- asking parents to record a 3–5 day food diary that can then be assessed in terms of food group content (see Chapter 5, page 58).

In most cases parents can be reassured that the child is eating adequately and growing

Table 13.1 Dos and Don'ts for managing challenging eating behaviour

Do	Reason
Make each meal a pleasant and social occasion with no coercion, bribery, stress or arguments.	Children don't eat well if they are anxious
Develop a daily routine of three meals and two to three snacks around your child's sleeping pattern.	Children don't eat well if they become over hungry or very tired.
Offer two courses at meals: one savoury course followed by a sweet course.	This gives two opportunities for your child to take in calories and nutrients and offers a wider variety of foods. It also makes the meal more interesting.
Eat with your child as often as possible and eat the foods you would like your child to eat.	Toddlers learn by copying their parents and others. Parents are their strongest role models.
Always offer something you know your child will eat at each meal. In addition, offer the foods you and others are eating.	Your child will be able to eat and enjoy some food while having the opportunity to become more familiar with the foods that others are eating but s/he is still wary of.
Offer foods in the way your child likes to eat them – maybe dry and each food kept separate from the other foods.	Your child will be more likely to eat foods served in the way s/he prefers them. This may be plain, dry foods of just one texture
Praise children when they eat well or try something new.	Children respond positively to praise.
Make positive comments about the food.	Parents and carers are strong role models. If you make positive comments about foods children will be more willing to try them.
Arrange for children to eat with other children as often as possible.	Some children eat better when they are with their own age group.
Give small portions. If these are finished, praise the child and offer more.	Children can be overwhelmed by large portions and lose their appetite.
Offer finger foods as often as possible.	Toddlers enjoy having the control of feeding themselves with finger foods.
Eat in a calm relaxed environment without distractions such as screens, games and toys.	Toddlers concentrate on one thing at a time. Distractions makes it more difficult to concentrate on eating.
Finish the meal after about 20–30 minutes and accept that is all your child is going to eat.	Dragging the meal on for a long time is unlikely to result in your toddler eating much more. It is better to wait for the next snack or meal and offer more nutritious foods then.
Take away uneaten food without comment.	Accept that your child has eaten enough and doesn't need any more.

(Continued)

Table 13.1 (Continued)

Do	Reason
Change the venue of meals and have an impromptu picnic with everyone in the garden or on the playroom floor.	This will break the link with any of your toddler's unpleasant memories and anxieties of eating in the usual place and will make eating and food a fun experience for your toddler.
Outside of mealtimes play games using real foods e.g. counting games.Involve children in food shopping and preparing for the meal such as putting things on the table.	Handling and touching foods without pressure to eat them will help your toddler become familiar with the touch and feel of new foods and more likely try eating them in the future.
Involve toddlers in simple cooking and food preparation without any pressure to eat the foods prepared.	

Don't	Reason
Rush a meal	Some toddlers eat quite slowly and rushing a toddler to eat can reduce their appetite
Insist a toddler finishes everything on his or her plate	Toddlers should be allowed to eat to their appetite and parents and carers need to respect this
Coerce toddlers to eat more when they have indicated that they have had enough	
Take away a refused meal and offer a completely different one in its place	Toddlers will soon take advantage if you do this. In the long run it is better to offer family meals and accept that your child will prefer some foods to others. Always offer one food at each meal that he or she will eat
Offer the sweet course as a reward	That will make the sweet course seem more desirable
Offer large drinks of milk, squash or fruit juice within an hour of the meal	Large calorific drinks will reduce appetite for food. Give water instead
Offer snacks just before a meal	Snacks will reduce appetite
Give a snack very soon after a meal if a toddler hasn't eaten well at the meal	Many parents may do this just to ensure their toddler has eaten something. However, it is best to have a set meal pattern and wait until the next snack or meal before offering food again
Assume that because a toddler has refused a food, he or she will never eat it again	Tastes change with time. Some toddlers need to be offered a new food up to 12–15 times before they feel confident to try it

normally. If the child is not eating a balanced diet, a vitamin and mineral supplement can be given to cover the low intakes of specific nutrients until the child eventually widens their intake of different foods.

Avoidant Restrictive Food Intake Disorder *(ARFID)* is the diagnosis where there are nutritional or growth concerns with a restrictive eating pattern (Mammel and Ornstein, 2017). If growth is faltering, then a child needs a referral to a paediatrician for assessment. Referral to a specialist feeding team may be possible where a multidisciplinary team can support parents to manage the feeding problem.

A very small number of children do not grow out of this phase and continue to restrict the foods they eat throughout their childhood years. If they eat enough of their preferred foods to meet their energy requirements and take a vitamin and mineral supplement to address any nutrient deficiencies, they will grow and develop normally despite a very restricted diet.

Faltering growth

When children do not eat enough their growth may falter. This is defined as weight or height crossing down through 2 centile spaces on a growth chart.

Causes of faltering growth are:

- malnutrition through not eating enough food;
- diseases involving malabsorption or decreased appetite;
- hormonal syndromes (e.g. hypothyroidism, Turner syndrome, growth hormone insufficiency);
- physical or emotional neglect.

Most faltering growth in children 1–4 years old is due to poor eating. Only 5 per cent is due to disease or hormonal disorders. It is estimated that a further 5 per cent is due to neglect and will need the support of those involved in child protection.

If faltering growth is due to ARFID as described above, then:

1. a strategy for managing meal and snack times should be agreed so that the child does not become anxious around mealtimes and is allowed to decide what and how much they eat. Often the appetite is suppressed and so strict healthy eating guidelines should be put aside until the child is gaining weight and has an improved appetite;
2. energy intake needs to be increased and this is best achieved by giving more of the foods the child is happy to eat along with a vitamin and mineral supplement to cover any nutrient deficiencies;
3. if possible, increasing the energy content of foods and meals that the child is happy to eat however this may change the appearance and taste of the foods which may result in them being rejected by the child.

Increasing fat intake using oil, butter, cream and mayonnaise are the most effective ways of increasing energy content:

- Foods can be roasted or fried in butter or oil rather than grilled, steamed or boiled.
- Butter or oil can be added or mixed into hot foods such as pasta, rice, vegetables and mashed potatoes.
- Mayonnaise can be added to dishes in larger quantities.
- Butter and fat spreads can be spread more thickly on bread or crackers.
- Cream can be added to puddings, fruit and breakfast cereals.

Increasing carbohydrate is usually most effective by adding extra sugar to cold foods, drinks, puddings and breakfast cereals.

If children enjoy high-calorie foods such as cheese, peanut butter, fatty meats, puddings, cakes and biscuits, these can be offered more frequently and in larger portions.

Powdered supplements for adding to food and supplement drinks are available on prescription but should only be used as a second choice and with medical and dietetic supervision. They are an expensive item for GPs' budgets and their use and effectiveness needs to be carefully monitored to justify the cost.

If improving mealtime management and increasing the calorie content of foods is not successful in restoring normal growth velocity then the child should be referred to a paediatrician and on to a specialist feeding clinic.

Specialist feeding clinics

Children with ARFID whose health is compromised by their eating behaviour may be referred to a feeding clinic if one exists in their NHS area. Such clinics provide a coordinated multidisciplinary approach to helping families decide how to change the way they manage mealtimes and feeding children with feeding difficulties. Before referral, a child should have been seen by a doctor and have had any relevant medical investigations.

Feeding assessments may be done by one or two trained health professionals in the home or within a specialist clinic. The combination of specialized healthcare professionals that see patients within a clinic usually includes:

- community paediatrician/paediatric gastroenterologist;
- clinical psychologist;
- paediatric dietitian;

- paediatric speech and language therapist;
- paediatric occupational therapist.

Vitamin D deficiency and rickets

The main source of vitamin D is not food but cutaneous synthesis when outside in sunlight (see Chapter 1 page 8). Genetic inheritance determines how efficient cutaneous synthesis is in each child and synthesis is less efficient in children of Asian, African and Middle eastern origin with dark skins. Current indoor lifestyles do not always allow adequate skin synthesis even in summer for all under-fives.

Julies et al. (2020) found 116 reported cases in the UK in children under five years over the 2 years 2015–2017. The majority were not taking a vitamin supplement. Deficiency not only affects growth and bone health but has also been implicated in certain forms of cancer, cardiovascular disease, tuberculosis, multiple sclerosis and type 1 and 2 diabetes.

The specific effects of vitamin D deficiency include:

- decreased calcium absorption from diet, low plasma calcium, increased plasma bone alkaline phosphatase activity (commonly measured in blood tests);
- raised parathyroid hormone concentration to mobilize calcium from bone;
- rickets: swelling of rib junctions giving a characteristic lumpy appearance ('rachitic rosary'); 'bowlegs' in weight-bearing children; swelling over the ends of long bones (e.g. wrist);
- cardiomyopathy;
- enamel hypoplasia and delayed appearance of teeth;
- deformity of spine (kyphoscoliosis) and pelvis in longstanding cases.

Vitamin D deficiency can only be diagnosed by a blood test and these are not done routinely. Risk factors that make vitamin D deficiency more likely include:

- Asian, African and Middle Eastern ethnic origin
- prolonged exclusive breastfeeding with late introduction of complementary feeding
- not taking the recommended daily supplement of vitamin D (see Chapter 12, page xx)
- limited options for being outside with some bare skin exposed
- excess use of sunscreen which prevents cutaneous synthesis of vitamin D.

Once diagnosed, vitamin D deficiency or rickets is treated with high doses of vitamin D until symptoms resolve.

References and further reading

Atkins LA, McNaughton SA, Spence AC, Szymlek-Gay EA (2020) Adequacy of iron intakes and socio-demographic factors associated with iron intakes of Australian pre-schoolers. *Eur J Nutr.* **59**(1): 175-184. doi:10.1007/s00394-019-01897-7.

Capozzi L, Russo R, Bertocco F *et al.* (2010) Diet and iron deficiency in the first year of life: a retrospective study. *Hematology* **15**(6): 410–413. doi: 10.1179/102453310X12647083621588.

Cooke L (2004) The development and modification of children's eating habits. *Nutrition Bulletin* **29**: 31–35.

Cowin I, Emond A, Emmett P *et al.* (2001) Association between composition of the diet and haemoglobin and ferritin levels in 18-month-old children. *Eur J Clin Nutr.* **55**: 278–286.

Food Standards Agency and Public Health England (2018) *Results of the National Diet and Nutrition Survey (NDNS) rolling programme for 2014 to 2015 and 2015 to 2016.* www.gov.uk/government/statistics/ndns-results-from-years-7-and-8-combined Accessed 01November2018.

Fildes A, van Jaarsveld CH, Llewellyn CH, Fisher A, Cooke L, Wardle J (2014) Nature and nurture in children's food preferences. *Am J Clin Nutr.* **99**(4): 911-917. doi:10.3945/ajcn.113.077867.

Gordon M, MacDonald JK, Parker CE, Akobeng AK, Thomas AG (2016) Osmotic and stimulant laxatives for the management of childhood constipation. *Cochrane Database Syst Rev.* **2016**(8): CD009118. Published 2016 Aug 17. doi:10.1002/14651858.CD009118.pub3.

Greenhalg J, Dowey AJ, Horne PJ, Fergus Lowe C, Grifffiths JH and Whittaker CJ (2009) Positive and negative peer modelling effects on young children's consumption of novel blue foods. *Appetite* **52**: 646–653.

Guarino A, Ashkenazi S, Gendrel D, et al. (2014) European Society for Pediatric Gastroenterology, Hepatology, and Nutrition/European Society for Pediatric Infectious Diseases evidence-based guidelines for the management of acute gastroenteritis in children in Europe: update 2014. *J Pediatr Gastroenterol Nutr.* **59**(1): 132-152. doi:10.1097/MPG.0000000000000375.

Hoekstra, JH. 1998 Toddler diarrhoea: more a nutritional disorder than a disease. Archives of Disease in Childhood 79: 2–5.

Ivan der Merwe LF, Eussen SR (2017) Iron status of young children in Europe. *Am J Clin Nutr.* **106**(Suppl 6): 1663S–1671S. doi:10.3945/ajcn.117.156018. Epub 2017 Oct 25.

Julies P, Lynn RM, Pall K, *et al.* (2020) Nutritional rickets under 16 years: UK surveillance results. *Archives of Disease in Childhood* Published Online First 105(6): 587–592. 16 January. doi: 10.1136/archdischild-2019-317934.

Kerzner B, Milano K, MacLean WC Jr, Berall G, Stuart S, Chatoor I. (2015) A practical approach to classifying and managing feeding difficulties. *Pediatrics* **135**(2): 344-353. doi:10.1542/peds.2014-1630.

Łoboś P, Januszewicz A. (2019) Food neophobia in children. Neofobia żywieniowa u dzieci. *Pediatr Endocrinol Diabetes Metab* **25**(3): 150–154. doi:10.5114/pedm.2019.87711.

Mammel KA, Ornstein RM (2017) Avoidant/restrictive food intake disorder: a new eating disorder diagnosis in the diagnostic and statistical manual 5. *Curr Opin Pediatr.* Aug; **29**(4): 407–413. doi: 10.1097/MOP.0000000000000507.

Moynihan P and Petersen PE (2004) Diet, nutrition and the prevention of dental diseases. *Public Health Nutrition* 7(1A): 201–226.

National Institute of Care and Clinical Excellence (2017) Constipation in children and young people: diagnosis and management Clinical guideline [CG99] (July) https://www.nice.org.uk/guidance/cg99/chapter/1-Guidance#clinical-management.

Public Health England (2017) *National Dental Epidemiology Programme for England: oral health survey of five-year-old children* https://assets.publishing.service.gov.uk/government/uploads/system/uploads/attachment_data/file/708157/NDEP_for_England_oral_health_survey_5yr_2017_report.pdf Accessed 01November2018.

Thane CW, Walmsley CM, Bates CJ *et al.* (2000) Risk factors for poor iron status in British toddlers: further analysis of data from the National Diet and Nutrition Survey of children aged 1.5–4.5 years. *Pub Health Nutr.* **3**: 433–440.

Thorisdottir AV, Ramel A, Palsson GI *et al.* (2013) Iron status of one year-olds and association with breast milk, cow's milk or formula in late infancy. *Eur J Nutr.* **52**(6): 1661.

Wardle J, Herrera ML, Cooke L and Gibson EL (2003) Modifying children's food preferences: the effects of exposure and reward on acceptance of an unfamiliar vegetable. *European Journal of Clinical Nutrition* **57**: 341–348.

Wardle J, Cooke L. (2008) Genetic and environmental determinants of children's food preferences. *Br J Nutr.* **99**(Suppl 1): S15–S21.

Resources

Infant and Toddler Forum (www.infantandtoddlerforum.org) Factsheets

Public Health England: Delivering Better Oral Health https://assets.publishing.service.gov.uk/government/uploads/system/uploads/attachment_data/file/605266/Delivering_better_oral_health.pdf Accessed 01 November 2018.

Specialist feeding support for faltering growth and feeding difficulties. London Evelina Hospital: https://www.evelinalondon.nhs.uk/our-services/hospital/feeding-clinics/clinics.aspx

14

Feeding preschool children in childcare settings

Summary

- Food intake of preschool children may change on entering nursery or childcare settings.
- Childcare settings are not required to adopt any monitored nutritional standards but there are several guidance documents available.
- Childcare settings can teach healthy eating habits to children who do not encounter a healthy diet in their home.

Opportunities and challenges for children eating in childcare settings

When young children begin nursery or attend daycare it is an opportunity for them to encounter a wider range of foods and different ways of having foods prepared and presented. For some children this will be a positive opportunity as they will see a large peer group eating and will be able to watch and copy their behaviour and may have more control over feeding themselves than they do at home.

Toddlers who do not eat well at home may eat much better at nursery. They may have had negative experiences around eating at home and prefer the eating environment at nursery where there may be less pressure and stress at mealtimes. Toddlers who eat better at nursery may include:

- those who have often been fed on their own – if they see very few people eating different foods at home they may try new foods at nursery where they see a large group of other toddlers eating different foods;
- those who have experienced some of the negative actions of parents as described in Chapter 13; for example they may have been pressured to eat more than they wanted to.

For other children, particularly very faddy or selective eaters, being offered only unfamiliar foods in an unfamiliar environment will be a disadvantage for them. Some will eat very little and others may refuse new foods altogether. They need time to become more familiar with the new environment and the foods served. They may need to watch the other children eating a snack or a meal several times before they are prepared to try it. With time, as they become familiar with the foods served there and as they watch the other children and staff eating the foods, they will gradually gain the confidence to try the foods and then begin to learn to like them.

Feeding very selective eaters who will only eat a narrow range of foods requires a management plan agreed between the childcare setting and the parents. A food that they will eat must be offered at each meal so that they are able to join in the mealtime, sit with the other children and eat something. This might be a food the childcare setting can provide, such as bread or plain cooked pasta, but it may have to be food that the parents send in from home (e.g. a marmite sandwich). While eating his or her familiar food the toddler can also be offered the foods the other children are eating. However, undue pressure put on a very selective eater to eat the foods served by the childcare setting will have a negative effect.

Toddlers who eat poorly at nursery may leave feeling tired and hungry. Parents or carers need to be advised that their toddler has eaten very little so that a nutritious meal or snack can be offered immediately on arrival at home. It may be more appropriate to offer a quick snack if they are ready for a sleep and then a nutritious meal after the sleep.

Examples of nutritious snacks for a toddler who has not eaten well at nursery include:

- slices of fruit with a small cup of milk;
- ham sandwich with cherry tomatoes and a cup of water;
- peanut butter and banana sandwich and a cup water;
- slices of apple spread with cream cheese;
- pancakes spread with fruit puree and a cup of milk;
- pancakes spread with chocolate spread and a cup of water;
- breadsticks or crackers with cubes of cheese and celery sticks with a cup of water;
- pitta bread with hummus and apple slices and a cup of water;
- muffin with grapes and a small cup of milk;
- crumpet spread with butter and honey and a cup of water;
- scone with butter and jam, clementine segments and a cup of milk;
- yogurt or fromage frais and fruit slices;
- small piece of fruit cake and a cup of milk;
- small slice of pizza and a cup of water;
- small bowl of breakfast cereal with banana slices and milk;
- toast with peanut butter, carrot sticks and a cup of water.

Nutritional standards for food and drinks offered in childcare settings

There are currently no monitored nutritional standards governing the food that is served to under-fives in childcare: a nursery or other childcare setting can serve whatever foods they choose. There are voluntary guidelines but they are not monitored and enforced. This is a failing of our education system as a nutritious diet is very important for preschool children to:

- ensure they eat nutrient-rich foods to fulfil their high requirement for nutrients;
- teach them healthy eating habits.

Some nurseries will have had expert nutritional input in developing a food and drink policy and planning their menus, however, others may not. Ideally, a working group to develop a food policy and plan menus will include:

- the catering staff;
- community dietitians or nutritionists;
- teaching staff;
- parents.

Asking the children about their likes and dislikes will be helpful.

Menu planning for nurseries should be based on the principles of healthy eating for under-fives outlined in Chapters 2 and 12.

Poor menu planning can lead to a non-nutritious diet being offered, particularly a diet low in iron, thus exacerbating the common occurrence of iron deficiency in this age group.

Case Study

The pupils in a nursery in north-east London come from a wide variety of cultural backgrounds and parents of many children requested specific dietary restrictions. Many requests were for the children not to be given certain types of meat. Some requested

→

no meat as the family only ate halal meat. Other parents were concerned about previous food scares and preferred their children not to have red meat. Some were from vegetarian families. The nursery thought they had solved the problem by deciding to have a vegetarian menu only so that all the children could eat the same food. However, the vegetarian dishes were made up from vegetables only with cheese and eggs being included sometimes. The menu contained very few high-iron foods as no dishes containing pulses or nuts had been included to provide high-iron alternative foods in place of the excluded meat and fish. Consequently, the menu offered was low in iron for preschool children who have very high iron requirements.

By working with a paediatric dietitian, the nursery incorporated lentils, dhal, beans and other pulses into many of the savoury vegetarian dishes so that food with higher levels of iron and zinc was offered to the children. Most nurseries may have a nut free food policy but if not, chopped and ground tree nuts can be incorporated into some of the desserts to further increase the nutrient content of the menu.

Nutritional guidance available for nurseries

The UK countries have all developed nutritional guidance that can be used as the basis of a food policy and they can all be accessed online:

- England. Updated in 2017: *'Eat Better Start Better' Voluntary Food and Drink Guidelines for Early Years Settings in England -A Practical Guide* (www.schoolfoodtrust.org.uk/parents-carers/for-parents-carers/eat-better-start-better). https://www.foundationyears.org.uk/wp-content/uploads/2017/11/Eat-Better-Start-Better1.pdf
- Scotland: Setting the Table: Nutritional guidance and food standards for early years childcare providers in Scotland. http://www.healthscotland.com/documents/30341.aspx
- Wales: Food and nutrition for childcare settings. https://gov.wales/food-and-nutrition-childcare-settings-fullguidance
- Northern Ireland: Nutrition matters for the early years: Guidance for feeding under-fives in the childcare setting. https://www.publichealth.hscni.net/publications/nutrition-matters-early-years-guidance-feeding-underfives-childcare-setting

Food for celebrations at nurseries

This is usually covered within the food policy if a nursery has one.

Nurseries that celebrate festivals with some traditional foods for the meal and snacks on the day of the festival offer children the opportunity to learn about the festivals that cultures other than their own celebrate.

Birthday celebrations need to be covered carefully within a food policy. If children are allowed to bring in cakes and confectionery on their birthday to share with their classmates then this can become more than an occasional celebration in a large nursery group. With up to 30 young children in a group there may be a birthday every week. It would be preferable for the nursery to ban confectionery altogether and to offer another way of celebrating each child's birthday. For example:

- allow the birthday child to bring in non-food items such as balloons or pencils instead;
- allow candles on a small cake like structure at lunchtime for that day for the child whose birthday it is;
- allow a birthday cake to be brought in from home but served with some fruit as the second course of the main meal.

Packed lunches

Ideally, packed meals should include something from each of the four main food groups so that

Table 14.1 Ideas for lunchbox foods for children who like their different foods separated

Food groups	Food items
1: Bread, rice, potatoes, pasta and other starchy foods	Bread, breadsticks, crispbreads, crackers, plain popcorn, sliced pitta bread, cooked pasta pieces, plain scones
2: Fruit and vegetables	Sticks or slices of carrot, cucumber, celery, courgette
	Cherry tomatoes or grapes cut in half
	Berries (e.g. strawberries, raspberries, blueberries, blackberries)
	Slices of apple, pear, banana, peach, plum, apricot – these need to be wrapped to stop them going brown
	Orange, tangerine or clementine segments
	Cubes of melon
	Small packets of dried fruit
3: Milk, cheese and yogurt	Milk to drink, cubes of cheese, pot of yogurt or fromage frais
4: Meat, fish, eggs, nuts and beans	Cold sliced meat – bought or that may have been cooked the day before (e.g. roast chicken, turkey, lamb, beef or pork)
	Ham, pepperoni, cocktail sausages or frankfurters
	Fish cakes
	Boiled egg – whole or quarters
	Mini falafel
Fluids	Water, milk

preschool children have a balanced, nutritious meal. Foods need to be easy for toddlers to eat and not require preparation by time-pressured staff.

Some ideas for children who like their foods all separate are listed in Table 14.1. One or 2 items from each food group can be put into the lunchbox.

For children who are happy to eat mixed foods, savoury items for a lunchbox could include:

- finger food pieces of pizza or quiche;
- small bhajis made with lentil or chickpea flour;
- sandwiches, filled rolls or wraps;
- dips with vegetable sticks;
- salads.

Sandwich fillings for sliced bread, bread rolls, bagels, pitta bread or wraps

- cold meat such as ham, lean salami or cold roast meat with lettuce, tomato or cucumber;
- liver pâté or liver sausage – limit to once per week;
- peanut butter with mashed banana or jam;
- 1 tbsp drained tinned tuna mixed with 1 tsp mayonnaise and 1 tsp plain yogurt;
- 1 tbsp tinned sardines with a squeeze of lemon juice;
- 1 tbsp of smoked fish such as smoked mackerel or smoked trout mixed with ½ tbsp of plain yogurt and ½ tbsp of mayonnaise;
- fish pâtés such as mackerel or salmon pâté;
- slices of smoked salmon;
- 1 tbsp hummus mixed with ½ tbsp finely diced red pepper;
- bean spreads such as black bean spread;
- mashed avocado or guacamole or tofu;
- grated hard cheese with sliced tomatoes;
- 1 tbsp cream cheese with ½ tsp chopped herbs such as chives or parsley;
- 1 tbsp cream cheese with a scrape of marmite.

Cut sandwiches made with sliced bread diagonally into four triangles so that only 1 side of the sandwich has a crust. Toddlers find it easier to eat the sandwich and can leave the crusts if they prefer.

Dips to go with breadsticks or vegetable sticks

- hummus;
- cucumber, mint and yogurt dip;
- avocado dip such as guacamole;
- fish or meat paté mixed with some extra plain yogurt or mayonnaise to make them a suitable consistency for a dip.

Salads

Salads can be based on any of the following with an added mix of vegetables. A fork or spoon will need to be provided.

- rice;
- pasta;
- bean;
- lentil;
- potato.

Pudding or second course

Fruit pieces, yogurt or fromage frais are a nutritious second course. The following cakes and biscuits all contain nutrients and can also be included as a nutritious second course, served with some fresh fruit:

- fruit cake;
- carrot cake;
- muffins containing fruit;
- biscuits with dried fruit (e.g. Garibaldi biscuits);
- mini tarts with ground nuts (e.g. Bakewell tarts);
- cereal bars with added fruit or crushed nuts;
- rice pudding.

Promoting healthy lifestyles and healthy eating habits in childcare settings

When a childcare setting adopts a healthy eating policy and offers nutritious meals and snacks to the children, they will be teaching those children healthy eating habits. This will be a valuable learning experience for children who do not encounter a healthy diet in their home, such as those never offered vegetables or fruit.

In addition, other activities could be offered, such as:

- a range of interactive parental education sessions to prevent obesity;
- interactive cookery demonstrations;
- videos and group discussions on practical issues such as healthy eating, meal planning and local shopping for nutritious foods;
- sessions to promote ideas for family activities involving physical activity, opportunities and local facilities for active play;
- discussion of safety concerns that limit physical activity of young children;
- encouraging more walking instead of always using the car or pushing toddlers around in a stroller.

Reference

Hodder RK, Stacey FG, O'Brien KM, et al. (2018) Interventions for increasing fruit and vegetable consumption in children aged five years and under. *Cochrane Database of Systematic Review* **1**(1): CD008552. Published 2018 Jan 25. doi:10.1002/14651858.CD008552.pub4.

Section 6
School-age children

15 **Primary school-age children 5–11 years**

16 **Nutrition for Adolescents**

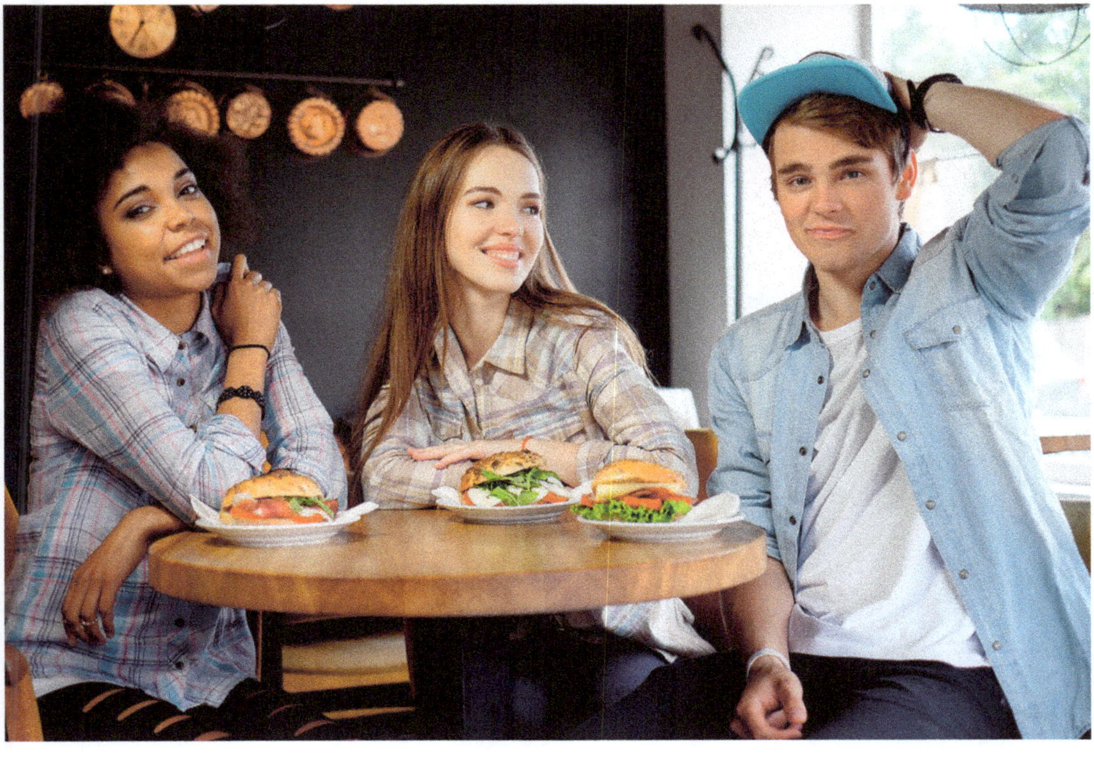

15

Primary school-age children 5–11 years

Summary

- Children prefer familiar foods and most need to be motivated to try new foods.
- Children innately prefer sweet, salty and energy-dense foods.
- Parents and carers are responsible for food offered to primary school-age children and have the power and influence to change eating habits.
- Primary school children generally satisfy their nutrient needs.
- School meals make a nutritious contribution to children's dietary intake, especially those entitled to free school meals.
- Food group based standards for school meals are in place in England, Wales and Northern Ireland. Scotland also has nutrient standards.

A diet broadly in line with a balance of food groups as discussed in Chapter 2 along with a vitamin D supplement will provide primary school children with a nutritionally adequate intake.

Influences on food tastes and preferences

From the age of about 5 years, children tend to eat from social cues, as adults do, rather than regulating their energy intake according to their needs as do the vast majority of infants and under-fives. That is, they eat when others are eating even when they are not hungry and eat more of the foods they particularly like.

Many children continue to prefer foods with which they are familiar rather than trying new foods. They need to be motivated to taste new foods. Work in this field (Sick et al. 2019, Hill 2002, Cooke 2007, Brug et al. 2008, Scaglioni et al. 2008) continues to show evidence for the following factors:

- Children innately prefer sweet, salty and energy-dense foods.
- Taste, smell, texture and appearance along with food availability and accessibility are the most important determinants of children's choice and consumption of particular foods.
- As parents and carers are responsible for the foods offered to children, they have the power to influence and change children's eating habits.
- Parental control over what and how much children can eat influences food preferences but sometimes in a counterproductive way. Restricting a food such as chocolate can make it even more attractive and likely to be selected and eaten in situations where parents are not present.
- Parents are key role models – children model their own eating behaviour from their observations of their parents' eating.
- From around 7 years of age, preferences and behaviours of peer groups begin to have a stronger influence on children's food choices.

- The number of times children are exposed to a food increases the likelihood they will try the food and then learn to like it, for example children eat more fruit and vegetables at schools where more fruit and vegetables are offered.

Energy and nutrient intakes of children 5–10 years

Average dietary intakes in this age group in the UK are provided by the National Diet and Nutrition Survey (NDNS) rolling programme with data from four-day reported food diaries. The macronutrient intakes compared to the Scientific Advisory Committee on Nutrition (SACN) recommendations are shown in Table 15.1. Indications published in 2018 are (Food Standards Agency and Public Health England 2018):

- Primary school-aged children have a more nutritious diet than those 11 years and over.
- Energy intakes are below the estimated average requirement, which probably indicates under reporting and/or of lower physical activity levels.
- Protein intakes are adequate, being above the RNI.
- Percentages of energy derived from total fat and total carbohydrate are close to recommendations: 35 per cent and 50 per cent, respectively.
- Saturated fat and free sugar intakes exceed recommendations. Soft drinks and confectionery were the main source of free sugars.
- Fibre and vitamin A intakes are low.
- Other vitamin and mineral intakes are generally adequate in primary school-age children.

A survey by a school meals caterer in 2005 reported that eating breakfast is at its highest in the pre-pubertal years, tending to decline, especially in girls, as adolescence approaches. Thirteen per cent of 8–16 year-old school children leave home in the morning having not eaten beforehand. Many buy sweets, crisps, chocolate and sweetened drinks on the way to school, but 8 per cent have nothing to eat before school (Sodexho 2005).

Portion sizes

Energy intakes and portion sizes depend on size, gender and activity. Excessively large portion sizes will contribute to obesity. Eating the number of portions of each food group each day and within the ranges in Table 15.2 will provide an average energy intake and nutrient sufficiency. The recommended number of portions per day from each food group is also discussed in Chapter 2 (see Table 2.1, page 18). Shorter and less active children would be expected to eat the portion sizes at the lower end of the range and taller and more active children from the upper end of the range. For general advice the midpoint of the range can be given.

Malnutrition in school children

Obesity is the most common form of malnutrition in school-age children in the UK. This is discussed in Chapter 18.

Table 15.1 Macronutrient intakes of children aged 4–10 years compared to SACN recommendations (Food Standards Agency and Public Health England 2018)

	Average intakes	SACN Recommendations
Total Fat (% of total energy)	33.4	35
Saturated Fat (% of total energy)	13	<10
Carbohydrate (% of total energy)	51.6	About 50
Free Sugars (% of total energy)	13.5	<5
Fibre (g)	14	20

Table 15.2 Portion size ranges and number of portions per day for children 4–10 years (Adapted from More et al. 2021.)

Food groups	Foods	Portion size range	
		4–6 years	7–10 years
1. Bread, rice, potatoes, pasta and other starchy foods *4 portions per day*	Bread	40–75 g (1–2 medium slices)	50–105 g (1½–3 medium slices)
	Potato	65–115 g	85–175 g
	Pasta (cooked)	65–115 g	85–175 g
	Rice (cooked)	60–110 g	85–175 g
	Dry breakfast cereal	20–35 g	25–50 g
	Weetabix	20–40 g (1–2 biscuits)	27–55 g (1½–3 biscuits)
	Porridge, cooked	100–175 g	105–220 g
2. Fruit and vegetables *3 portions of fruit and 3 portions of vegetables per day*	Apple/pear/orange	70–125 g	70–170 g
	Banana	65–115 g	65–130 g
	Berries/grapes	45–80 g	50–100 g
	Kiwi/plums/apricots	45–80 g (1–2 fruit)	50–100 g (2–3 fruit)
	Vegetables	25–50 g	35–60 g
3. Milk, cheese and yoghurt *3 portions per day*	Milk	110–150 ml	130–200 ml
	Yoghurt /Lassi	100 –150 g	125–200 g
	Cheese/paneer	20–35 g	25–45 g
	Custard	70–120 g	70–145 g
	Rice pudding	70–120 g	85–175 g
4. Meat, fish, eggs, nuts and pulses *2 portions per day* *2 portions fish per week – 1 of oily fish*	Meat	30–60 g	45–80 g
	Fish/fishcakes/ fishfingers	35–60 g	45–85 g
	Eggs	35–65 g (1 medium)	40–85 g (1–1½ large)
	Nut butter	20–35 g	25–50 g
	Nuts/Bombay mix	20–35 g	25–50 g
	Baked beans	55–100 g	65–140 g
	Pulses/beans (cooked)	45–90 g	60–130 g
5. Oils, butter and fat spreads *2 portions per day*	Butter/fat spread	6–10 g (1–2 tsp)	7–15 g (1½–3 tsp)
	Oil	2–4 g (1 tsp)	4–9 g (1–3 tsp)
	Mayonnaise	6–11 g (1–2 tsp)	8–17 (½–1 tbsp)
	Double cream	15–20 g (1–1½ tbs)	15–30 g (1–2 tbsp)
6. Cake, biscuit, pudding *1 portion per day*	Biscuits	15–25 g (1–2 plain)	20–45 g (2–3 plain)
	Cake/croissant	20–40 g	30–65 g
	Fruit based pudding	45–80 g	55–115 g
	Ice cream	45–80 g	55–110 g

(Continued)

Table 15.2 (Continued)

Food groups	Foods	Portion size range	
		4–6 years	7–10 years
7. Sauces, and sweet/savoury spreads	Jam/honey/syrup	7–12 g (1–2 tsp)	8–17 g (1½–3 tsp)
	Gravy	20–35 g 1½–2 tbsp	25–45 g (1½–3tbsp)
2 portions per day	Tomato or curry sauce	35–60 g (2–3 tbsp)	45–85 g (2½–4½ tbsp)
	Ketchup/savoury sauce	15–25 g (1–1½ tbsp)	20–40 g (1–2 tbsp)
8. Sweet drinks, confectionery, savoury snacks	Fruit juices/sweet drinks	100–150 ml	105–220 ml
1 portion per week	Sweets	20–35 g	25–50 g
	Chocolate/Indian Sweets	20–35 g	25–50 g
	Crisps/other packet snacks	½ small (25 g) packet	1 small packet (25 g)

Underweight or faltering growth

Children below the 2nd centile line on a body mass index (BMI) for age centile chart are considered underweight however for some of them this will be their normal stature and parental stature should be considered. Faltering growth is usually defined as crossing 2 centile spaces downwards on a weight-for-age or height-for-age centile chart.

Both these conditions are less common in school-age children than those below the age of 5 years and in school-age children they are usually due to an underlying medical condition, poor appetite, early satiation, family problems, concern about body image or self-imposed dietary restriction. Poor appetite and early satiation can be addressed by offering 5-6 small meals per day rather than 3 larger meals and small snacks. If increasing food intake does not rectify any of these conditions, a child should be referred to a paediatrician for investigation.

Anorexia nervosa (see Chapter 16, p. 200) should always be considered as a cause for poor growth or weight loss as although rare, cases have been noted in children as young as 7 years. Eating disorders can be a way of coping with feelings or situations that are making the child unhappy, angry, depressed, stressed or anxious. Maintaining a regular meal and snack routine and eating together as a family reduces the risk of eating disorders (Loth et al. 2015).

Inappropriate dieting among children

When children choose to restrict their food intake to control weight, they are unlikely to meet their nutrient requirements. They often reduce their intake of nutritious foods such as milk, cheese and meat.

Girls as young as 9 years old, and some younger, indicate body dissatisfaction and a desire to be thinner. Hill (2006) found both overweight boys and girls desire weight loss and are unhappy with their body shape. He suggested this body dissatisfaction was a result of picking up on parental attitudes to weight and shape, the idealization of thinness promoted in the media and peer behaviour.

Dental caries

Children are more susceptible to dental caries than adults, although the incidence of caries in children in the UK decreased following the introduction of fluoride toothpaste in the 1970s. However, high and frequent consumption of sweet and acidic drinks contributes to figures from the last dental survey of 12 year olds in 2013/2014 (NHS Digital 2015):

- 46 per cent of 8 year olds had decay in their primary teeth;
- 34 per cent of 12 year olds had dental decay in their permanent teeth.

When sugary food and drinks are limited to four eating occasions per day (e.g. 3 meals and 1 snack), the risk of dental caries is much lower (Moynihan and Petersen 2004).

Anaemia

Iron-deficiency anaemia is much less common in children over 5 years than in preschool children but does occur, particularly in:

- children who are vegetarian;
- girls after menarche;
- children with malabsorption due to an underlying disease;
- children with a poor dietary intake due to dietary restriction.

Increasing the iron content of a diet is described in Chapter 13, page 168.

Non-haem iron uptake from eggs, nuts, pulses, cereals and vegetables can be maximized by including a good source of vitamin C with meals, such as citrus fruit, other fruits and tomatoes, and avoiding drinking tea with meals, which reduces iron absorption.

Low vitamin D levels

The NDNS 2019 reported in January to March, 19 per cent of 4–10 year olds with blood levels of vitamin D below 25 nmols/L indicating deficiency. Very few children in this age group meet the RNI of 10 ug per day as average daily intakes from food and supplements is below 3 ug/day (Food Stadards Agency and Public Health England 2018). SACN recommend a supplement of 10 ug per day during autumn and winter and but only recommended the supplement in spring and summer for children who do not spend time outside each day or wear concealing clothing when outside. However, there is no harm in all school-aged children taking the 10 ug/day supplement all year round as the European UL of 50 ug/day is very unlikely to be exceeded.

School food and drinks

Food and drinks consumed at school can make a large contribution to a child's nutrient intake. The children of parents who can claim means tested benefits are entitled to free school meals. In 2020 the government policy is that all children in Key Stage 1 in England and Scotland are entitled to a free school lunch.

School food standards

Historically, school meals had to comply with set nutritional standards but, following the abolition of school meal standards in 1980, cheap, low-nutrient foods were often served to children to keep costs down. From 2001, school meal standards based on the food groups and/or nutrients were introduced but there has never been any statutory monitoring by an outside body and it is up to the Board of Governors or Trustees for each school to ensure they are followed. Currently Ofsted are expected to assess healthy eating and nutrition teaching in schools but school food monitoring will only change if governments change policies.

Standards and guidance apply to school lunches and food and drinks provided by the school at other times, on and off the school food premises. They specify foods allowed and not allowed, the number of portions of each food group to be offered and frequency of offering fried and high fat, high sugar foods. Standards vary across the four countries in the UK:

England has food-based standards

https://assets.publishing.service.gov.uk/government/uploads/system/uploads/attachment_data/file/788884/School-food-in-England-April2019-FINAL.pdf

They apply to:

- all local-authority-maintained schools;
- pupil referral units;
- academies and free schools;
- non-maintained special schools (a school for children with special educational needs that the Secretary of State for Education has approved under section 342 of the Education Act 1996).

Wales has food-based standards (http://learning.gov.wales/docs/learningwales/publications/160226-healthyeating-maintained-schools-en-v2.pdf).

Scotland has nutrient- and food-based standards (https://www.gov.scot/publications/healthy-eating-schools-guide-implementing-nutritional-requirements-food-drink-schools/).

Northern Ireland has food-based standards (www.education-ni.gov.uk/sites/default/files/publications/de/de1-09-125640-nutritional-standards-for-school-lunches-aguide-for-implementation-3-2.pdf).

Popular school lunches

School children responding to The Sodexho School Meals and Lifestyle Survey in 2005 cited the following as the most popular school meals: pizza, pasta, burgers, chicken and filled jacket potatoes. Cakes, buns, doughnuts, ice cream, chocolate sponge, other sponges and yogurt were the most popular desserts.

Activity 1

Write a 1-week menu for school lunches for a primary school. Allocate appropriate portion sizes and check whether your menu has satisfied the school meal standards. Use a dietary analysis programme to assess whether your menu has met one third of daily energy and nutrient requirements.

Changing school meals

As children prefer familiar food, radically changing school meals from 1 term to another has been unsuccessful. A step wise change combining the classroom curriculum, school food services, tasting sessions with pupils and discussion forums with parents, appear to be most effective in making acceptable changes or nutritional improvements.

Activity 2

Plan the key components to be included in a school intervention to increase the variety of foods the pupils will eat. Plan a programme to oversee such an intervention.

Packed lunches

Many children bring a packed lunch rather than have school meals they dislike or that their parents either cannot afford or, of which they disapprove. Packed lunches can also be of poor nutritional content: a survey of primary school lunchboxes showed that only 1 per cent met all the food-based standards for school meals (Evans et al. 2010): 85 per cent contained a sandwich; 82 per cent contained confectionery and/or crisps; 54 per cent contained fruit; 19 per cent contained vegetables.

Ideally, lunchboxes should include foods from each of the food groups and include a drink (Table 15.3). A small ice pack or a frozen drink will keep a closed lunchbox cool for a few hours.

Table 15.3 Suggestions for healthy packed lunchboxes

Food group	Suitable foods
1: Bread, rice, potatoes, pasta and other starchy foods	Bread, bread rolls, tortilla wraps and pittas can be filled or used for sandwiches
	Crispbreads, crackers, oatcakes or breadsticks
	Cooked pasta, couscous, rice or potatoes as the base for a salad
2: Fruit and vegetables	Vegetables sliced in sandwiches or combined in a salad
	Sticks of raw vegetables e.g. celery, carrots, cucumber, peppers
	Cherry tomatoes
	Pieces of fruit or small packets of dried fruit
	Vegetable soup

(Continued)

Table 15.3 (Continued)

Food group	Suitable foods
3: Milk, cheese and yogurt	Cheese is a popular sandwich filling
	Cubes, triangles, strings of cheese as finger foods
	Pots of yogurts, fromage frais or rice pudding make popular desserts
	Cartons of milk or flavoured milk as the drink
4: Meat, fish, eggs, nuts and pulses	Cold meats or flaked fish can be included in sandwiches or salads
	Chicken drumsticks or cold sausages
	Hard boiled eggs
	Falafels
	Nuts or nut butters – if allowed in school
Foods combining more than 1 food group	Slices of quiche or pizza
	Samosas or bhajis
	Vegetable soups with lentils or other beans, meat or fish
Cakes, biscuits and puddings	Small cakes or muffins (e.g. fruit cake or fruit muffins)
	Biscuits and cakes containing dried fruit or ground or chopped nuts
	Buns, scones, tea breads are a lower fat alternative
Drinks	Water, milk, flavoured milk

School breakfasts

School breakfasts have the potential to improve nutrient intakes in the large numbers of school children who leave home without breakfast. Government funded schemes are now offered in many schools through the National School Breakfast Programme run by family-action.org.uk. Anecdotal claims have been made that school attendance, behaviour and performance all improve when school breakfasts are provided. However, a systematic review found that although a school breakfast is better than no breakfast, this only makes a difference in children who are malnourished. Any improved academic performance noted may be due in part to the increased school attendance that a school breakfast encourages (Hoyland et al. 2009). Children say they enjoy the social side of school breakfasts.

The National Fruit and Veg Scheme

The School Fruit and Vegetable Scheme is designed to encourage fruit and vegetable consumption. All 4–6-year-old children in fully state-funded infant, primary and special schools are entitled to a free piece of fruit or vegetable each school day (www.nhs.uk/live-well/eatwell/school-fruit-and-vegetable-scheme). It is usually offered at the mid-morning break.

Subsidized school milk

Through the EU Milk Subsidy Scheme, subsidies are provided to schools and other educational establishments so that they can provide their pupils with selected milk and milk products. The aim of the scheme is to encourage consumption of milk and milk products to establish a nutritious balanced diet by making them available in schools at a reduced cost to pupils. Schools choose whether they wish to sign up to this scheme and offer it. If they do, children entitled to free school meals are entitled to free milk. In England, Scotland and Northern Ireland ⅓ pint of milk (189 ml) daily is available free to children up to the age of 5 years. Children up to 7 years of age in Wales are entitled to ⅓ pint milk free per day.

References and further reading

Bevelander KE, Anschutz DJ and Engels RC (2012) The effect of a fictitious peer on young children's choice of familiar v. unfamiliar low- and high-energy-dense foods. *British Journal of Nutrition* 7: 1–8.

Brug J, Tak NI, te Velde SJ, Bere E and de Bourdeaudhuij I (2008) Taste preferences, liking and other factors related to fruit and vegetable intakes among schoolchildren: results from observational studies. *British Journal of Nutrition* **99**(suppl 1): S7–S14.

Cooke L (2007) The importance of exposure for healthy eating in childhood: a review. *Journal of Human Nutrition and Dietetics* **20**(4): 294–301.

Evans CE, Cleghorn CL, Greenwood DC, Cade JE (2010). A comparison of British school meals and packed lunches from 1990 to 2007: meta-analysis by lunch type. *British Journal of Nutrition* **104** (4): 474–487.

Evans CEL and Harper CE (2009) A history and review of school meal standards in the UK. *Journal of Human Nutrition and Dietetics* **22**: 89–99.

Food Standards Agency and Public Health England (2018). *Results of the National Diet and Nutrition Survey (NDNS) rolling programme for 2014 to 2015 and 2015 to 2016.* www.gov.uk/government/statistics/ndns-results-from-years-7-and-8-combined Accessed June 2020.

Hill AJ (2002) Developmental issues in attitudes to food and diet. *Proceedings of the Nutrition Society* **61**: 259–266.

Hill AJ (2006) The development of children's shape and weight concerns. In: Jaffa T and McDermott B (eds) *Eating Disorders in Children and Adolescents.* Cambridge: Cambridge University Press.

Hoyland A, Dye L and Lawton CL (2009) A systematic review of the effect of breakfast on the cognitive performance of children and adolescents. *Nutrition Research Reviews* **22**(2): 220–243.

Loth K, Wall M, Choi CW, et al. (2015) Family meals and disordered eating in adolescents: are the benefits the same for everyone?. *International Journal of Eating Disorders* **48**(1): 100–110. doi:10.1002/eat.22339.

Martin-Biggers J, Spaccarotella K, Berhaupt-Glickstein A, Hongu N, Worobey J, Byrd-Bredbenner C. (2014) Come and get it! A discussion of family mealtime literature and factors affecting obesity risk. *Advances in Nutrition* **5**(3): 235-247. Published 2014 May 14. doi:10.3945/an.113.005116.

More JA, Lanigan J & Emmett PA (2021) The development of food portion sizes suitable for 4-18-year-old children used in a theoretical meal plan meeting energy and nutrient requirements. *Journal of Human Nutrition and Dietetics* 00: 1–16. doi:10.1111/jhn.12852.

Moynihan P and Petersen PE (2004) Diet, nutrition and the prevention of dental diseases. *Public Health Nutrition* 7(1A): 201–226.

NHS Digital (2015) Children's Dental Health Survey 2013 https://digital.nhs.uk/data-and-information/areas-of-interest/public-health/children-s-dental-health-survey (Accessed June 2020).

Rooney E, Davies G, Neville J, Robinson M, Perkins C, Bellis MA (2010) *NHS Dental Epidemiology Programme for England Oral Health Survey of 12 year old Children 2008/2009* https://assets.publishing.service.gov.uk/government/uploads/system/uploads/attachment_data/file/773897/Oral_health_survey_of_12_year_olds_2008.pdf (accessed June 2020).

Scaglioni S, Salvioni M and Galimberti C (2008) Influence of parental attitudes in the development of children eating behaviour. *British Journal of Nutrition* **99**(suppl 1): S22–S25.

Sick J, Højer R, Olsen A. (2019) Children's Self-Reported Reasons for Accepting and Rejecting

Foods. *Nutrients* **11**(10): 2455. Published 2019 Oct 14. doi:10.3390/nu11102455.

Sodexho (2005) *The Sodexho School Meals and Lifestyle Survey*. London: Sodexho Ltd.

Resources

British Nutrition Foundation www.nutrition.org.uk/foodinschools

Dairy UK (www.milk.co.uk): Information on Dairy, Nutrition and Health

Food in Schools Programme (www.foodinschools.org)

School fruit and vegetables scheme (www.nhs.uk/Livewell/5ADAY/Pages/Schoolscheme.aspx)

Subsided school milk: www.coolmilk.com/

School Food Standards: Resource for schools: https://www.gov.uk/government/publications/school-food-standards-resources-for-schools (Accessed June 2020)

School Food Standards A practical guide for schools their cooks and caterers: https://assets.publishing.service.gov.uk/government/uploads/system/uploads attachment_data/file/847621/School-Food-Standards-Guidance-FINAL-V3.pdf (Accessed June 2020)

Government leaflet on suggestions for healthy lunchboxes is available at www.healthylunch.org.uk/government.

16

Nutrition for adolescents

Summary

- Adolescents have more control over their food choices than younger children.
- They conform increasingly to peer pressure and less to their parents' role modelling.
- Nutritional intakes and status are poorer than in younger children.
- Dieting or a diet high in fast food, sugar and soft drinks and low in milk and milk products, fruit and vegetables are mainly responsible for the nutrient deficiencies common in this age group.
- Appetite and energy intake increase during the pubertal growth spurt.
- Psychological changes and emotional difficulties at this age can lead to eating disorders in both girls and boys.
- Committed physical training for sport requires an individual plan to cover energy needs for growth and training, competition and recovery afterwards.
- Pregnancy is usually unplanned and increases nutrient requirements.

Adolescence is a period of transition between childhood and adulthood, and involves both physical and emotional change, along with increasing independence and making more personal choices. The food choices of adolescents impact on their nutritional intake and status.

Physical development

During adolescence the onset of the sexual characteristics of puberty is a better marker of the stage of adolescence and the pubertal growth spurt – and thus nutritional requirements – than age. Normal age limits of pubertal progress are shown on the growth charts in Appendix 2 and physiological characteristics showing stages of puberty are shown in Table 4.4 p. 51.

Emotional changes and food choices

Over the teenage years adolescents develop their own autonomy, often rejecting their parents' values in order to develop their own. Values relating to food and meals are no exception to this and many teenagers change their eating habits to be different from the rest of their family. They may:

- avoid family meals to avoid parental control, scrutiny and gifts of food – they may say they are not hungry or 'I'll make something for myself later';
- adopt different eating patterns such as vegetarianism or diet to manage weight.

It is also a time of experimentation, with little regard for long-term consequences such as health problems in middle age. Hence they may be drawn to junk food for its taste appeal and to fall in with their peer group with no regard for nutritional consequences.

Their food choices are most likely to be based on or influenced by:

- convenience – particularly when eating outside the home;

- preference;
- taste;
- brand name;
- fashion and peer group pressure or influence;
- personal ideology, such as the choice of a low carbohydrate, vegetarian or vegan diet;
- a preoccupation with control of body weight or of body shape -whether justified or not;
- choosing less healthy foods as an act of parental defiance and peer solidarity;
- following specific diets to enhance muscle development or sporting prowess.

Nutritional requirements in adolescence

During rapid growth, energy and nutrient needs are higher, as shown in Tables 1.1 (page 4) and 1.4–1.6 (pages 12–13). Appetite increases and parents often report boys being hungry about an hour after a large meal. If this increase in appetite is met with nutrient-dense food, then the extra energy and nutrients required will be supplied. However, extra snacks are often high-energy, low-nutrient foods which may meet energy needs but not the increased need for essential nutrients.

Boys have higher energy and protein requirements than girls due to their greater gain in height and lean body mass during puberty. Undernutrition in both sexes at this time can inhibit bone development, resulting in a lower peak bone mass and lower height increase velocity, leading to stunting. Severe undernutrition can also delay puberty or halt its progression, as is seen in cases of severe anorexia nervosa.

Vitamins

Reference Nutrient Intakes (RNIs) for vitamins are generally similar to those recommended for adults except those for niacin and vitamin B6, which are slightly higher for 15–18 year olds than for adults. The higher requirements will be provided within a higher energy and balanced diet.

Since pregnancies in this age group are usually unplanned, all girls who could become pregnant are recommended to take a supplement of:

- 400 µg of folic acid to reduce the risk of fetal neural tube defects;
- 10 µg of vitamin D to prevent hypocalcaemia in new-born infants and rickets in older infants and toddlers.

Minerals

The RNIs for calcium, phosphorus and iron in both genders, and magnesium in girls, are higher for adolescents than for adults. This reflects the increased needs for growth and development.

Calcium and phosphorus

Calcium and phosphorus are important for the rapid accretion of bone tissue. A large US study reported over one third of adult bone mineral content is gained during the 2 years before and 2 years after the peak height velocity growth spurt. Another 7–11 per cent of bone mineral content is incorporated after linear growth has ceased (McCormack et al. 2017). Peak bone mass is reached at most bone sites from 16 to 30 years. Although 70–80 per cent of peak bone mass is determined by genetic factors, the remaining 20–30 per cent can be influenced by diet and exercise. In the United Kingdom, white and Asian teenagers are more susceptible to poor bone mass than other races. The risk of bone fractures is highest in 10-14 years olds but fairly high throughout adolescence. Adequate calcium intakes at this age will protect against osteoporosis in later life, especially females (Weaver et al. 2016).

High intakes of carbonated drinks are associated with a lower bone density and bone fractures in teenage girls (Libuda et al. 2008, McGartland et al. 2003). The reason may be due to the high phosphate content of carbonated drinks disturbing bone physiology along with the low-calcium diets adolescents tend towards by not having 3 daily portions of milk, cheese and yogurt.

Iron

Iron is a key nutrient during growth since it is a component of muscle and blood. The RNI of 11.3 mg/day set for boys 11–18 years old is higher than that for either younger or adult males. The iron requirement for girls 11–18 years old is even higher, at 14.8 mg/day to allow for menstrual losses. Achieving adequate iron stores becomes important for girls as menstrual periods become more regular and heavier as they mature.

Healthy eating

The guidelines on healthy eating for adolescents are based on a number of daily portions from each of the food groups (see Chapter 2). Three large portions of milk, cheese or yogurt will ensure that calcium, iodine and phosphorus requirements are met to ensure bone deposition and brain development. Consuming 2 portions per day, or 3 for vegetarians, from the meat, fish, eggs, nuts and pulses food group each day will ensure the extra iron requirement is met.

Portion sizes vary depending on size, gender and activity levels. Table 16.1 provides a guide to the portion size ranges for different age groups over the wide range of weights of children in each age group. Portions may need to increase to the upper limit during the pubertal growth spurt and for physical training. Limiting intakes to within these portion size ranges will help address overweight and obesity.

Nutritious snacks will provide extra energy and boost nutrient intake and should be encouraged – particularly fortified foods such as breakfast cereals and bread (see Chapter 2 p. 18). However, adolescents tend to snack outside the home and advice on healthier convenience and take-away foods with less fat, sugar and salt is appropriate. Some suggestions are provided in Table 16.2.

Nutritional intakes and status as reported in surveys

Despite their high requirements for nutrients, the food choices of adolescents in the United Kingdom tend to be poor compared to the food eaten by younger children. The National Diet and Nutrition Surveys (NDNS) in the United Kingdom (Food Standards Agency and Public Health England 2018) show:

- macronutrient intakes are high in free sugars and low in fibre compared to the recommendations from the Scientific Advisory Committee on Nutrition (SACN) (Table 16.3);
- intakes of key vitamins and minerals are very poor in a large percentage of adolescents. Only 3 per cent of a population are expected to eat less than the Lower Reference Nutrient Intake (LRNI), but the percentages of adolescents in the United Kingdom who eat less than the LRNI for several vitamins and minerals are very high (Table 16.4).

NDNS also reported over 50 per cent of girls 11–18 years old had folate intakes below the RNI of 200 μg/day and 9 per cent of girls over 11 years had a red cell folate level indicative of deficiency. The risk of low folate status is significant in this age group where unplanned pregnancies can occur. Young women who do not consume fortified breakfast cereals and have low intakes of other important dietary sources of folate, such as green leafy vegetables, pulses, citrus fruits and yeast extract are particularly at risk.

Blood analyses from the latest NDNS (Food Standards Agency and Public Health England 2018) revealed that:

- 24 per cent of girls had low serum ferritin levels indicating low body stores, and 9 per cent had low haemoglobin levels indicating iron deficiency;
- during January to March 37 per cent had vitamin D plasma levels below 25 nmols/L indicating deficiency. This decreased to 6 per cent during July to September when levels are at their highest for the year. During October to December the percentage with deficiency rose to 20 per cent.

Table 16.1 Portion size ranges of foods and number of portions per day for adolescents (Adapted from More et al. 2021)

Food groups	Foods	11-14 years	15-18 years	
			Girls	Boys
1. Bread, rice, potatoes, pasta and other starchy foods	Bread	75–145 g (2-4 medium slices)	85–135 g (2½–4 medium slices)	120–220g (3–6 medium slices)
4 portions per day	Potato	105–205 g	120–185 g	125–230 g
	Pasta (cooked)	105–205 g	120–185 g	140–260 g
	Rice (cooked)	105–205 g	120–185 g	130–240 g
	Dry breakfast cereal	30–55 g	30–50 g	35–65 g
	Weetabix	35–65 g (2–3½ biscuits)	40-60 g (2–3 biscuits)	55–100 g (3–5 biscuits)
	Porridge, cooked	150–300 g	200–310 g	210–390 g
2. Fruit and vegetables	Apple/pear/ orange	75–150 g	95–150 g	85–155 g
3 portions of fruit and 3 portions of vegetables per day	Banana	65–130 g	85–140 g	75–145 g
	Berries/grapes	55–110 g	65–100 g	60–105 g
	Kiwi/plums/ apricots	55–110 g	65–100 g	60–105 g
	Vegetables	40–80 g	65–100 g	55–105 g
3. Milk, cheese and yoghurt	Milk	140–275 ml	165–315 ml	230–250 ml
	Yoghurt /Lassi	105–205 g	120–185 g	140–260 g
3 portions per day	Cheese/paneer	25–50 g	30–45 g	30–50 g
	Custard	90–180 g	100–160 g	105–195 g
	Rice pudding	105–205 g	120–180 g	125–235 g
4. Meat, fish, eggs, nuts and pulses	Meat	55–110 g	65–100 g	65–120 g
	Fish	60–115 g	65–150 g	70–130 g
2 portions per day	Fishcakes/fingers	60–115 g	70–105 g	70–130 g
2 portions fish /week – 1 of oily fish	Eggs	60–125 g (1–2 eggs)	70–110 g (1–2 eggs)	85–155 g (2–2 ½ eggs)
	Nut butter	30–60 g	35–55 g	45–80 g
	Nuts /Bombay mix	30–60 g	35–55 g	40–80 g
	Baked beans	85–165 g	95–150 g	95–180 g
	Pulses/ beans (cooked)	80–165 g	100–150 g	95–180 g
5. Butter, oils and fat spreads	Butter/fat spread	10–20 g (2–4 tsp)	10–20 g (2–4 tsp)	15–25 g (3–5 tsp)
	Oil	6–12 g (2–4 tsp)	7–11 g (2–4 tsp)	6–12 g (2–4 tsp)
2 portions per day	Mayonnaise	10–20 g (2–4 tsp)	15–20 g (1–1½ tbsp)	15–25 g (1–1½ tbsp)
	Double cream	30–55 g (2–4 tbsp)	30–50 g (2–3 tbsp)	30–55 g (2–3 tbsp)

(Continued)

Table 16.1 (Continued)

Food groups	Foods	11-14 years	15-18 years	
			Girls	Boys
6. Cake, biscuit, pudding *1 portion per day*	Biscuits	30–65 g	30–65 g	30–65 g
	Cake/croissant	40–80 g	45–75 g	65–120 g
	Fruit based pudding	70–130 g	80–120 g	85–155 g
	Ice cream	60–115 g	65–105 g	70–125 g
7. Sauces, and sweet/ savoury spreads *2 portions per day*	Jam/honey/syrup	(10–15 g) 1–2 tsp	9–15 g (1–2 tsp)	13–23 g (2–3 tsp)
	Gravy	30–60 g (2–4 tbsp)	35–55 g (2–4 tbsp)	40–80 g (3–5 tbsp)
	Tomato or curry sauce	50–105 g (3–6 tbsp)	60–95 g (3½–5½ tbsp)	65–120 g (4–7 tbsp)
	Ketchup/savoury sauce	25–50 g (2–3 tbsp)	30–45 g(2–3 tbsp)	35–60 g (2–4 tbsp)
8. Sweet drinks, confectionery or savoury snacks *1 portion per week*	Fruit juices/sweet drinks	175–340 ml	200–310 ml	210–390 ml
	Sweets	30–50 g	30–50 g	30–60 g
	Chocolate/Indian Sweets	30–50 g	30–50 g	30–60 g
	Crisps/other packet snacks	1 small packet (25 g)	1 small packet (25 g)	1 packet (37.5 g)

tbsp, tablespoon (15 ml); tsp, teaspoon (5 ml).

Food choices

The NDNS and other dietary surveys suggest that factors contributing to nutritional imbalances in this age group include the following:

- Snacking or 'grazing' is a common pattern of eating in this age group, with most adolescents eating on at least six occasions during the day. The snacks are more likely to comprise crisps, biscuits, confectionery and carbonated drinks than fresh fruit, sandwiches or milk-based products.
- Savoury snacks such as crisps, potato chips, biscuits and chocolate confectionery are among the most commonly consumed foods, with large numbers eating them every day.
- High consumption of sugar-containing foods and soft drinks provides a high intake of energy and free sugars but few micronutrients.
- Fruit and vegetable consumption is poor, with many adolescents eating less than 1 portion a day.
- Intake of milk-based foods is inadequate from the age of 11 years, with few drinking milk.
- High rates of dieting among teenage girls.
- Vegetarianism and veganism where suitable high-iron alternatives to meat and fish such as nuts and pulses are often not included.
- Breakfast is often not eaten which reduces nutrient intakes. A survey in 2005 found that 12 per cent of children aged 15–16 years did not eat anything before school (Sodexho Ltd 2005).
- Older boys have better nutrient intakes than girls as they eat larger quantities of food, including more biscuits, meat, fortified breakfast cereals, baked beans and potatoes.

Table 16.2 Guidance for choosing healthier snack foods and take-away meals

Choose less	Reason	Choose instead	Reason
Fizzy drinks	High in sugar and acid which damage tooth enamel and increase risk of dental caries	Plain or flavoured milks or yogurt drinks	Good for strengthening bone and preventing fractures during sport
Diet soft drinks	High in acid which dissolves tooth enamel May decrease bone density	Plain or sparkling water	Do not damage teeth or bones and good for hydrating the skin
Crisps and other savoury snacks	High in saturated fat and salt	Nuts or sandwiches with meat, fish, egg or hummus combined with salad fillings	More protein, iron and zinc for skin repair and building muscle rather than fat
Pan-fried pizzas	High in fat	Plain oven-baked pizza bases	Less fat and a good source of nutrients depending on toppings
Doner kebab	High in fat	Shish kebab	Less fat and a better source of protein, iron and zinc
Croissants, doughnuts, sweet pastries, flapjacks	High in fat	Hot cross buns, tea bread, fruit scones, pancakes	A convenient high-energy snack and a good source of a range of nutrients
Fries with a burger	High in fat	Burger in bun with salad without the fries	Less fat and more vitamins and minerals
Fried rice/noodles or naan	High in fat	Boiled or steamed rice or chapatti	Low-fat, high carbohydrate
Creamy and oily sauces with pasta	Sauces are high in fat	Tomato-based or vegetable sauces with pasta	Vegetables provide more vitamins and antioxidants which aid skin repair
Fried chicken and fish in batter	The batter coatings are high in fat with few nutrients	Eat the chicken and fish inside the batter and throw away most of the batter	Protein, iron, zinc and B vitamins from the meat or fish are good for muscle building

Table 16.3 Macronutrient intakes of children aged 11-18 years compared to SACN recommendations (Food Standards Agency and Public Health England 2018)

	Average Intakes	SACN Recommendation
Total Fat (% of total energy)	33.7	35
Saturated Fat (% of total energy)	12.4	<10
Carbohydrate (% of total energy)	50.3	About 50
Free Sugars (% of total energy)	14.1	<5
Fibre (g)	15.3	25 (11–16 years)
		30 (16+ years)

Table 16.4 Percentage of 11–18-year-old boys and girls eating less than the LRNI for certain nutrients (Food Standards Agency and Public Health England 2018)

Nutrient	Percentage eating less than the LRNI	
	Boys	Girls
Vitamin A	19	24
Riboflavin	13	26
Folate	2	15
Iron	12	54
Calcium	11	22
Magnesium	27	50
Potassium	18	38
Zinc	18	27
Selenium	26	45
Iodine	14	27

LRNI, Lower Reference Nutrient Intake.

Further causes of malnutrition

Obesity is discussed in Chapter 18.

Vegetarianism

Most dietary regimens are short lived but vegetarianism may be 1 way of sustaining a reduced energy intake. For some, dieting and vegetarianism are intertwined. In a US study (Neumark-Sztainer 1997) vegetarians were:

- twice as likely to report frequent dieting;
- four times more likely to vomit for weight control;
- eight times more likely to use laxatives.

Being vegetarian is not a problem in itself, but if the diets are poorly planned and unbalanced, the result can be an inadequate intake of some micronutrients, iron and vitamin B12 in particular. Common pitfalls are failure to consume foods which sufficiently compensate for the loss of haem iron from the diet.

Vegan diets need very careful planning including supplementation to ensure adequate intakes of protein, iron, iodine, calcium, zinc and vitamins A and B12. Even if adequate nutrient intake is assured, optimal growth and final adult height is not, as milk and meat proteins play a key role on growth in height by acting as positive influencers on the growth plates of the bones where growth occurs (Chapter 2 p. 24).

Inappropriate slimming

Adolescence is the peak age for body dissatisfaction, and surveys of UK teenagers consistently show that more than 50 per cent of girls feel fat and want to lose weight including those of a normal body weight. Through media sources adolescents come to believe that thinness is equated with beauty, success and health. Unfortunately adolescents frequently make very poor nutritional choices using media sources of dubious and unreliable information that are based in fad trends and financial incentives and not on scientific evidence. Factors leading to unhealthy weight control behaviours are (Canadian Paediatric Society 2004):

Individual factors	Female
	Overweight and obesity
	Body image dissatisfaction and distortion
	Low self-esteem
	Low sense of control over life
	Psychiatric symptoms: depression and anxiety
	Vegetarianism
	Early puberty
Family factors	Low family connectedness
	Absence of positive adult role models
	Parental dieting
	Parental endorsement or encouragement to diet
	Parental criticism of child's weight

Environmental factors	Weight-related teasing
	Poor involvement in school
	Peer group endorsement of dieting
	Involvement in weight-related sports
Other factors	Certain chronic illnesses, especially diabetes
	Presence of other risk behaviours: smoking, substance use, unprotected sex

Many boys are concerned that they are not muscular enough and seek ways to increase a muscular appearance which may also involve dieting alongside working out.

Unsupervised and unnecessary slimming can result in low micronutrient intakes as 'the diet' often involves missing meals, particularly breakfast. Body image can be improved by encouraging physical activity, but care must be taken when discussing diet with girls who are concerned about their weight in case an over-focus on food encourages a drift towards an eating disorder. Emphasis on variety and balance rather than restriction or 'good versus bad foods' is important.

Disordered eating

A concern about body image becomes more serious if an eating disorder develops. This can occur at any age but most commonly between 13 and 17 years of age (NICE 2017). Although eating disorders are more common in girls, boys also suffer.

Genetic make-up and the attitude of other family members to food may have some influence on susceptibility. It can occur in children with any cultural or racial background.

Eating disorders usually develop from a combination of many factors that make the child feel unable to cope with life. This includes events, feelings or pressures such as:

- low self-esteem;
- problems with friends or family relationships;
- peer pressure;
- the death of someone special;
- problems at school, college, university or work;
- high academic expectations;
- sexual or emotional abuse such as being bullied;
- feeling too fat.

Eating disorders have been divided into 3 different categories: anorexia nervosa, bulimia nervosa and eating disorder not otherwise specified but there can be an overlap between them.

Anorexia nervosa is a psychological eating disorder in which a child controls their food intake obsessively and reduces their intake below their needs in order to reduce their body weight. It is most common in females 15–19 years but can occur in younger children. It is characterized by:

- weight loss or no weight gain during a period of growth;
- intense fear of gaining weight;
- distorted body image;
- amenorrhoea in females – absence of at least 3 consecutive menstrual cycles.

Bulimia nervosa is characterized by:

- binge eating of abnormally large amounts of food along with a feeling of lack of control;
- compensatory behaviour after the binge, including vomiting, use of laxatives, fasting or excessive exercise.

Eating disorders not otherwise specified is a broad diagnostic category of abnormal eating behaviours including binge eating disorder, body dysmorphic disorder and the female athlete triad. These include aspects of anorexia and bulimia but do not meet the diagnostic criteria.

In ***Binge eating disorders***, binge eating is not followed by the compensatory behaviours seen in Bulimia nervosa.

Body dysmorphic disorder (BDD), is a preoccupation with an imagined defect in physical appearance. Within this classification ***Muscle dysmorphia*** or ***Bigorexia*** is increasing in teenage males aiming for a more muscled appearance and may involve:

- working out compulsively,
- prioritizing exercise over family and friends,
- abuse of anabolic steroids, supplements and protein shakes in place of normal eating.

The ***Female athlete triad*** is a syndrome of sportswomen with 3 characteristics (Mehta et al. 2018):

- low energy intake which may be a result of trying to lose weight for sports performance reasons, body image reasons or not understanding the energy and nutrient requirements of their lifestyle and training regime;
- menstrual dysfunction;
- low bone mineral density which can result in bone fractures during training or performance.

The long-term energy and nutrient depletion of eating disorders and the resulting malnutrition can have lasting effects on growth, sexual development, brain development and bone density. In the short term, dental erosion caused by self-induced frequent vomiting increases.

If an eating disorder is suspected in a child, the family should be alerted and encouraged to seek professional help from a specialized treatment centre with a multidisciplinary team. NICE guidelines encourage a family-based approach (NICE 2017). The first phase aim is for health professionals to establish a good therapeutic alliance with the person, their parents or carers and other family members as change cannot happen outside a therapeutic relationship. Early treatment results in the most positive outcomes. When the eating disorder develops into a chronic condition, even with treatment there may be frequent relapses throughout life. In about 10 per cent of cases it causes death.

Alcohol

Alcohol intakes tend to increase during the teenage years, reaching a peak at about the age of 19 years. In adolescence, alcohol intake is often limited to 1 or 2 days per week and intoxication and value for money are the key aims. The Health Survey for England 2017 reported lower rates of children drinking than previous years: 6 per cent of 10–12 year olds and 32 per cent of 13–15 year olds had experience of a full alcoholic drink. UK adolescents have 1 of the highest levels in Europe of alcohol use, binge drinking and getting drunk.

High alcohol intakes are a cause for concern for both health and social reasons. Teenagers have less ability to metabolize alcohol than fully mature adults and are more susceptible to its adverse effects. Under the influence of alcohol they are more likely to have accidents, unsafe sex because they are less likely to use contraception, and also more likely to have sex they later regret.

Regular heavy alcohol consumption and binge drinking:

- are associated with physical problems, antisocial behaviour, violence, accidents, suicide, injuries, road traffic accidents and criminal offences;
- affects school performance;
- can exacerbate existing mental health problems;
- may have adverse effects on health in later life.

Regular alcohol consumption can displace more nutrient-dense foods from the diet and, since alcohol has a high energy density but little impact on appetite, regular drinking can easily lead to over-consumption of energy.

If health advice on alcohol is over-negative it may be ignored. Emphasis is better placed on ensuring that young people:

- are aware of safe drinking limits;
- know how to assess the alcoholic strength of products, particularly some of the 'designer drinks' or special brews of lagers which may have a deceptively high alcohol content.

Conditions that increase nutritional requirements

Physical training for sport

Adolescents undertaking sports training at the same time as undergoing physical change and development may have very high energy requirements. Specialist input from a trained sports dietitian can ensure that nutrient and energy requirements to support growth as well as training needs are met. If energy needs are not met, growth can be compromised.

Monthly height measurements can be used to assess when the growth spurt is taking place. Individual energy needs can be calculated using basal metabolic rate and physical activity level and adding 60–100 kcal/day to allow for extra growth (Department of Health 1991).

Adolescents undertaking sports training should aim to:

- maintain good hydration by drinking sufficient fluid;
- be well hydrated before exercise and drink enough fluid during and after exercise to balance fluid losses as body weight loss of >2 per cent through dehydration can compromise cognitive ability and aerobic exercise performance;
- eat a high-carbohydrate diet with 60–70 per cent of energy from carbohydrate;
- eat sufficient protein to cover growth as well as muscle development and recovery after training or competing;
- follow a balanced diet with a minimum of the daily portions of the food groups (see Table 16.1) to make sure they meet their nutrient requirements to maintain health and a strong immune system;
- eat a high-carbohydrate snack or meal, containing some protein and sodium within an hour of finishing training or competing – to ensure repair of muscle tissue and the replenishment of glycogen stores within muscles.

Sports beverages containing carbohydrates and electrolytes may be consumed before, during and after exercise to help maintain blood glucose concentration, provide fuel for muscles and decrease risk of dehydration and hyponatraemia. Milk is an effective and nutritious recovery drink after exercise.

More precise recommendations on energy and nutrients intakes per kg body weight can be found (Thomas et al. 2016) and depend on:

- the sport;
- timing of fluid and food intakes throughout the day;
- timing of whether before, after or during a session of training or competition.

Pregnancy

Pregnancy and lactation during teenage years place extra nutritional requirements on girls who may not have finished growing themselves and who will not have attained their peak bone mass. Nutrient requirements have not been specified for these young mothers but a nutritious balanced diet with folic acid and vitamin D supplementation is a minimum requirement. For those eating poorly, a multivitamin and mineral supplement excluding the retinol form of vitamin A can be recommended. As part of the Healthy Start programme, all pregnant girls under 18 are entitled to benefits regardless of their financial circumstances, including free vitamins and vouchers for milk, fruit and vegetables.

(See also Chapter 7 p. 87–88).

Cooking and food preparation skills

Many adolescents leave home at the age of 18, or soon afterwards, and cooking skills enable them to prepare alternatives to convenience foods for themselves. Current school curricula do not ensure they will learn to cook and many parents and carers cannot or do not teach them. Health promotion activities could usefully address this problem.

References and further reading

Banna J, O'Driscoll J, Boushey CJ, et al. (2018) Parent and household influences on calcium intake among early adolescents. *BMC Public Health* **18**(1): 1390. Published 2018 Dec 19. doi:10.1186/s12889-018-6297-5.

Boutelle KN, Birkeland RW, Hannan PJ, Stat M, Story M and Neumark-Sztainer D (2007) Associations between maternal concern for healthful eating and maternal eating behaviors, home food availability, and adolescent eating behaviors. *Journal of Nutrition Education and Behavior* **39**: 248–256.

Canadian Paediatric Society (2004) Dieting in adolescence. *Paediatrics & Child Health* **9**(7): 487-503. doi:10.1093/pch/9.7.487.

Department of Health (1991) *Report No 41. Dietary Reference Values for Food Energy and Nutrients for the UK. Report of the Panel on Dietary Reference Values of the Committee on Medical Aspects of Food Policy*. London: HMSO.

Food Standards Agency and Public Health England (2018). *Results of the National Diet and Nutrition Survey (NDNS) rolling programme for 2014 to 2015 and 2015 to 2016*. www.gov.uk/government/statistics/ndns-results-from-years-7-and-8-combined Accessed 01 November 2018.

Gebremariam MK, Henjum S, Terragni L, Torheim LE (2016) Correlates of fruit, vegetable, soft drink, and snack intake among adolescents: the ESSENS study. *Food & Nutrition Research* **60**: 32512. Published 2016 Sep 20. doi:10.3402/fnr.v60.32512.

Gubbels JS (2020) Environmental Influences on Dietary Intake of Children and Adolescents. *Nutrients* **12**(4): 922. Published 2020 Mar 27. doi:10.3390/nu12040922.

Hermans RCJ, Smit K, van den Broek N, Evenhuis IJ, Veldhuis L (2020) Adolescents' Food Purchasing Patterns in The School Food Environment: Examining the Role of Perceived Relationship Support and Maternal Monitoring. *Nutrients* **12**(3): 733. Published 2020 Mar 11. doi:10.3390/nu12030733.

Larson NI, Neumark-Sztainer D and Story M (2009) Weight control behaviors and dietary intake among adolescents and young adults: longitudinal findings from Project EAT. *Journal of the American Dietetic Association* **109**: 1869–1877.

Libuda L, Alexy U, Remer T, Stehle P, Schoenau E, Kersting M. (2008) Association between long-term consumption of soft drinks and variables of bone modeling and remodeling in a sample of healthy German children and adolescents. *The American Journal of Clinical Nutrition* **88**(6): 1670-1677. doi:10.3945/ajcn.2008.26414.

Kerksick CM, Arent S, Schoenfeld BJ, et al. (2017) International society of sports nutrition position stand: nutrient timing. *Journal of the International Society of Sports Nutrition* **14**: 33. Published 2017 Aug 29. doi:10.1186/s12970-017-0189-4.

Loucks AB, Stachenfeld NS and DiPietro L (2006) The female athlete triad: do female athletes need to take special care to avoid low energy availability? *Medicine and Science in Sports and Exercise* **38**: 1694–1700.

Krebs G, Fernández de la Cruz L, Mataix-Cols D. (2017) Recent advances in understanding and managing body dysmorphic disorder. *Evidence-Based Mental Health* **20**(3): 71–75. doi:10.1136/eb-2017-102702.

McCormack SE, Cousminer DL, Chesi A, et al. (2017) Association Between Linear Growth and Bone Accrual in a Diverse Cohort of Children and Adolescents. *JAMA Pediatrics* **171**(9): e171769. doi:10.1001/jamapediatrics.2017.1769.

McGartland C, Robson PJ, Murray L, et al. (2003) Carbonated soft drink consumption and bone mineral density in adolescence: the Northern Ireland Young Hearts project. *Journal of Bone and Mineral Research* **18**(9): 1563–1569. doi:10.1359/jbmr.2003.18.9.1563.

Matthys C, De Henauw S, Bellemans M, De Maeyer M and De Backer G (2007) Breakfast habits affect overall nutrient profiles in adolescents. *Public Health Nutrition* **10**(4): 413–421.

Mehta J, Thompson B, Kling JM (2018) The female athlete triad: It takes a team. *Cleveland Clinic Journal of Medicine* **85**(4): 313-320. doi:10.3949/ccjm.85a.16137.

More JA, Lanigan J & Emmett PA (2020) The development of food portion sizes suitable for 4-18-year-old children used in a theoretical meal plan meeting energy and nutrient requirements. *Journal of Human Nutrition and Dietetics*. 00: 1–16. doi:10.1111/ jhn.12852

Moreno LA, Gonzalez-Gross M, Kersting M, *et al.* (2007) Assessing, understanding and modifying nutritional status, eating habits and physical activity in European adolescents: The HELENA (Healthy Lifestyle in Europe by Nutrition in Adolescence) study. *Public Health Nutrition* **11**(3): 288–299.

Neumark-Sztainer D, Story M, Resnick M, & Blum R (1997) Adolescent vegetarians. A behavioural profile of a school-based population in Minnesota. *Archives of Pediatric and Adolescent Medicine* **151**: 833–838.

NHS Health Survey for England (2017) https://digital.nhs.uk/data-and-information/publications/statistical/health-survey-for-england/2017.

NICE (2017) Eating disorders: recognition and treatment. National Institute of Clinical Excellence guideline [NG69]. https://www.nice.org.uk/guidance/ng69.

Robinson-O'Brien R, Perry CL, Wall MM, Story M and Neumark-Sztainer D (2009) Adolescent and young adult vegetarianism: better dietary intake and weight outcomes but increased risk of disordered eating behaviors. *Journal of the American Dietetic Association* **109**(4): 648–655.

Rodriguez NR, DiMarco NM, Langley S American Dietetic Association, Dietitians of Canada, American College of Sports Medicine (2009) Position of the American Dietetic Association, Dietitians of Canada, and the American College of Sports Medicine: Nutrition and athletic performance. *Journal of the American Dietetic Association***109**(3): 509–527.

Sjöberg A, Hallberg L, Höglund D and Hulthén L (2003) Meal pattern, food choice, nutrient intake and lifestyle factors in The Göteborg Adolescence Study. *European Journal of Clinical Nutrition* **57**(12): 1569–1578.

Smith AD, Fildes A, Cooke L, et al. (2016) Genetic and environmental influences on food preferences in adolescence. *The American Journal of Clinical Nutrition* **104**(2): 446–453. doi:10.3945/ajcn.116.133983.

Sodexho Ltd (2005) *The Sodexho School Meals and Lifestyle Survey*. London: Sodexho Ltd.

Thomas DT, Erdman KA, Burke LM (2016) Position of the Academy of Nutrition and Dietetics, Dietitians of Canada, and the American College of Sports Medicine: Nutrition and Athletic Performance [published correction appears in J Acad Nutr Diet. 2017 Jan;117(1):146]. *Journal of the Academy of Nutrition and Dietetics* **116**(3): 501–528. doi:10.1016/j.jand.2015.12.006.

Tumin R, Anderson SE (2017) Television, Home-Cooked Meals, and Family Meal Frequency: Associations with Adult Obesity. *Journal of the Academy of Nutrition and Dietetics* **117**(6): 937–945. doi:10.1016/j.jand.2017.01.009.

Weaver CM, Gordon CM, Janz KF, et al. (2016) The National Osteoporosis Foundation's position statement on peak bone mass development and lifestyle factors: a systematic review and implementation recommendations. *Osteoporosis International* **27**(4): 1281–1386. [PubMed: 26856587].

Resources

Body Dysmorphic Disorder Foundation: https://bddfoundation.org/

British Dietetic Association Clinical Guidelines for dietitians treating young people with anorexia nervosa: family focused approach. Request from: graeme.oconnor@nhs.net

Eating Disorders Association: https://www.beateatingdisorders.org.uk/

Healthy Start Programme (www.healthystart.nhs.uk

Section 7
Nutrition for chronic conditions

17 **Food Hypersensitivity – Food Allergies and Intolerances**

18 **Childhood Obesity**

19 **Nutrition for Children with Chronic Diseases and Syndromes**

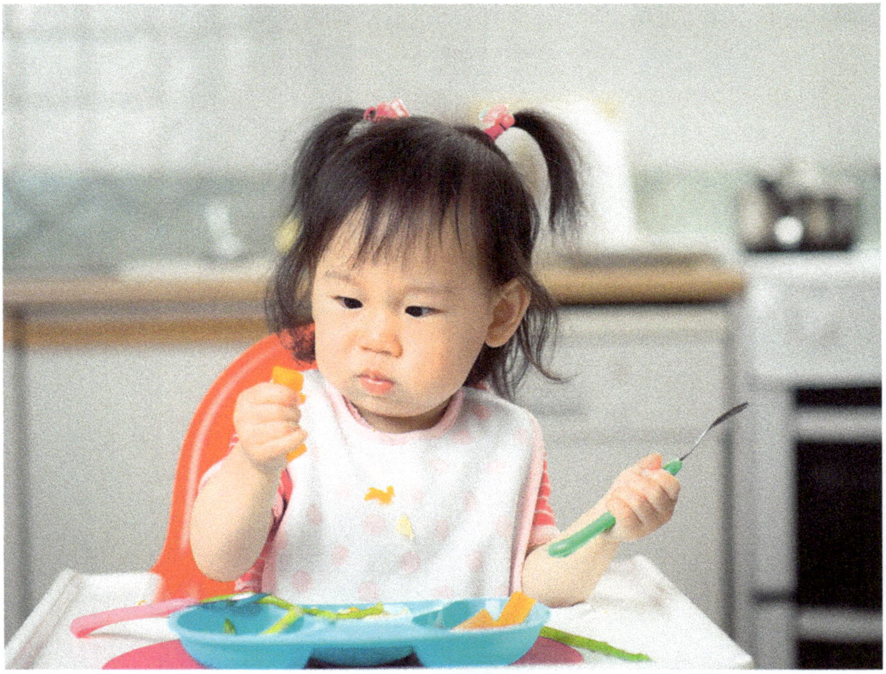

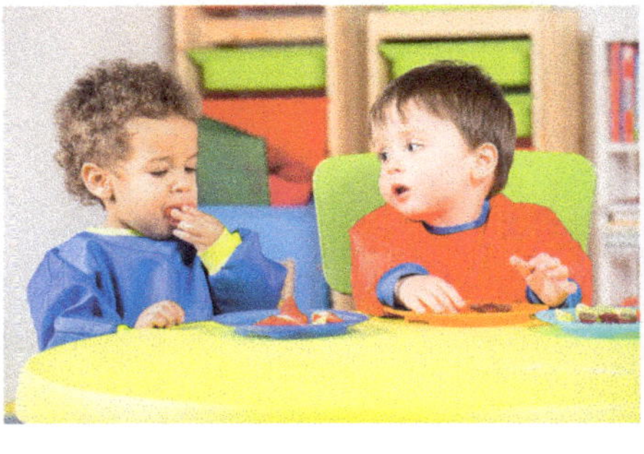

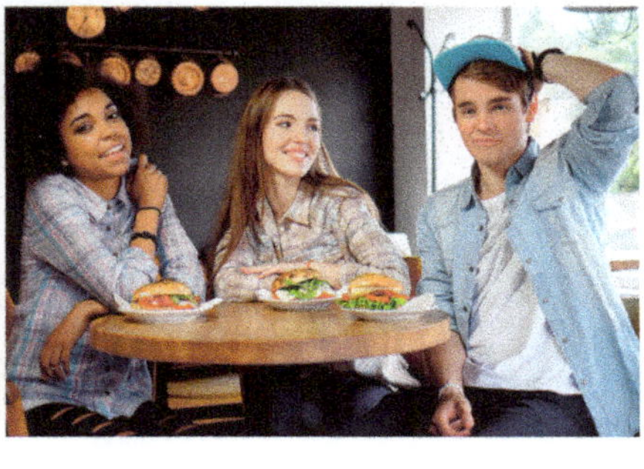

17

Food hypersensitivity – food allergies and intolerances

Summary

- Food hypersensitivity can be either an allergic reaction to a protein involving the immune system or an intolerance that is an adverse reaction to non-protein chemicals in food and does not involve the immune system.
- Infants with moderate to severe eczema are at highest risk of developing a food allergy.
- Symptoms of food allergy that appear rapidly involve the production of immunoglobulin E (IgE). A slower onset of symptoms at least 2 hours after eating the food may not involve IgE.
- Common foods that children in the United Kingdom have adverse reactions to are milk, eggs, peanuts, tree nuts and fish.
- Food hypersensitivity is less common than parents report and is diagnosed by clinical history with 1 or more of the following: skin prick tests, blood tests, food challenge or trial exclusion diet.
- Children need to avoid the foods to which they are allergic which lowers their quality of life and that of their whole family.
- Many children grow out of their food allergies but not all.
- Oral immunotherapy may increase tolerance of small quantities of the allergenic food which improves quality of life.
- European law requires that the following foods must be listed in the ingredients list on the label if they are present in a food: milk, cereals containing gluten, eggs, fish, shellfish, molluscs, peanuts or ground nuts, tree nuts, soybeans, celery, mustard, sesame seeds, lupin, sulphur dioxide and sulphites.

The number of children who become allergic or intolerant to foods is rising and the increase depends on the country they live in and the foods involved. For example, peanut allergy may be increasing in some countries and egg allergy increasing in other countries. The causes of increasing prevalence are still to be elucidated but involve genetic, epigenetic and environmental factors inducing more inflammatory responses. Environmental factors may include:

- air pollution;
- exposure to a wider range of chemicals in the environment, many of which have only been introduced in the last 50 or so years;
- exposure to a less diverse range of microorganisms due to lifestyle factors, including how clean homes are kept;
- improved public health measures such as immunisations that prevent infections in infants and toddlers;
- more processed food and drinks with additives to lengthen the shelf-life and less fresh food from a local producer.

In the United Kingdom, non-Caucasian children are at slightly higher risk of developing peanut allergy than Caucasian children.

Prevention in children

Infants with moderate to severe eczema are at highest risk of developing food allergies as parts of specific food proteins in the environment are believed to enter the blood stream via their broken skin and induce the immune system to react to those proteins. Introducing high allergen foods to infants, early in complementary feeding, will induce oral tolerance of the proteins in most infants, unless the infant is already sensitised to the protein, and prevent a food allergy developing. Avoiding any of the highly allergenic foods until a later age than around 6 months is more likely to induce development of a food allergy in susceptible infants (Du Toit et al. 2016, Perkin et al. 2016).

Recommendations on when to introduce the high allergen foods vary slightly from country to country but in general:

- around 4 months of age for those with moderate to severe eczema;
- around 6 months of age for other infants.

Once an allergenic food is introduced about 2g of the food protein/week should be given regularly, spreading the 2 g protein over 2–3 meals per week. For peanuts this would be 1½–2 tsp peanut butter over week or ½ tsp on 3 days per week (Lack 2020).

If a mother is eating high allergen proteins in her diet during pregnancy, peptides of these food proteins can be found in the amniotic fluid from about 22 weeks gestation. They are also found in the breastmilk of most mothers if they are in the mother's diet (Palmer et al., 2008). An hypothesis proposes that some oral tolerance may be built up and ongoing research is looking into whether including allergenic foods in pregnant mothers' diets at a reasonably high dose will decrease the risk of her child developing a food allergy (Palmer 2020). To date there is no convincing evidence that breastfeeding reduces the risk of children developing food allergies.

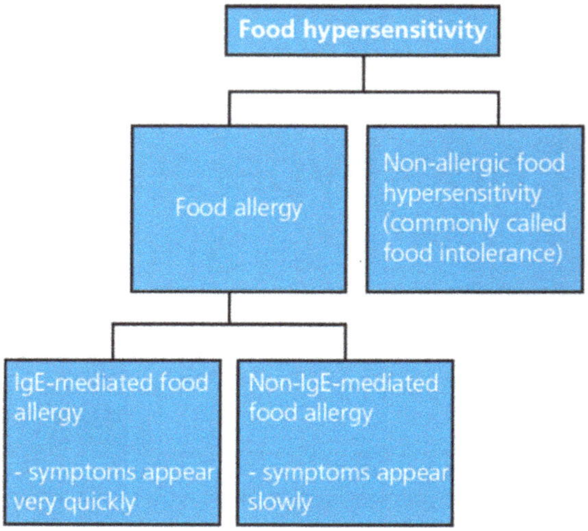

Figure 17.1 Classification of adverse reactions to food

Classification of food hypersensitivity

Although most people use the term 'food allergy' loosely to cover all unpleasant reactions to food, the current clinical classification is based on the type of adverse response to food (Johansson et al. 2004). 'Food hypersensitivity' is the umbrella term used to cover all the different types of physiological reactions to foods (Figure 17.1).

Food allergy triggers the immune system to respond to a food protein, whereas the term 'food intolerance' is used when the immune system is not involved and the reactions may be triggered by non-protein chemicals in a food that are either naturally occurring or have been added in the processing of that food.

Food allergy

The foods that are most likely to cause an allergic reaction vary between children and adults from country to country. Peanut and egg allergies are more common in northern Europe and North America while shellfish and fish are more common in southern and eastern Europe and Asia. In United Kingdom, children the more common allergenic foods are:

- cow's milk – more likely in infancy;
- eggs;
- peanuts, also called ground nuts;
- tree nuts – almonds, hazelnuts, walnuts, cashew nuts, pecan nuts, brazil nuts, pistachio nuts, macadamia nuts and Queensland nuts;
- fish;
- shellfish – prawn, shrimp, crab, lobster and crayfish;
- wheat;
- soya;
- sesame.

When an infant or child is allergic to a food, a protein in that food triggers their immune system to respond in a variety of ways. It may be a rapid, mainly severe response or a slower, less severe response depending on whether the antibody immunoglobulin E (IgE) is released by the immune system or not. Not all allergic reactions involve the production of IgE.

All children with food allergy should be under the care of a paediatrician or GP.

IgE-mediated food allergy

In infants and children who do make the specific antibody IgE to a food, a protein in the food reacts with the IgE and 1 or more of the following symptoms will appear immediately or up to 2 hours after eating the food:

Respiratory symptoms	asthma/wheeze
	breathing difficulties
	swelling of lips, tongue, face
Skin symptoms	eczema gets worse
	rashes
	redness – particularly a red facial flush in infants and young children
	hives (blotchy red rash) or urticaria
	itching
	pallor
Gastro-intestinal symptoms	diarrhoea
	abdominal pain, nausea and vomiting
	eosinophilic oesophagitis
Whole body	Falling blood pressure
	Anaphylaxis – usually seen as any of the symptoms above followed by a drop in blood pressure and then collapse and unconsciousness

Anaphylaxis is the most serious reaction and includes breathing problems, and a rapid drop in blood pressure. Children who suffer in this way need immediate medical attention to prevent death. Fatal allergic reaction to food is rare and is seen more in adolescents than young children. The risk factors are:

- the presence of asthma;
- failure to use adrenalin autoinjectors promptly;
- a history of severe reactions;
- known food allergy;
- denial of symptoms;
- adolescent and young adult age.

Adrenaline auto-injector pens can be prescribed by the medical team for all children at risk of anaphylaxis. Older children and the parents and carers of children need to be taught how to use them (Figure 17.2). The adrenaline reverses the allergic reaction and the dose of adrenalin needed depends on the age and weight of the child. Two adrenaline auto-injectors need to be with the child at all times so that it can be accessed rapidly and used in an emergency.

The 3 brands of autoinjector pens available in the United Kingdom are:

- Emerade;
- Epipen;
- Jext.

Each brand has a different mode of usage and parents and older children must be trained to use their brand.

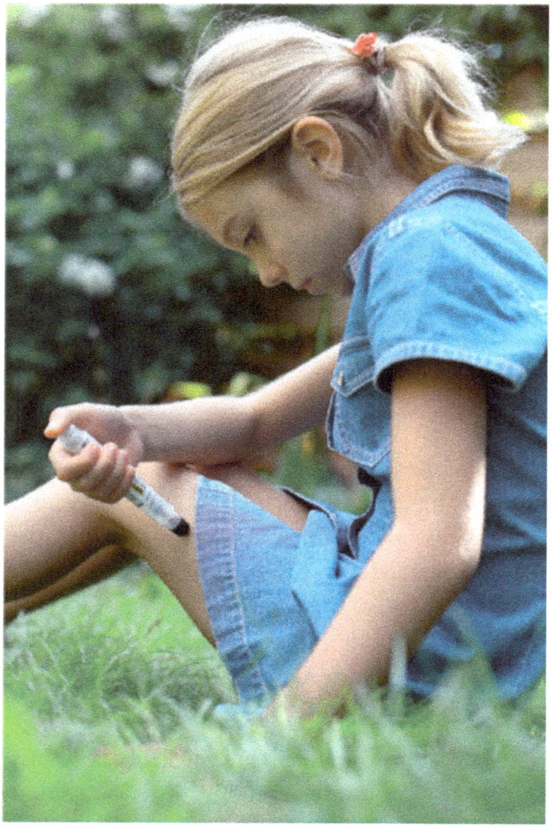

Figure 17.2 An adrenaline auto-injector pen

Non IgE-mediated food allergy

When immune cells other than IgE are involved in the reaction to a protein in the food, the symptoms appear more slowly – usually a few hours after eating the food. The typical symptoms are:

- wheeze and/or a worsening of asthma;
- eczema – a gradual increase in the number and size of the sites being affected;
- abdominal pain or colic, bloating and wind;
- constipation;
- diarrhoea;
- reflux;
- vomiting a few hours after meal.

Food Intolerance – non-allergic food hypersensitivity

When a child has a food intolerance, the immune system does not respond to the food but an unpleasant reaction to food still occurs. The symptoms usually appear a few hours or even days after eating the food and they are rarely life-threatening. Chemicals in food to which children can be intolerant include:

- ***Benzoic acid*** in citrus fruits can cause a harmless flare reaction around the mouth.
- ***Salicylates or histamines*** can cause reactions similar to food allergy such as hives and skin rashes, even facial swelling in some toddlers. They are found in fruit and vegetables such as strawberries, tomatoes (fresh, puree and ketchup), blueberries, blackberries, sharp green apples, cherries, dried fruit, fruit juices, tea (except fruit and camomile teas), coffee, dried herbs and spices, black pepper, cider, wine, peppermints and liquorice.
- ***Biogenic amines*** can cause headache, nausea and giddiness and are found in:
    - cheese, especially if matured;
    - fermented foods such as blue cheese, sauerkraut, fermented soya products;
    - yeast extracts;
    - fish, especially if stale or pickled;
    - microbial contaminated foods;
    - chocolate;
    - some fruits, especially citrus fruits, bananas and avocado pears.
- ***Lactose*** in milk and milk products – infants and children may sometimes become intolerant to this sugar in milk, for a short time following a bout of viral gastroenteritis. During this time they lack the enzyme lactase and consequently do not digest the lactose. This can cause loose stools and wind but usually resolves within a few weeks. After avoiding lactose to resolve symptoms it must be reintroduced gradually so that the production of lactase in the small intestine is built up and not overwhelmed.

- ***Monosodium glutamate (MSG)*** – a flavour enhancer. Large amounts may cause flushing, headache and stomach ache.

Whether additives in food such as artificial colours and preservatives cause reactions is currently unclear and needs further investigation. The Food Standards Agency advises that any foods, drinks or medicines containing the following should not be given to infants and children, and any food products containing them should carry a warning that it may affect children's behaviour:

Colours:	
Tartrazine	E102
Ponceau 4R	E124
Sunset yellow	E110
Carmoisine	E122
Quinoline yellow	E104
Allura red AC	E129
Preservative:	
Sodium benzoate	E211

Coeliac disease

This autoimmune disease is not a food allergy or intolerance but children with this condition cannot tolerate the protein gluten which is found in the 3 cereals: wheat, rye and barley. All food and drinks made from these 3 cereals need to be eliminated from the diet. Some children may also need to avoid oats if they are also sensitive to the protein in oats which is similar in structure to gluten. Often oats are contaminated with traces of wheat, rye or barley and so very sensitive children may be advised to avoid oats along with wheat, rye and barley as a matter of course.

Coeliac disease is discussed further in Chapter 19.

How common are food allergies?

Food allergy is more likely to develop in infants with moderate to severe eczema but may develop in older children (Venter et al. 2016).

Many parents suspect their child has a food allergy but it is only clinically diagnosed in about 10 per cent of these children. Allergy symptoms may be caused by other environmental substances such as dust mites or pollen rather than food. Studies on the Isle of Wight show that food allergy was only responsible for allergic sensitivity in about half of children up to ten years of age who had allergic reactions. Over the first ten years life 6.8 per cent of children had a diagnosed food allergy but about half had grown out of it by 10 years (Venter, Patil et al. 2016). Those with slow onset symptoms are more likely to outgrow their food allergies than those who experience rapid appearance of symptoms. In general (Venter and Arshad 2011):

- 80–90 per cent of infants will outgrow their milk allergy by 3 years;
- 50 per cent of infants will outgrow their egg allergy by 3 years;
- 20 per cent of children may outgrow their peanut allergy.

Only about 4 in 100 toddlers remained allergic to 1 or more foods at the age of ten years. Even an adolescent may become tolerant to a food that had caused symptoms previously. Therefore children should be retested with the allergen to which they allergic in a food reintroduction schedule or a food challenge at an appropriate age to check if they have out grown their allergy, as quality of life is lower in children with allergies and their parents than in children without allergies.

Diagnosing food allergies and intolerances

There is no simple diagnostic test for food allergy or food intolerance. A detailed history is an important part of the diagnosis, and the National Institute for Health and Clinical Excellence (NICE) recommends the following points are included (National Institute for Health and Clinical Excellence 2011, 2016, 2020):

- individual and family history of atopic disease – eczema, asthma, allergic rhinitis and also food allergy – in parents or siblings;
- any personal history of atopic disease especially eczema;
- the suspected allergen;
- details of any foods that are avoided and why;
- presenting symptoms and other symptoms that may be associated with food allergy, including age of first onset, speed of onset, duration, severity and frequency, reproducibility of symptoms on repeated exposure and what food and how much exposure to it causes a reaction;
- feeding history (e.g. beginning complementary feeding in infancy);
- details of any previous treatment or exclusions and the response.

A paediatrician or allergy clinic can organise additional investigations that may be helpful, including:

- specific IgE testing;
- skin prick tests (SPT);
- patch tests;
- endoscopy and biopsy.

There is no clinical or scientific evidence to support the use of various other tests including hair analysis, kinesiology and bioresonance (National Institute for Health and Clinical Excellence 2011). However, many alternative therapists use them.

Specific IgE tests measure the level of food-specific IgE levels in the blood and are highly predictive of foods causing allergic reactions. However, a child with a high food-specific IgE level will not always have an adverse reaction to that food.

A positive SPT causes redness and swelling of the skin. The size of the skin wheal formed is graded. SPTs are:

- rarely negative in someone with true IgE-mediated allergic reactions;
- almost always negative in non-IgE-mediated reactions.

However, a positive blood or skin test indicates sensitisation but can be seen in the absence of food allergy. The positive blood or skin response merely means that the child is making IgE to the proteins in that food. There is no need to avoid a food that a child is regularly eating without symptoms even if the SPT or blood test to that food is positive.

If the child has a history of a reaction to a food, however, and the SPT or blood test is positive, that would mean a clinical allergy in most cases and the food needs to be avoided. A food challenge may be needed for a definitive diagnosis in some cases.

If the SPT or blood test is positive and the child has never knowingly eaten the food, a food challenge will be needed to diagnose or rule out food allergy.

Food challenges are the most definitive part of diagnosis but are not always necessary if the clinical history is convincing. They will either:

- detect a specific food which causes symptoms and needs to be excluded from the diet; or
- confirm that a specific food is not responsible for symptoms and does not need to be restricted.

They are also used to determine if, and when, a child has outgrown their food allergy.

The gold standard test is the placebo-controlled double blind food challenge. In clinical practice, however, open challenges are usually performed. A paediatric or allergy specialist dietitian needs to be involved as the food suspected to be the cause of symptoms must be consumed by the child and the response monitored.

Challenges must be carried out in appropriately staffed and equipped settings because of the risk of a severe reaction. For children with any level of specific IgE or any size SPT to the food or who have developed symptoms to a food less than 2 hours after eating it in the past, the food challenge should be done in hospital where the necessary medication can be administered to reverse any severe symptoms.

For children with no specific IgE levels to a food or negative SPT and a history of only slow onset symptoms, food challenges can usually be carried out at home (National Institute for Health and Clinical Excellence 2011).

A food challenge for non-severe, slower onset symptoms of non-IgE-mediated food allergy and non-allergic food hypersensitivity usually involves:

1. recording the symptoms and foods eaten while on a normal diet for 1 or 2 weeks;
2. recording the symptoms and foods eaten while on a diet excluding the suspected food – usually for 1 or 2 weeks;
3. recording the symptoms and foods eaten for a further period of time with the suspected food eaten to see if the symptoms reappear if they have disappeared in step 2.

Expert advice is needed from a dietitian to cut out a suspected food completely as parents and children may not be aware of all the foods that can contain traces of a suspected food.

Grading the severity of the symptoms to be recorded helps make the parent or carer recording the symptoms more objective. For example, diarrhoea can be graded as follows:

Severity of symptoms	Diarrhoea
0	Formed stool
1	Slightly loose stool
2	Very loose stool
3	Liquid stool

During the period of investigation the parent/carer records the timings of all the food and drinks consumed by the infant or child along with the time of any symptoms and the grade of severity. For example:

Time	Food and drinks consumed	Symptoms
7:30	Small bowl Cheerios with full-fat milk + banana slices 1 cup milk	
8:30		Diarrhoea 2
10:30	120 mL cup of apple juice diluted 50 per cent with water 1 digestive biscuit	
12:00	2 tbsp pasta 1 tbsp meat sauce 3 carrot sticks 2 cauliflower florets 1 flavoured fromage frais 6 grapes 120 mL cup of water	
13:00		Diarrhoea 1

The dietitian can then assess the diary and discuss with the parents whether the suspect food is likely to be causing the adverse reaction or not.

Managing diagnosed food hypersensitivity

Current clinical management of food hypersensitivity is to exclude the culprit food or foods causing the problem, but the degree of avoidance needed is very individual. It is important to monitor the condition so that foods are not excluded for longer than is necessary as young children may grow out of their food hypersensitivity.

Some infants and children with IgE-mediated food allergies need to completely avoid the food – even in trace amounts. Others may be able to tolerate small amounts of the food or the cooked food but not the raw food. Quality of life in these children, adolescents and families through fear and anxiety is lower than in the general population (Warren et al. 2020). From time to time food challenges will be arranged to test whether the child has outgrown the food allergy.

All children should know which foods they need to avoid and should be encouraged to tell others about their food allergy or intolerance.

Clothes, stickers, t-shirts, watches and jewellery that alert people to food allergy are available from certain websites (e.g. www.allergylifestyle.com).

Oral immunotherapy (OIT) is now being tested in clinical trials (Bégin et al. 2020). It involves exposing children to a minutely small, measured quantity of the food protein to which they are allergic and increasing that quantity daily by an infinitesimally small amount. This is done through pharmacological preparations as the miniscule quantities of the protein must be very precisely measured. Over time tolerance of very small amounts of the food protein increases such that some peanut allergic children may be able to tolerate a whole peanut without reacting (Cavaliere et al. 2019, Kim et al. 2019). This can improve quality of life by reducing some of the anxiety in parents and children. Parents report a greater improvement in quality of life than the children (Epstein-Rigby et al. 2020).

Exclusion diets

Children may be hypersensitive to more than one food. Exclusion diets which exclude the food or foods to which the child is hypersensitive can lead to a nutritional inadequacy and therefore all children should see a paediatric or allergy specialist dietitian for nutritional assessment and advice.

An excluded food can often be substituted with other foods from the same food group (see Chapter 2). However, if the food suspected of causing a reaction is milk then that whole food group must be excluded. A dietitian can recommend suitable alternatives to milk which may be prescribable by a doctor.

The responsibilities of a dietitian managing any exclusion diet are to advise:

- which foods a child can eat and which foods he or she will have to avoid;
- which family foods to use in place of excluded foods;
- how to check food labels for food ingredients that must be avoided;
- on any food products or milks a child may be entitled to have prescribed;
- on supplements that may be required to ensure nutritional adequacy;
- where to buy certain foods;
- which organisations can give extra advice and support;
- on menu planning and recipe modification;
- a nursery or school about the special diet the child needs.

Useful advice for parents and children is summarized in Table 17.1.

Cutting out eggs

Many foods (e.g. cakes, some biscuits, some ice cream, mayonnaise, quiche, pancakes and some pasta) contain eggs as an ingredient. Often eggs are used to glaze baked goods.

Some children may be able to eat very small quantities of egg in cooked foods such as cakes as cooking denatures some of the protein, making it less likely to cause a reaction (Lemon-Mule et al. 2008).

Cutting out peanuts and tree nuts

Peanuts are from a different biological family to tree nuts and children may not be allergic to both peanuts and tree nuts. However, whatever the nut allergy it is prudent to avoid both types of nuts as they are often processed in the same factories, which can lead to cross-contamination of tree nuts with traces of peanuts or vice versa.

Cutting out sesame

Many foods contain sesame or tahini: particularly hummus, halvah and many Turkish, Greek, Chinese and Japanese foods. Sesame can also be present in bread, biscuits, salad dressings and sauces.

Cutting out milk

Because this involves the elimination of a whole food group, a child needs to have a substitute food to provide the same nutrients that milk, cheese and yogurt provide.

Table 17.1 Foods to avoid and suggested alternatives

Food to be excluded by the child	Other foods and ingredients to avoid	Foods to replace the excluded food
Milk	Butter, casein, cheese, cow/sheep/goat's milk, evaporated or condensed milk, cream, yogurt, fromage frais, cheese, ice cream, curd, ghee, lactoglobulin, lactose, milk solids, whey, yogurt, milk proteins	GP can prescribe a replacement milk for infants. Children can use a prescribed replacement milk or calcium-enriched soya or oat milks, soya-based yogurts and desserts and tofu
Egg	Albumin, dried egg, egg powder, egg protein, egg white and yolk, frozen egg, globulin, lecithin (E322), livetin, ovalbumin, ovoglobulin, ovomucin, ovovitellin, pasteurized egg, vitellin	Meat, fish, nuts and pulses
Wheat	Bran, breadcrumbs, bulgur wheat, cereal filler, couscous, durum wheat, farina, flour, rusk, semolina, starch, vegetable protein, wheatgerm and wheatgerm oil	Rice, potatoes, wheat-free breads, pasta and flours, sago, tapioca, quinoa and millet, buckwheat
Foods containing gluten	Bran, breadcrumbs, bulgur wheat, cereal filler, couscous, durum wheat, farina, flour, rusk, semolina, starch, vegetable protein, wheatgerm and wheatgerm oil, rye, barley and oats, spelt	Rice, potatoes, corn, maize, sago, tapioca, quinoa, millet and gluten-free cereals, breads and flour Gluten-free products can be prescribed by a GP for children diagnosed with coeliac disease
Fish or shellfish	Anchovy, Worcestershire sauce, aspic, caviar, fish stock and fish sauce	Meat, eggs, nuts and pulses To replace the omega 3 fats in fish: walnuts and walnut oil, rapeseed oil
Peanuts – also known as ground nuts	Peanuts, ground nuts, peanut oil which could also be called arachis oil or hypogaea, peanut flour, peanut protein. It is best to avoid all other nuts as well as they may be contaminated with small amounts of peanuts	Meat, fish, eggs and pulses
Other nuts which are called tree nuts	Almonds, hazelnuts, walnuts, cashews, pecan nuts, Brazil nuts, pistachio nuts, macadamia nuts and Queensland nuts (You do not need to avoid coconut, pine nuts, nutmeg and butternut squash) Pesto often contains cashew nuts	Meat, fish, eggs and pulses
Soya	Hydrolysed vegetable protein, soya lecithin, soya sauce, miso, soya albumin, soya beans, soya flour, soya milk, soya nuts, soya oil, soya proteins, soya sprouts, tempeh, texturized vegetable protein, tofu	Meat, fish, eggs and nuts
Sesame	Sesame seeds, sesame oil, tahini	–

Most infants and children who are allergic to cow's milk will also be allergic to goat, buffalo, camel and sheep milk so these cannot be used instead. Hydrolysed infant formulas are prescribable for infants. Soya formula milk is not considered appropriate for infants less than 6 months of age (see Chapter 8, page 113). Soya or oat drinks which are fortified with extra calcium and vitamins are often the substitute milk for children over 12 months. However some infants and children have an allergy to both milk and soya. Nut, cereal and soya drink substitutes for milk are not uniformly fortified with iodine and the iodine RNI will not be met without a supplement.

Rice drink is not recommended for children under 5 years as it may contain small amounts of arsenic.

Cutting out wheat

Cutting out wheat is very difficult as many foods are based on wheat flour. This includes bread, pasta, couscous and almost all biscuits and cakes. Wheat flour is often used as an ingredient for thickening sauces and wheat rusks are added to sausages and other processed meats.

There are a variety of pastas, breads and crispbreads based on flours made from other cereals or foods, such as maize, polenta, rye, oats, chickpeas, gram, lentil, bean, potato, rice, millet, arrowroot and buckwheat. Labels need to be checked carefully to make sure they are 100 per cent wheat free as some may contain a small percentage of wheat flour, making them unsuitable. For example, rye bread may be made from 90 per cent rye flour and 10 per cent wheat flour and oat flapjacks often contain some wheat flour.

Cutting out soya

Soya flour is used along with wheat flour in many foods – most breads have some soya flour in them. Naan breads, breakfast muffins and pancakes are usually soya free.

Reintroduction of excluded foods to test whether a food allergy has been out-grown

Allergens can be re-introduced slowly to test the level of tolerance that the child now has. Usually this begins with a graded introduction of a food containing the protein to which the child is allergic with decreasing levels of the denaturing of the protein. The iMap Milk Ladder (Figure 17.3) is used for milk reintroduction. A similar ladder for egg allergy is shown in Figure 17.4, but any protein can be reintroduced in the same way following the same principles on introducing small but increasing amounts of:

1. the protein baked at a high temperature of about 180° centigrade such as biscuits or cakes baked at this temperature;
2. the protein cooked a lower temperature – such as pancakes cooked on frying pan;
3. the protein in a fermented food;
4. the protein in a non baked, non fermented state.

It is usual to stay on each step of the ladder for 2–4 weeks and having the food daily before progressing to the next step.

The foods introduced can be adapted by a dietitian to the food availability, preferences and food preparation abilities of the family. Some families may be happy to cook from recipes while others may prefer to buy commercially available foods.

Food labels

Parents, carers and older children need to check food labels very carefully by reading the list of ingredients to check for anything that needs to be avoided – even when the food product is well used. Sometimes the manufacturer may change the recipe slightly and include new ingredients. The label will not always be modified to say 'new' or 'improved'.

European legislation now requires that all prepacked food must be clearly labelled if it contains any of the following foods:

- cereals containing gluten (i.e. wheat, rye, barley, oats, spelt, kamut or their hybridized strains);
- eggs;
- fish;
- shellfish;
- peanuts or ground nuts;

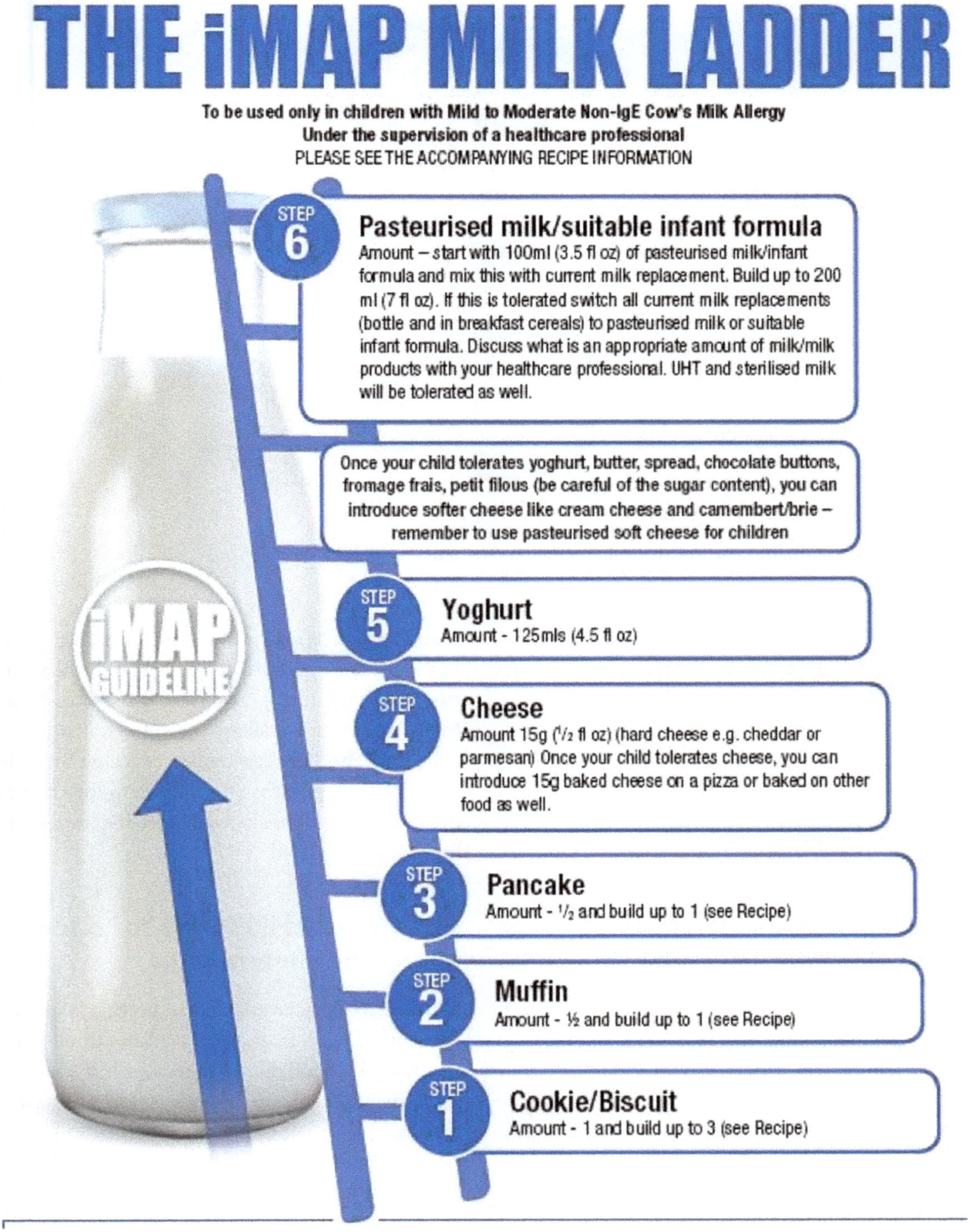

Figure 17.3 iMAP Milk Ladder

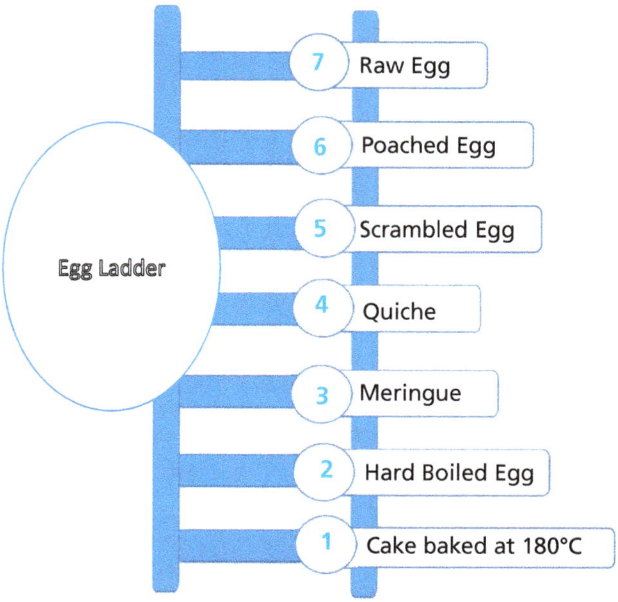

Figure 17.4 Ladder for re-introducing eggs into a diet (Palmer 2020)

- soybeans;
- milk and lactose;
- nuts;
- celery;
- mustard;
- sesame seeds;
- sulphur dioxide and sulphites;
- lupin;
- molluscs.

If these foods are included in a product they must be included in the ingredients list so that they stand out using a different font, style or background colour. Since 2019 the UK legislation requires food prepared and sold on the same premises must also carry a similar full list of ingredients.

However, foods sold loose, in small packages and bottles and catering packages are exempt from this guidance and will not usually display this information.

'Free-from' foods and lists

Some supermarkets and manufacturers also produce 'free-from' lists on which all their own-brand products are listed according to their suitability for various diets. Clients can telephone customer care lines to request a list of 'free-from' foods for the food allergy or intolerance that a child has. This does not replace checking the food labels prior to purchase or offering to the child as the recipe may have changed since the 'free-from' list was last updated.

Adapting family foods for a food allergy or intolerance

Many recipes can be adapted and recipe books for particular food allergies are available in all good bookshops. Dietitians or others with a food allergy may be able to provide some well-tested recipes.

To prevent cross-contamination of foods that need to be avoided by a child:

- cooking utensils must be washed thoroughly;
- special care taken when washing chopping boards or work surfaces;
- hands must be washed thoroughly before

preparing special foods for the food-allergic child;
- oil for cooking different foods must not be re-used;
- the same spoon must not be used when dishing up different foods.

Eating outside the home

Eating outside the home presents several challenges, especially if a child has an IgE-mediated allergy. It is best to avoid foods if the full list of ingredients is not known rather than taking risks.

In the United States it has become common for people to carry a 'chef card' that outlines the foods that a child must avoid. The card can be presented to the chef or manager and serves as a reminder of the food allergy. However the reliability depends on the training, understanding and attitudes of the chef and other staff.

At nursery and school

Parents may perceive that their child has a food allergy but with no formal diagnosis. This creates extra work for staff where it may not be necessary and staff are entitled to ask for a doctor's letter to confirm the child has a diagnosed allergy.

Teaching staff and carers need written information about a child's food allergy or intolerance that includes what to avoid and which foods can be offered in their place. Nursery staff need information and/or training on:

- how to check food labels;
- how to ascertain ingredients in catering packs even if it means that the company should be contacted;
- what degree of food avoidance is required for each food for each child;
- any other allergic conditions;
- how to deal with severe allergic reactions.

Travel to non-English-speaking countries

When travelling abroad to foreign countries, families who do not speak the local language will need accurate translations of the key foods and ingredients that a child needs to avoid. Various websites provide a series of translation sheets for various allergies (www.allergyaction.co.uk, www.allergyuk.org, www.kidsaware.co.uk, www.yellowcross.co.uk).

> **Activity**
>
> Devise a 1-day menu for a 2–year-old child who is allergic to wheat, milk, fish and soya protein. Research a suitable supplement to address any nutrient deficiencies.

References and further reading

Bégin P, Chan ES, Kim H, et al. (2020) CSACI guidelines for the ethical, evidence-based and patient-oriented clinical practice of oral immunotherapy in IgE-mediated food allergy. *Allergy, Asthma & Clinical Immunology* **16**: 20. Published 2020 Mar 18. doi:10.1186/s13223-020-0413-7.

Cavaliere C, Masieri S, Miranda V, et al. (2019) Clinical and immunological effects of a treatment with desentizating low-dose multicomponents in IgE mediated and non IgE mediated food allergies: observational retrospective pilot study. *Clinical Therapeutics* **170**(1): e10–e15. doi:10.7417/CT.2019.2102.

De Martinis M, Sirufo MM, Suppa M, Ginaldi L (2020) New Perspectives in Food Allergy. *International Journal of Molecular Sciences* **21**(4): 1474. Published 2020 Feb 21. doi:10.3390/ijms21041474.

Du Toit G, Sayre PH, Roberts G, et al. (2016) Effect of Avoidance on Peanut Allergy after Early Peanut Consumption. *New England Journal of Medicine* **374**(15): 1435–1443.

Epstein-Rigbi N, Goldberg MR, Levy MB, Nachshon L, Elizur A (2020) Quality of life of children aged 8-12 years undergoing food allergy oral immunotherapy: Child and parent perspective *Allergy* **75** (10): 2623–2632.

Hill DA, Dudley JW, Spergel JM (2017) The Prevalence of Eosinophilic Esophagitis in Pediatric Patients with IgE-Mediated Food Allergy. *The Journal of Allergy and Clinical Immunology: In Practice* **5**(2): 369–375. doi:10.1016/j.jaip.2016.11.020.

Johansson SG, Bieber T, Dahl R, et al. (2004) Revised nomenclature for allergy for global use: Report of the Nomenclature Review Committee of the World Allergy Organization, October 2003. *Journal of Allergy and Clinical Immunology* **113**(5): 832–836.

Kim EH et al. (2019) Long-term sublingual immunotherapy for peanut allergy in children: Clinical and immunologic evidence of desensitization. *Journal of Allergy and Clinical Immunology* **144** (5): 1320–1326, DOI: 10.1016/j.jaci.2019.07.030.

Lack, Gideon (2020) Allergy to Peanuts Presentation at Nutrition and Growth Conference, London.

Lemon-Mule H, Sampson HA, Sicherer SH, Shreffler WG, Noone S, & Nowak-Wegrzyn A (2008) Immunologic changes in children with egg allergy ingesting extensively heated egg. *Journal of Allergy and Clinical Immunology* **122** (5): 977–983.

National Institute for Health and Clinical Excellence (NICE) (March 2016) Food Allergy Quality Standard 118 https://www.nice.org.uk/guidance/qs118 (Accessed June 2020).

National Institute for Health and Clinical Excellence (NICE) Food Allergy in Under 19's overview 2020. https://pathways.nice.org.uk/pathways/food-allergy-in-under-19s (Accessed June 2020).

NICE (2011) Clinical Guidance 116. Diagnosis and assessment of food allergy in children and young people in primary care and community settings. https://www.nice.org.uk/guidance/cg116 (Accessed June 2020).

Palmer, Debora (2020) Allergy to Eggs Presentation at Nutrition and Growth Conference, London.

Palmer DJ, Gold MS, Makrides M (2008) Effect of maternal egg consumption on breast milk ovalbumin concentration. *Clinical & Experimental Allergy* **38**(7): 1186–1191. doi:10.1111/j.1365-2222.2008.03014.x.

Perkin MR, Logan K, Tseng A, et al. (2016) Randomized Trial of Introduction of Allergenic Foods in Breast-Fed Infants. *New England Journal of Medicine* **374**(18): 1733–1743.

Peters RL, Koplin JJ, Gurrin LC, et al. (2017) The prevalence of food allergy and other allergic diseases in early childhood in a population-based study: HealthNuts age 4-year follow-up. *The Journal of Allergy and Clinical Immunology* **140**(1): 145–153.e8. doi:10.1016/j.jaci.2017.02.019.

Rigbi NE, Goldberg MR, Levy MB, Nachshon L, Golobov K, Elizur A (2017) Changes in patient quality of life during oral immunotherapy for food allergy. *Allergy* **72**(12): 1883–1890. doi:10.1111/all.13211.

Smeekens JM, Kulis MD (2020) Evolution of Immune Responses in Food Immunotherapy. *Immunology and Allergy Clinics of North America* **40**(1): 87–95. doi:10.1016/j.iac.2019.09.006.

Venter C and Arshad SH (2011) Epidemiology of food allergy. *Pediatric Clinics of North America* **58**(2): 327–349.

Venter C, Maslin K, Patil V, et al. (2016) The prevalence, natural history and time trends of peanut allergy over the first 10 years of life in two cohorts born in the same geographical location 12 years apart. *Pediatric Allergy and Immunology* **27**(8): 804–811. doi:10.1111/pai.12616.

Venter C, Patil V, Grundy J, et al. (2016) Prevalence and cumulative incidence of food hypersensitivity in the first 10 years of life. *Pediatric Allergy and Immunology* **27**(5): 452–458. doi:10.1111/pai.12564.

Warren CM, Jiang J, Gupta RS (2020) Epidemiology and Burden of Food Allergy. *Current Allergy and Asthma Reports* **20**(2): 6. Published 2020 Feb 14. doi:10.1007/s11882-020-0898-7.

Resources

The Anaphylaxis Campaign (www.anaphylaxis.org.uk)

Allergy UK: https://www.allergyuk.org/

The British Society for Allergy and Clinical Immunology https://www.bsaci.org/

The iMap Milk Ladder: https://www.allergyuk.org/assets/000/001/297/iMAP_Final_Ladder-May_2017_original.pdf?1502804928

The iMap Recipes for the UK: https://www.allergyuk.org/assets/000/001/767/iMAP-Recipes_%28Final%29_original.pdf?1524663093

Wright T (2001) *Food Allergies – enjoying life with a severe food allergy*. London: Class Publishing Ltd.

18

Childhood obesity

Summary

- Overweight and obesity are measured by body mass index (BMI), which is calculated by dividing a person's weight in kilograms by the square of their height in metres.
- BMI varies throughout childhood, decreasing from about 1 year to 5–7 years and then slowly increasing throughout the rest of childhood.
- BMI-for-age centile charts are used in clinical settings to classify children as overweight or obese – above the 91st centile is considered overweight and above the 98th centile is classified as obese.
- Organic causes of obesity are very rare and family lifestyle is the most common cause of childhood obesity.
- Limiting food intake to age appropriate food portion sizes is key addressing obesity.
- Families first need to acknowledge that their child is overweight or obese and be motivated to address this through lifestyle changes if interventions are to be successful.
- Making lifestyle changes is very difficult for families who may need considerable support to achieve change.

Definitions of overweight and obesity in children

In children, overweight and obesity are defined by body mass index (BMI) for age centile. As discussed in Chapter 4, BMI is a measure of weight relative to height and is calculated by dividing the weight in kilograms by the square of the height in metres:

$$\mathbf{BMI} = \frac{\textbf{weight in kg}}{(\textbf{height in m})^2}$$

BMI varies throughout childhood and this variation is slightly different between boys and girls. Hence there are gender-specific BMI-for-age centile charts (See Appendix 3). BMI:

- increases during infancy;
- decreases from around 1 year of age or when the toddler becomes increasingly mobile until about 5–7 years of age – the average BMI at 1 year is 17.5, falling to about 15.5 at 5–7 years of age;
- steadily increases from about 6–7 years of age until adulthood - also known as the adiposity rebound;
- may rise just before the pubertal growth spurt begins as height gain slows temporarily.

BMI is only considered accurate as a measure of whether a child is a normal or abnormal weight for their height from about 2 years of age.

Clinical definitions of overweight and obesity in the United Kingdom

Once a child's weight and height have been measured accurately on calibrated equipment the BMI is calculated and then plotted on a BMI-for-age centile chart. In clinical settings a child is:

- overweight if they are between the 91st and 98th centile lines;
- obese if they are on or above the 98th centile line;
- severely obese on or above the 99.6th centile line.

Definitions of overweight and obesity for national statistics

To date, UK government statistics use the 85th BMI for age centile as the cut-off for overweight and the 95th BMI for age centile as the cut-off for obesity. As these 2 centile lines are not marked in the BMI charts in clinical use, they are not used in clinical practice.

Definitions used in other countries vary and the International Task Force on Obesity set cut-offs that are similar to those used clinically in the United Kingdom but not exactly the same.

Assessing overweight or obesity

Studies have shown that neither healthcare professionals nor parents can reliably assess, just by eye, whether a child is overweight or obese. The assessment must be carried out more objectively, using the BMI for age centile.

Waist circumference centile charts (See Appendix 3) can be used to estimate truncal fat stores and the consequent risks to health. Waist circumference has increased at a greater rate than BMI over the last few decades.

Where an adolescent is in relation to their pubertal growth spurt should be taken into consideration as full height may not have been reached and some adolescents become overweight for their height just before their pubertal growth spurt. With the rapid growth in height during the growth spurt they may slim down into a lower BMI category.

Prevalence of childhood obesity in the United Kingdom

The prevalence of childhood overweight and obesity has been increasing in developed countries over the last few decades. In the UK, rates have risen from around:

- 8 per cent in 1974 to
- 25 per cent in 1995 and remained
- around 30 per cent since 2000

The National Child Measurement Programme in UK schools measures children when they enter Reception, age 4–5 years, and again in their final year of primary school – Year 6, age 10–11 years. About 93 per cent of children take part, not 100 per cent as they are able to opt out. The figures (Table 18.1) show an increase in the percentage of children overweight, obese and severely obese over the primary school years. They may be a slight underestimate as parents of obese children are more likely to request that their children are not measured.

Figures from the Health Survey for England show similar figures but are over a wider age range (Table 18.2).

Factors associated with childhood obesity

The vast majority of overweight and obesity is caused by a higher energy intake (consumed in

Table 18.1 Percentage of children classified as obese in National Child Measurement Programme

Age	Percentage of children classified as obese			Percentage of children classified as severely obese
	2006/07	2010/11	2018/19	2018/19
4–5 year olds in Reception	9.9	9.4	9.7	2.4
10–11 year olds in Year 6	17.5	19	20.2	4.4

Table 18.2 Percentage of children classified as overweight or obese in Health Survey for England 2018

	Percentage of children	
Age range	Overweight	Obese
2–4 years	13	7
5–7 years	12	12
8–10 years	12	20
11–12 years	14	19
13–15 years	15	21

food and drinks) than energy expenditure through growth, development and activity. The excess energy intake is stored as extra adipose tissue which contributes to the physical and metabolic changes seen in obesity.

Medical causes of obesity in children are extremely rare and include:

- endocrine disorders often signalled by short stature such as hypothyroidism, Cushing's syndrome and growth hormone deficiency;
- single-gene defects (e.g. leptin deficiency and melanocortin 4 receptor (MC4R) deficiency);
- chromosomal disorders, such as Prader-Willi syndrome, Bardet Biedl syndrome, Alstrom syndrome and Cohen syndrome.

Obesity rates vary across the country and are more prevalent in deprived areas, urban environments and lower socio-economic groups. Genetics, epigenetics, ethnicity, low socio-economic status, environment, eating patterns, food portion sizes, activity levels and sleep duration all play a part in the development of obesity. Early life factors include: pre pregnancy maternal obesity, paternal obesity, excess gestational weight gain, diabetes during pregnancy, high birth weight of over 4 kg and rapid weight gain in infancy and the toddler years.

Genetic and epigenetic differences make some children more susceptible to obesity in an obesogenic environment.

Excess weight gain in preschool children is of particular concern as a UK study found that most of the excess weight in 9-year-old children had been gained as excess weight before 5 years of age (Gardner et al. 2009). As part of the Avon Longitudinal Study of Parents and Children (ALSPAC), Reilly et al. (2005) identified the following risk factors for childhood obesity at age 7 years irrespective of whether the child was overweight at 3 years or not:

- parental obesity of one or both parents;
- high birthweight;
- rapid weight gain in the first year – crossing upwards across weight for age centile lines after 8 weeks of age;
- catch-up growth between birth and 2 years;
- an early adiposity rebound at 3–4 years of age when the BMI does not continue to decrease as expected on BMI for age centile charts;
- sedentary behaviour: more than eight hours watching TV per week at 3 years;
- less than 10½ hours sleep/24 hours at 3 years – normally 3 year olds sleep for about 12 hours in every 24 hours.

Similar factors were found in the Born in Bradford Study (Fairley et al. 2015)

Parental obesity

Having one obese parent increases the risk, and if that parent is the mother the risk is higher. The highest risk is in children with two obese parents (Reilly et al. 2005). This could be due to a combination of factors: genetic, social or environmental.

Rapid weight gain in infancy

Whether breastfeeding in early infancy plays a role in preventing obesity in childhood or not remains controversial. Formula-fed infants lose less weight in the first few days after birth and their overall growth pattern is different to that of exclusively breastfed babies. As discussed in Chapter 8 it is easier to overfeed a baby by bottle feeding than by breastfeeding. However, there are many lifestyle factors throughout the toddler years and early childhood, in addition to the mode of milk feeding during infancy, that may contribute to the development of obesity. Low birth weight followed by rapid weight gain in the first 6 months is also related to low socioeconomic status (Wang et al. 2018), which is in turn associated with a higher risk of obesity.

Adiposity rebound

'Adiposity rebound' is the term given to the time when BMI begins to increase after falling to a low point at around 5–7 years. Children with an early adiposity rebound (i.e. whose BMI begins to increase earlier than 5–7 years) are at higher risk of obesity (Aris et al. 2019).

Consequences of obesity

The health risks associated with obesity in childhood are:

- increased severity of asthma and other respiratory disease;
- lower levels of fitness;
- social discrimination, such as bullying, victimization and social exclusion that can lead to low self-esteem, lower quality of life and lower academic achievement;
- orthopaedic and musculoskeletal problems;
- increased risk of insulin resistance and type 2 diabetes;
- higher incidence of atherosclerosis;
- increased risk of cardiovascular disease;
- non-alcoholic fatty liver disease;
- kidney disease;
- several cancers.

Obese adolescents may also develop one or more of the following:

- sleep apnoea;
- hypertension and dyslipidaemia – found in 80 per cent;
- type 2 diabetes;
- gallstones;
- encopresis;
- steato-hepatitis;
- gastro-oesophageal reflux.

An overweight child has a 40–70 per cent chance of becoming an obese adult. The older an overweight child is, the more likely they will remain overweight or obese as an adult.

Preventing obesity

Initiatives to improve lifestyles in families at risk of obesity need to be undertaken sensitively and should involve support for parents to improve their parenting skills. Preschool children learn by copying, so parents need to adopt healthy lifestyle patterns themselves. Home visits during pregnancy and infancy may be a time when parents are receptive to advice on healthy eating for young children and may have more incentive to change behaviours.

Changing eating habits is usually difficult but particularly so for parents who:

- do not understand the principles of healthy eating and age appropriate food portion sizes;
- do not have the cooking skills necessary to prepare simple home-cooked food and instead rely on convenience foods which are usually higher in energy, fat, sugar and salt;
- do not have set mealtimes either as a family or for their children so that frequent snacking forms part of their eating pattern.

Prenatal prevention, discussed in Chapters 6 & 7, requires a healthy weight for both parents pre-conception, normal gestational weight gain and avoiding lifestyle factors which lead to a low birth weight.

Postnatal prevention: responsive feeding, ideally breastfeeding, should prevent early life rapid weight gain. However infants with poor appetite control due to genetic or epigenetic changes can overconsume due to the pleasure and comfort in feeding and eating and consequently gain weight rapidly and cross upwards on their weight for age centiles. It is seen in breastfeeding infants, though more commonly in bottle fed infants. Weight gain monitoring and limits on milk and complementary feeding intakes will be needed.

Preschool and primary school children are dependent on parents and carers for their food and opportunities for physical activity, so it is the parents and carers who must take responsibility for a healthy family lifestyle. Multicomponent family based interventions are the most effective and parents are likely to enjoy programmes which involve group learning with the ability to compare notes with other parents, sessions that are fun, interactive and practical and lead by enthusiastic leaders (Lanigan 2018). Issues to include are:

- cultural sensitivity;
- active engagement of the parents in the programme and as role models of healthy living;
- responsive parenting (see Parenting Styles Chapter 3, Figure 3.3);
- controlling food portion sizes to those in Chapters 12 and 15 – Tables 12.1 and 15.2;
- sustained moderate to vigorous physical activity;
- active engagement of the children in nutrition education;
- acknowledgement of the issues faced by parents and support for their role directly, through making healthy and active behaviours easily available, and indirectly, through providing local services, including early childhood services.

Secondary school children make more of their own lifestyle decisions and the responsibility for preventing obesity is a shared responsibility between themselves and their parents and carers. However, the lifestyle habits and preferences of secondary school children, particularly around food and physical activity, will have been largely learned by parental role modelling when they were younger. Environmental factors and marketing will also influence lifestyle choices of adolescents.

Portion sizes of food and drinks

Adopting the principles of nutritious balanced diets as discussed in Chapter 2 and limiting food portion sizes to those in Tables 12.1, 15.2 and 16.1 are a key part of obesity prevention. Although most infants and preschool children tend to regulate their energy intakes to their needs, some young children do not regulate their energy intake well and some derive considerable pleasure from sweet, high-energy foods. From 5 years of age children tend to eat to social cues and can easily override their feelings of satiety. Portion control becomes most important for children who do not regulate their intake according to their feelings of satiety.

However, providing food is an emotional issue for parents and many show their love through giving food. Research has found that more parents are concerned about their young children being underweight than overweight (Pagnini et al. 2007). Some parents:

- coerce children to finish up larger portions than the child wants to eat;
- give high-energy, low-nutrient foods as treats, rewards or for comfort.

Small amounts of foods high in fat and sugar are acceptable but children often eat these foods to excess – particularly sweetened drinks, confectionery and high-fat snack foods such as crisps. The rise in obesity is parallel to the increase in consumption of sweetened drinks by children. Restricting these foods and drinks to one item once per week as detailed in Chapter 2 p21 in today's environment requires discipline, as children naturally prefer energy-dense foods (Cooke 2004).

Family meals and planned snacks with age appropriate food portion sizes are preferable to allowing unplanned snacking and grazing throughout the day as unplanned snacks tend to include higher energy, lower nutrient foods than planned meals and snacks.

Physical activity

Physical activity accounts for about 25–35 per cent of children's energy expenditure.

When toddlers and preschool children are encouraged and given the opportunities for active play, they will develop coordination and skills that will allow them to enjoy sport as they

Table 18.3 Types of physical activity

	Activity	Moderate-intensity activities	Vigorous-intensity activities that enhance muscle and bone strength:
Infants	30 minutes of tummy time spread throughout the day	Once moving around encourage as much safe activity as possible	
Children under five	playing with blocks and other objects messy play playground activities outdoor activities throwing and catching	jumping walking dancing swimming climbing active play, like hide and seek scooting riding a bike skipping	
Children over five		walking to school playground activities riding a scooter skateboarding rollerblading walking the dog cycling on level ground or ground with few hills	games such as tug of war skipping with a rope swinging on playground equipment bars gymnastics and dance basketball and netball football, rugby and hockey tennis and badminton sit-ups, press-ups and other similar exercises aerobics climbing or rock climbing martial arts resistance exercises with exercise bands, weight machines or handheld weights

get older. Most preschool children do not need encouragement for active play but opportunities depend on their housing situation and the local environment. Older children may need more motivation to take part in physical activity.

The Department of Health recommends:

Children under 5 years:

- are physically active for at least 3 hours each day. Short periods of activity can be spread out over the day;
- should not be inactive for long periods, except when they are asleep. Watching TV, travelling by car, bus or train, or being strapped into a

buggy for long periods are not good for a child's health and development.

Children 5–18 years:

- engage in moderate to vigorous intensity physical activity for at least 60 minutes and up to several hours every day;
- take part in a variety of types and intensities of physical activity across the week to develop movement skills, muscles and bones;
- reduce the time spent sitting or lying down and break up long periods of not moving with some activity;
- activities should make them breathe faster and feel warmer.

Studies show that physical activity tends to decrease in girls after the age of 10–12 years, whereas boys remain more active although activity levels are lower in those aged 15–18 than in 11–14 year olds. Girls aged 15–18 years are the least active. Few adolescents achieve the recommended 60 minutes or more of physical activity of at least moderate intensity. Adolescents cite greater embarrassment and self-consciousness about their bodies – along with lack of time – as barriers to physical activity.

The role of physical activity in obesity prevention remains controversial as when children become overweight, they reduce their activity and that inactivity is less implicated in causing obesity than a high energy intake through food and drinks.

Limiting sedentary behaviour

The same Department of Health guidelines recommend that all children and young people should minimize the amount of time spent being sedentary (sitting) for extended periods. In the United States and elsewhere watching television is not recommended for the under-twos, and for those aged 3 and over the American Academy of Pediatrics recommends no more than 2 hours per day in sedentary behaviours such as TV viewing. Video games and computers do not represent such a high risk compared to watching TV (Rey-López et al. 2008).

Many toddlers and young children spend a lot of time being babysat by a screen such as TV/DVD/computer games when parents are busy doing chores.

Getting enough sleep

Several studies have reported an association between inadequate sleep and obesity (Chaput et al. 2011). The mechanism by which less sleep might affect growth and predispose young children towards obesity is not clear but it may be via hormonal influences on growth.

Childcare settings

National Institute for Health and Care Excellence Guidance CG43 (2015) recommends that all nurseries and childcare facilities should:

- minimize sedentary activities during play time, and provide regular opportunities for enjoyable active play and structured physical activity sessions;
- implement government guidance on food procurement and healthy catering;
- ensure that children eat regular, healthy meals in a pleasant, sociable environment free from other distractions (such as television). Children should be supervised at mealtimes and, where possible, staff should eat with children.

Activity 1

Plan a community-based obesity-prevention programme for families with young children.

Treating obesity

Most NHS Trusts have a locally agreed protocol for treating childhood obesity. Scottish guidance recommends that children with a BMI over the 99.6th centile should be referred to a paediatrician for investigation.

In pre-pubertal obese and overweight children, weight loss may not be required but weight gain can be slowed or stopped temporarily through lifestyle changes so that BMI declines as the child grows taller. Any weight loss should be limited to about 1kg/month. Older children who have already been through their pubertal growth spurt and very obese pre-pubertal children will require weight loss to reduce their BMI. Bariatric surgery is available in some areas for post-pubertal children who have unsuccessfully tried lifestyle change.

The most effective way of managing overweight and obesity in children remains uncertain as the evidence base is limited (Colquitt et al. 2016). Successful interventions include a combination of:

- change in dietary habits to reduce energy intake through limiting food and drink portion sizes to those appropriate for age (see Tables 12.1 p. 164, Table 15.2 p. 197, Table 16.1 p. 208);
- increase in physical activity;
- decreasing sedentary behaviour;
- ensuring adequate sleep for growth;
- family-based behavioural therapy.

Engaging parents

Most parents do not recognize that their children are overweight or obese so healthcare professionals need to be sensitive when discussing the issue. Parents could be asked how they feel about their child's weight as a way of beginning a discussion. A measurement of the child's weight and height/length could then be offered. Showing a parent how the BMI of their overweight/obese child relates to the normal range by using the BMI for age centile chart is a good way to continue the discussion.

Unless parents acknowledge that there is a problem and are ready to change their lifestyle there is little that can be achieved for an overweight or obese preschool or primary school child.

Supporting parents to make lifestyle changes

Lifestyle changes for the whole family are preferable to just targeting the behaviour of the overweight or obese child on their own. When lifestyle changes become a normal part of their family life they are more likely to be maintained long term. Each family will probably have a preference for either:

- a single family intervention or;
- a multi-family group programme although accessibility to group programmes may be limited.

In most cases the cause of the obesity will be multifactorial and a single solution will not suit every family. Parents are likely to be aware of factors but they may involve emotional issues, making change seem more difficult.

Discussion points to explore with a family with an overweight or obese child:
Weight change – what are the aims for this child/family?
Adolescent growth spurt – has this occurred yet and how does this affect weight change goals?
Planned meal and planned snack routine rather than allowing grazing on food and drinks
Snacks – changes towards low energy, higher nutrient planned snacks
Portion sizes eaten by child – are they age appropriate or do they need to be reduced?
Speed of eating – children who eat quickly tend to eat larger quantities of food
Lifestyle role modelling by parents and siblings – the overweight child must not be expected to do anything the other family members are not also doing
Child's enjoyment of food vs. enjoyment of non-food activities
Family attitude to food and food as rewards, treats or for comfort
Family activities that can be introduced to replace food and drink-based activities
Current family lifestyle balance between physical activities and sedentary activities
Overweight child's aspirations to try new non-food-related activities
Increasing children's self-esteem around non-weight-related activities or skills. Praise from parents when achievements are made is important.
Finding a physical activity that the child enjoys – this may be available within their school but it may not, and parents may have to investigate other activities within the community and/or while on holiday

Once contributing factors have been identified, families can explore which of these factors they feel they may be able to change. The barriers to making changes may be considerable for some families because of:

- the family lifestyle;
- lack of knowledge of appropriate portion sizes and the principles of a nutritious diet;
- lack of cooking skills or facilities to prepare appropriate meals;
- housing and facilities in the local environment;
- limited finances.

There will be pros and cons, and solutions may not always be clear cut. For instance, excess sedentary behaviour and lack of physical activity could be a major factor for a family living in a cramped flat in a high-rise building with no access to a playground or garden. Taking a young child to play outside would impact on the time a busy mother might have to prepare ideal meals and snacks. A carefully structured assessment of need will enable healthcare professionals to support parents in balancing needs and priorities.

Behavioural intervention programmes should incorporate the following aspects:

- stimulus control;
- self-monitoring;
- goal setting;
- rewards for reaching goals;
- problem solving.

Although not strictly defined as behavioural techniques, giving praise and encouraging parents to role-model desired behaviours are also recommended.

Stimulus control

This involves removing inconsistencies in the family environment. Parents can limit the availability of foods and triggers that lead to overeating, for example:

- ideally, not bringing high-calorie, low-nutrient foods into the house at all;
- buying an individual packet rather than multipacks of snack foods or biscuits that must be stored somewhere in the house;
- not going to 'all you can eat for £x' buffet style restaurants;
- having set mealtimes, preferably with all the family eating together;
- having readily available healthy snacks to use in between meals.

Goal setting

Families can agree simple goals for behaviour change and what benefits they will achieve. Three or less goals are ideal. They should not lead to conflict between family members and should be SMART (Table 18.4).

When these changes have been made and sustained, the family can be encouraged to consider another set of lifestyle changes.

Self-monitoring

By keeping records of the goals and the achievements the family can review them.

Table 18.4 Making goals SMART

Aspect of goal	Good examples	Poor examples
Specific	Have sugar-free squash in place of ordinary squash	Choose healthy drinks
Measurable	Have 1 packet of crisps each week	Eat fewer crisps
Achievable	Walk to school twice next week	Walk to school every day from now on
Relevant	Reduce the number of sweets I eat to 1 portion per week	No candyfloss at the funfair
Time-limited	Play football with Dad in the park once this weekend	Play more football in the park with Dad this year

When goals are not achieved, it can be an opportunity to re-evaluate motivation and the complexity or effort required to achieve that goal.

Reward systems

Children are more willing to repeat behaviours that are rewarded. The degree of the reward should match the magnitude of the effort required by the child to achieve that goal. A star chart can be used to work towards a larger reward in several stages. If a goal is not achieved then the reward agreed for it should not be given; however, earned rewards should not be withdrawn to punish poor behaviour. Rewards should not be food or drinks. More suitable non-food rewards include playing games with children, reading books to them, taking them on a swimming trip or other outing.

Problem solving

Through reviewing how difficult lifestyle changes are to make, problems can be identified and possible solutions explored.

Other solutions

Drug therapy and bariatric surgery are sometimes considered for older adolescents who are morbidly obese but not for those who:

- are pregnant;
- have an eating disorder;
- have failed to adopt healthy living principles.

Support for parents who are not ready to make lifestyle changes

Parents need to understand that obesity is a clinical condition with health implications rather than just a question of how someone looks. Discuss the benefits of making changes to physical activity and eating patterns and give them details of someone they can contact when they are ready to consider making changes.

Activity 2

Decide on a lifestyle change you would like to make yourself. Set yourself a goal making it adhere to all the SMART aspects of a goal. List the challenges and barriers to making those changes and any problem solving required to overcome those barriers.

Acknowledgements

With thanks to Dr Paul Chadwick, Clinical Psychologist, Centre for Behaviour Change University College London; Dr Helen Croker, Clinical Research Dietitian, Population, Policy and Practice Dept University College London and Dr Julie Lanigan, Research Dietitian, Childhood Nutrition Research, Population, Policy and Practice, University College London, United Kingdom.

References and further reading

Agarwal P, Morriseau TS, Kereliuk SM, Doucette CA, Wicklow BA, Dolinsky VW (2018) Maternal obesity, diabetes during pregnancy and epigenetic mechanisms that influence the developmental origins of cardiometabolic disease in the offspring. *Critical Reviews in Clinical Laboratory Sciences* **55**(2): 71–101. doi:10.1080/10408363.2017.1422109

Agosti M, Tandoi F, Morlacchi L, Bossi A (2017) Nutritional and metabolic programming during the first thousand days of life. *La Pediatria Medica e Chirurgica* **39**(2): 157. Published 2017 Jun 28. doi:10.4081/pmc.2017.157

Aris IM, Rifas-Shiman SL, Li LJ, et al. (2019) Patterns of body mass index milestones in early life and cardiometabolic risk in early adolescence. *International Journal of Epidemiology* **48**(1): 157–167. doi:10.1093/ije/dyy286

Chaput JP, Lambert M, Gray-Donald K, *et al.* (2011) Short sleep duration is independently associated with overweight and obesity in Quebec children. *Canadian Journal of Public Health* **102**(5): 369–374.

Colquitt JL, Loveman E, O'Malley C, et al. (2016) Diet, physical activity, and behavioural interventions for the treatment of overweight or obesity in preschool children up to the age of 6 years. *Cochrane Database of Systematic Reviews* **3**(3): CD012105. Published 2016 Mar 10. doi:10.1002/14651858.CD012105

Cooke L (2004) The development and modification of children's eating habits. *Nutrition Bulletin* **29**: 31–35.

Egan KB, Ettinger AS & Bracken MB (2013) Childhood body mass index and subsequent physician-diagnosed asthma: a systematic review and meta-analysis of prospective cohort studies. *BMC Pediatrics* **13**: 121.

Fairley L, Santorelli G, Lawlor DA, et al. (2015) The relationship between early life modifiable risk factors for childhood obesity, ethnicity and body mass index at age 3 years: findings from the Born in Bradford birth cohort study. *BMC Obesity* **2**: 9. Published 2015 Feb 24. doi:10.1186/s40608-015-0037-5

Gardner DS, Hosking J, Metcalf BS, Jeffery AN, Voss LD and Wilkin TJ (2009) Contribution of early weight gain to childhood overweight and metabolic health: a longitudinal study (EarlyBird 36). *Pediatrics* **123**(1): e67–e73.

Gregory JW (2019) Prevention of Obesity and Metabolic Syndrome in Children. *Front Endocrinol (Lausanne)* **10**: 669. Published 2019 Oct 1. doi:10.3389/fendo.2019.00669

Hemmingsson E. (2018) Early Childhood Obesity Risk Factors: Socioeconomic Adversity, Family Dysfunction, Offspring Distress, and Junk Food Self-Medication. *Current Obesity Reports* **7**(2): 204–209. doi:10.1007/s13679-018-0310-2

Kong AP & Chow CC (2010) Medical consequences of childhood obesity: a Hong Kong perspective. *Research in Sports Medicine* **18**: 16–25.

Kracht CL, Chaput JP, Martin CK, Champagne CM, Katzmarzyk PT, Staiano AE (2019) Associations of Sleep with Food Cravings, Diet, and Obesity in Adolescence. *Nutrients* **11**(12): 2899. Published 2019 Nov 30. doi:10.3390/nu11122899

Lanigan J. (2018) Prevention of overweight and obesity in early life. *Proceedings of the Nutrition Society* **77**(3): 247–256. doi:10.1017/S0029665118000411

Martin A, Booth JN, Laird Y, Sproule J, Reilly JJ, Saunders DH (2018) Physical activity, diet and other behavioural interventions for improving cognition and school achievement in children and adolescents with obesity or overweight. *Cochrane Database of Systematic Reviews* **3**(3): CD009728. Published 2018 Mar 2. doi:10.1002/14651858.CD009728.pub4

Mead E, Brown T, Rees K, et al. (2017) Diet, physical activity and behavioural interventions for the treatment of overweight or obese children from the age of 6 to 11 years. *Cochrane Database of Systematic Reviews* **6**(6): CD012651. Published 2017 Jun 22. doi:10.1002/14651858.CD012651

Mead E, Atkinson G, Richter B, et al. (2016) Drug interventions for the treatment of obesity in children and adolescents. *Cochrane Database of Systematic Reviews* **11**(11): CD012436. Published 2016 Nov 29. doi:10.1002/14651858.CD012436

National Institute for Health and Care Excellence (2015) NICE guideline 7 [NG7] *Preventing excess weight gain*. Available at: https://www.nice.org.uk/guidance/ng7.

National Institute for Health and Care Excellence (2015) NICE public health guidance 47: *Managing overweight and obesity among children and young people: lifestyle weight management services.* Available at https://www.nice.org.uk/guidance/qs94.

National Institute for Health and Care Excellence (2015) Clinical Guideline 43 [CG43] *Obesity Prevention*. Available at: https://www.nice.org.uk/guidance/cg43.

Oude Luttikhuis H, Baur L, Jansen H, et al. (2019) Interventions for treating obesity in children. *Cochrane Database of Systematic Reviews* **3**(3): CD001872. Published 2019 Mar 7. doi:10.1002/14651858.CD001872.pub3

Pagnini DL, Wilkenfeld RL, King LA, Booth ML and Booth SL (2007) Mothers of pre-school children talk about childhood overweight and obesity: The Weight of Opinion study. *Journal of Paediatrics and Child Health* **43**(12): 806–810.

Psaltopoulou T, Tzanninis S, Ntanasis-Stathopoulos I, et al. (2019) Prevention and treatment of childhood and adolescent obesity: a systematic review of meta-analyses. *World Journal of Pediatrics* **15**(4): 350–381. doi:10.1007/s12519-019-00266-y

Redsell SA, Edmonds B, Swift JA et al. (2016) Systematic review of randomised controlled trials of interventions that aim to reduce the risk, either directly or indirectly, of overweight and obesity in infancy and early childhood. *Maternal & Child Nutrition* **12**: 24–38.

Reilly JJ, Armstrong J, Dorosty AR, *et al.* (2005) Early life risk factors for obesity in childhood: cohort study. *British Medical Journal* **330**: 1357–1359.

Rey-López JP, Vicente-Rodr¡guez G, Biosca M and Moreno LA (2008). Sedentary behaviour and obesity development in children and adolescents. *Nutrition, Metabolism and Cardiovascular Diseases* 18 (3), 242–251.

Scottish Intercollegiate Guidelines Network (SIGN) (2010) Guideline 115. Management of obesity. https://www.sign.ac.uk/assets/sign115.pdf (Accessed June 2020)

Sjöberg RL, Nilsson KW, Leppert J (2005) Obesity, shame, and depression in school-aged children: a population-based study. *Pediatrics* **116**(3): e389–e392. doi:10.1542/peds.2005-0170

Styne DM, Arslanian SA, Connor EL, et al. (2017) Pediatric Obesity-Assessment, Treatment, and Prevention: An Endocrine Society Clinical Practice Guideline. *The Journal of Clinical Endocrinology and Metabolism* **102**(3): 709–757. doi:10.1210/jc.2016-2573

van Vuuren CL, Wachter GG, Veenstra R, et al. (2019) Associations between overweight and mental health problems among adolescents, and the mediating role of victimization. *BMC Public Health* **19**(1): 612. Published 2019 May 21. doi:10.1186/s12889-019-6832-z

Wang L, van Grieken A, Yang-Huang J, et al. (2018) Relationship between socioeconomic status and weight gain during infancy: The BeeBOFT study. *PLoS One* **13**(11): e0205734. Published 2018 Nov 2. doi:10.1371/journal.pone.0205734

Physical Activity and Health

Leppänen MH, Henriksson P, Henriksson H, Delisle Nyström C, Llorente-Cantarero FJ, Löf M (2018) Physical Activity Level Using Doubly-Labeled Water in Relation to Body Composition and Physical Fitness in Preschoolers. *Medicina (Kaunas)* **55**(1): 2. Published 2018 Dec 27. doi:10.3390/medicina55010002

Ubago-Guisado E, Mata E, Sánchez-Sánchez J, Plaza-Carmona M, Martín-García M, Gallardo L (2017) Influence of different sports on fat mass and lean mass in growing girls. *Journal of Sport and Health Science* **6**(2): 213–218. doi:10.1016/j.jshs.2015.06.001

Park J, Ishikawa-Takata K, Lee S, et al. (2018) Comparison of daily physical activity parameters using objective methods between overweight and normal-weight children. *Journal of Sport and Health Science* **7**(2): 210–217. doi:10.1016/j.jshs.2017.01.008

Hussey J, Bell C, Bennett K, O'Dwyer J, Gormley J. (2007) Relationship between the intensity of physical activity, inactivity, cardiorespiratory fitness and body composition in 7-10-year-old Dublin children. *British Journal of Sports Medicine* **41**(5): 311–316. doi:10.1136/bjsm.2006.032045

Resources

HENRY Programme for Family behaviour change: https://www.henry.org.uk/henryapproach

National Obesity Observatory (www.noo.org.uk)

NHS Physical Activity Guidelines for Children: https://www.nhs.uk/live-well/exercise/physical-activity-guidelines-children-and-young-people/ Accessed June 2020

Planet Munch Healthy Lifestyle Programme http://www.trimtots.com/

19

Nutrition for children with chronic diseases and syndromes

Summary

- Various medical conditions require dietary modification and to ensure nutritional adequacy to support health and normal growth, advice from a paediatric dietitian is required.
- Nutritional support is necessary for several conditions and may be delivered using higher energy family foods or prescribable sterile nutritional supplements.
- Some or all of a child's nutritional requirements may be provided by tube feeding when a child is unable to consume their energy and nutrient requirements orally.
- Pumps and plastics for home enteral tube feeding can be delivered directly to the home or a holiday destination.
- Children with coeliac disease need to eat a gluten-free diet and entitlement to a monthly allowance of gluten-free products on prescription is at the discretion of the local health authrority.
- Children with cystic fibrosis usually need a diet higher in energy and certain nutrients and usually take pancreatic enzymes with each meal and snack.
- Children with cancer may need nutritional support when their appetite is decreased.
- Children with insulin-dependent diabetes may need to control the carbohydrate content of their diet and the distribution of the carbohydrate throughout each day.

Medical conditions requiring dietary modifications

Several medical conditions in infants and children require a modified nutritional intake to treat or ameliorate either the condition itself or the consequences of some medical treatments. Table 19.1 lists the dietary modifications required for several medical conditions, the more common of which are discussed in further detail in the rest of this chapter. For a comprehensive guide to the treatment for all paediatric conditions requiring dietary modification, students and practitioners should use the 5th edition of *Clinical Paediatric Dietetics* edited by Vanessa Shaw and published by Wiley Blackwell (Shaw 2020).

Considerations when advising and supporting parents and carers

When an infant or child is diagnosed with a medical condition, it can be very traumatic for the family and they may need time to come to terms with the diagnosis before they can embark on a programme of learning about the extra responsibility of following the dietary modifications required of them. Parents may have to deal with

Table 19.1 Medical conditions and the main dietary modifications

Medical condition	Dietary modifications
Autistic spectrum disorders including attention deficit hyperactivity disorder (ADHD) and Asperger's syndrome	Extra nutrient supplementation to address any nutritional deficiencies in children with very selective eating.
	Parents can be supported when they wish to trial various dietary modifications to ascertain if this will improve symptoms in their child.
Burns	Increased energy, protein nutrient or fluid requirements depending on the extent of the injury, mobility and albumin levels.
	Early enteral feeding in children with major burns. Increased intake of prebiotics and probiotics in those with diarrhoea.
Cancer	Varies according to symptoms. Frequently nutritional support to address poor growth or a poor appetite as a result of cachexia or drug treatments.
Carbohydrate intolerances such as lactose, sucrose, glucose, fructose or galactose intolerance	Avoidance or limited intake of the sugar causing the intolerance.
Coeliac disease	A gluten-free diet avoiding the protein gluten found in wheat, rye and barley. Some children may also need to avoid the protein avenin in oats.
Congenital heart disease	Increased energy requirements and/or energy to be provided in smaller volumes of food or fluid.
Cystic fibrosis (CF)	Increased energy, protein and nutrient requirements to address malabsorption. Nutritional support is frequently needed to promote growth and an adequate BMI.
	About 90 per cent of children with cystic fibrosis take oral pancreatic enzyme treatments to improve their digestion and absorption of protein, fat and some vitamins
Diabetes – type 1	Controlled carbohydrate intakes to coordinate with insulin treatment.
Epilepsy	When patients do not respond to medication, a ketogenic diet, which is very high in fat and low in carbohydrate, may be tried.
Fat malabsorption	Reduced fat intake or a modified fat intake.
HIV and AIDS	Healthy eating to optimise immune system as even with undetectable viral loads, these children are more vulnerable to infection. Nutritional support when appetite is reduced or growth faltering. Limited saturated fat intake if cholesterol levels are raised.
Inherited metabolic disorders	Can affect metabolism of protein, fat or carbohydrate. Varies with the disorder – likely to be the restricted intake of one or more nutrients (e.g. specific amino acids).
Inflammatory bowel diseases: Crohn's disease	Varies according to symptoms of intestinal inflammation, nausea, poor appetite, malabsorption and malnutrition. Some centres use periods of a specified formula feed in place of all food to induce remission of symptoms followed by a diet excluding any foods that induce symptoms in that particular child.
Kidney disease	Nutritional support to address poor appetite and malnutrition. High-energy diet with modified fluid, protein, phosphate, sodium, potassium, calcium intakes may be required depending on the severity and type of disease and mode of renal replacement.
Liver disease	Nutritional support to address malnutrition and poor appetite. High-energy diet using specialised feeds, modified fat to address fat malabsorption, addition of branched chain amino acids and fat-soluble vitamins depending on the severity and type of disease.

(Continued)

Table 19.1 (Continued)

Medical condition	Dietary modifications
Neurological impairment, e.g. cerebral palsy and Down's syndrome	Food texture modifications or nutritional support to address feeding difficulties resulting from impaired oral motor functions such as poor chewing and swallowing.
	Decreased energy requirements if there is limited mobility.
	Portion control where there is a tendency towards obesity as in Down's syndrome.
	Increased energy requirements when there are frequent unwanted movements or congenital heart defects.
Poorly functioning or non-functioning gastrointestinal tract (gastrointestinal dysmotility or intestinal failure or feed intolerance)	Parenteral nutrition.
	Minimal enteral (trophic) feeding to maintain brush border integrity of the gastrointestinal tract may be appropriate.
Phenylketonuria	Controlled low intake of the amino acid phenylalanine.
Physical disabilities	Food texture modifications to address feeding difficulties.
	Decreased energy requirements if there is limited mobility.
Prader-Willi syndrome	Nutritional support for faltering growth in the first 2 years followed by controlled energy intake to prevent or minimise obesity.

guilt feelings, particularly if their child's condition was genetically inherited.

Individualised advice from a paediatric dietitian with experience of the medical condition is needed for any dietary modification. The aims of dietary treatment are to meet the nutritional and energy requirements for each child. This can sometimes be achieved using family foods and extra nutrient supplementation using over-the-counter supplements found in supermarkets and pharmacies. However, for more complex dietary needs, specialist dietary products are prescribable for specific conditions (listed in British National Formulary for Children: Borderline Substances).

When giving individualised advice to families, the paediatric dietitian needs to consider:

- family routines and food and drink preferences;
- family budget for food, drinks and supplements;
- family's knowledge of food and cooking skills;
- how well the parents and child understand the dietary treatment aims;
- the facilities available to the family for managing the dietary modifications.

The impact of dietary modifications on family lifestyle and the quality of life of the child or whole family should not be underestimated. Some modifications may make it difficult or even prevent the child from eating at school, at friends' homes, on school trips or other trips away from home.

Non-compliance with dietary treatment may occur for several reasons:

- young children may refuse foods if they do not like the taste, texture or appearance;
- older children may refuse to follow the dietary modifications in social settings rather than appear different to their peer group;
- adolescents may refuse to comply with both dietary and medical treatments to assert their independence;
- children may realise that by refusing to comply they are able to manipulate their parents or carers.

Nutritional support for children with an inadequate appetite to satisfy their energy and nutrient requirements

Malnutrition develops when children are unable to eat sufficient quantities of food and drink to satisfy their energy and nutrient requirements in the long term. This may begin to impact on health and growth if it is not addressed. The main causes of an inadequate oral intake are:

- decreased appetite due to the medical conditions and/or treatments;
- malabsorption increases the energy and nutrition requirements above that for healthy children;
- increased nutrient requirements due to altered metabolism, chronic illness, fever or a high level of physical activity.

The options available to increase energy and nutrient intakes are:

- more energy-dense foods and drinks so that more energy is taken within the same volume of food/drink;
- prescribable high-energy drinks or sip feeds to supplement or replace oral intake;
- supplementary tube feeding by bolus during the daytime or by pump during the day or overnight;
- 100 per cent of energy and nutrient requirements via tube feeding.

Increasing the energy density of the normal diet by adding extra carbohydrate and/or fat

Advice needs to be tailored to foods normally eaten and may include:

- adding extra sugar or syrups to breakfast cereals, puddings, drinks and other sweet foods;
- stirring extra cream or powdered milk into milk drinks and puddings;
- frying foods rather than grilling or baking them;
- adding extra oil or butter to vegetables, pasta, rice, sauces and gravies;
- adding a prescribable supplement containing carbohydrate and/or fat. These are much less sweet than sugar and should not greatly alter the taste of the food/drink. Suitable products include: Maxijul, Polycal, Vitajoule (carbohydrate), Calogen (fat) and Duocal (combined carbohydrate and fat).

Prescribable high-energy drinks or sip feeds

Several companies make a wide variety of these prescribable products which are either milk-based or juice-style drinks. A variety of flavours are available and it is a matter of trial and error to find which flavours each individual child will drink. Volumes vary and 200–250 ml bottles or cartons for drinking are usual. One such drink per day may be adequate or a child may need to try and drink 2 or 3. When they are drunk at the end of a meal or snack they are less likely to reduce the appetite for normal foods.

As they are an expensive item for a GP's budget, care should be taken to review the prescription frequently to make sure they are not being wasted by being thrown away once a child has begun to refuse them through taste boredom.

Tube feeding

When children are not able to eat or drink as much as they need to maintain a normal growth rate, feeding via a tube may be recommended (Martinez-Costa et al. 2019). Tube feeding may provide:

- some of their nutrient requirements to supplement a limited oral intake;
- all their energy and nutrient requirements where no oral intake is possible;
- specialised formulas for various disease states that may be unpalatable to the child who refuses to take them orally.

Tube feeding can be either continuous or bolus feeding:

- In continuous feeding the food is supplied over a long period of time via a pump. The flow rate can be adjusted. This is usual for overnight feeding when a child is in bed. For daytime tube feeding a child can wear a small backpack containing a small portable pump. The child can carry on with most daily activities while being tube fed this way.
- Bolus feeding can also use a pump or can be administered using gravity for the feed to drain down the tube.

Children who may need to be tube fed for some time are those who:

- are critically ill and require ventilation;
- have severe developmental delay;
- have malformations around the mouth;
- have faltering growth.

The routes of tube feeding can be via:

- a nasogastric tube or much less commonly an orogastric tube;
- a nasojejunal tube when the stomach needs to be bypassed;
- a tube connected to a gastrostomy or jejunostomy button – used for longer term feeding.

Nasogastric tube feeding

This route is used when a child initially requires tube feeding or requires it for a short time. A thin tube is passed through the child's nose down into the stomach so that liquids can be slowly pumped into the stomach. The tube is usually held in place by being taped to the child's cheek. They are easily pulled out and can be re-passed quite easily if the child is cooperative.

Orogastric tube feeding

In orogastric tube feeding, the tube is passed via the mouth down into the stomach.

Gastrostomy feeding

If tube feeding continues to be necessary for a longer period of time (about 6 weeks or more), gastrostomy feeding may be used (Martínez-Costa et al. 2019). A gastrostomy is formed which requires a minor surgical procedure: a short tube is passed directly through the child's skin and stomach wall and into the stomach. It is held in position with a plastic clamp or a button with a small inflatable balloon that sits inside the stomach. The feeding tube can then be connected directly to the gastrostomy device without having to go via the nose/mouth. When this form of feeding is no longer needed, the gastrostomy device can be removed and the small hole in the skin and stomach wall will close over and heal. A tiny scar may be the only indication that this route of feeding was ever used.

Jejunostomy feeding is either via a nasojejunostomy tube or a jejunostomy button. Jejunostomy feeding must be slow and continuous using a pump so that the jejunum does not receive large volumes of feed over a short period of time which can result in malabsorption. Bolus feeding is not appropriate when the natural reservoir of the stomach is bypassed. The pump flow rate will depend on the child's tolerance.

Feeds available for tube feeding

Several companies make a variety of sterile tube feeds that are 'ready to feed'. They can provide either complete nutrition or partial nutrition. Standard feeds have an energy content of 1 kcal/ml and are designed for different age groups to provide adequate energy, nutrients and fibre within a suitable fluid load for that age range: 0–1 year, 1–6 years and 7–12 years. Children over 12 years are usually given feeds formulated for adults.

Non-standard feeds include those providing complete nutrition:

- in lower volumes;
- with lower or higher energy content;
- with varying levels of fibre;
- with varying fat content such as different combinations of long and medium chain triglycerides;
- with varying protein type such as complete protein, hydrolysed protein or simple amino acids.

Although there is a choice of brands, commonly an NHS Hospital Trust will have a contract with one of the companies and use their products exclusively, where possible, at a lower cost. Feeds for children at home are prescribed by their GP usually on the advice of a paediatric dietitian or paediatrician.

Blended diets for gastrostomy feeding

Increasingly parents with children on long term tube feeding are keen to use blended family foods to be used in place of the synthetic feeds discussed above. This gives parents the opportunity to take more control over feeding their child in a less medical way (Coad et al. 2017). Parents can be supported to do this with advice on:

- hygienic preparation of the blended foods – as the acidic stomach is not bypassed food safety is not compromised;
- avoiding tube blockage and how to clear a blocked tube;
- combining foods in meals as they would for a balanced nutritious diet to meet their child's nutrient and energy needs;
- meeting nutritional needs within the fluid volume the child can tolerate – this may involve using an over the counter nutrient supplement.

If parents are not supported, they are likely to try this type of feeding on their own.

Selecting a feed and feeding regimen

A paediatric dietitian can assess a child's nutritional needs and advise on the type of feed and feeding regimen that meets their nutritional requirements. The assessment will include an estimation of their:

- energy requirements, taking into account mobility, activity level, body temperature and the need for catch-up growth or energy restrictions to address obesity;
- fluid requirements;
- nutrient and fibre requirements.

Requirements are usually based on a child's weight so, as the child grows, requirements and the feeding regime need to be regularly reassessed and recalculated.

Considerations when initiating tube feeding

If a child has not been eating for some time a feed may need to be started slowly and increased over several days according to how the child tolerates an increased flow rate or increased energy density. Stomach pain, vomiting and diarrhoea are all indications that the child is not tolerating the feed. However, these symptoms need to be interpreted according to the clinical condition of the child.

The gradual introduction of feed over several days will also protect against the risk of 'refeeding syndrome' in those children who have had very little nutrition for some time.

Support for home tube feeding

When infants and children are tube fed at home, parents and carers need to be trained in:

- operating the pump using appropriate flow rates or bolus volumes;
- frequency and method of changing the plastic tubes (giving sets and reservoirs);
- appropriate flushing of tubes before and after feeding episodes;
- cleaning the gastrostomy site;
- clearing blocked tubes.

Companies making the feeds all have home delivery services to deliver both the sterile plastic tubes (giving sets and reservoirs) and the feeds either to a local pharmacy or directly to the home. They can usually arrange deliveries to holiday accommodation as well. They also have 24-hour helplines to answer carers' queries and offer support to cope with any problems.

Parenteral feeding for critically ill children with poor gut function

This is an expensive treatment and usually only used in hospital. The child is fed directly into a vein with a combination of sterile solutions prepared by a pharmacy. The solutions must be calculated carefully and prescribed for each child. Together these solutions provide fat, carbohydrate, protein, vitamins and minerals. Children can be fed at home by this method but parents require considerable support and training to do this safely and effectively.

Common medical conditions requiring dietary modifications

Autistic spectrum disorders, including attention deficit hyperactivity disorder (ADHD) and Asperger's syndrome

Some children with these disorders only eat a narrow range of foods. This selective eating may be related to either over- or under-sensory perception with tastes, smells, texture and temperature of foods as well as the visual appearance of food. Diaries of foods normally eaten can be assessed by a paediatric dietitian for nutritional adequacy and a supplement recommended for any deficiencies.

Parents often wish to try a variety of dietary modifications for which there is varying anecdotal evidence of symptom improvement in some children. A dietitian can support parents to do this safely so that there is no nutritional risk to the children. Such dietary interventions requested include:

- supplements of zinc, iron, magnesium, omega 3 fatty acids (eicosapentaenoic acid (EPA) in particular), vitamin A, methyl sulphonyl methane/magnesium sulphate, folinic acid, betaine and/or methylcobalamine;
- excluding phenolic compounds, salicylates, aspartame, monosodium glutamate (MSG), artificial colours or benzoates;
- casein and gluten-free diet;
- ketogenic diet – very high-fat and low-carbohydrate.

To assess the effectiveness of any dietary intervention for a particular child, an objective record of symptoms must be kept during a baseline period of the regular diet, the intervention period and then a return to the regular diet as described for open food challenges (see Chapter 17, page 225).

Before embarking on an exclusion diet with a child who eats very selectively it is advisable to assess whether excluding any key foods they normally eat will compromise their energy or nutrient intake, as once foods have been excluded for a while the child may refuse to begin eating them again.

Cancer

Children with cancer may have a reduced appetite due to:

- pain;
- repeated infections when the immune system is compromised due to chemotherapy and radiotherapy;
- nausea and vomiting caused by chemotherapy and radiotherapy;
- diarrhoea because of antibiotic treatments or because of cancer treatments;
- changes to their taste buds making food less enjoyable.

Children eating poorly can become malnourished quite quickly, which will further lower their immune system and they may begin to lose weight.

Considerations for nutritional support

- Small frequent snack-style meals about 5 or 6 times each day may be preferable to 3 big meals and 2–3 small snacks.
- If the child has a sore mouth, very soft foods may be preferable.
- If nausea occurs, cold food may be preferred to hot food.
- Increasing energy intake using extra oil, butter and cream may not be suitable when a child is feeling nauseous. It may be better to try the prescribable high-calorie/high-nutrient drinks. They can be taken as drinks or frozen to make an ice cream substitute.
- Overnight tube feeding is often recommended as it can help to maintain growth, boost the immune system and prevent weight loss.

Coeliac disease

In children with this autoimmune disease, the protein gluten causes the production of destructive antibodies which damage the tissue of the small intestine, causing malabsorption of food.

Gluten is found in the 3 cereals: wheat, rye and barley. All food and drinks made from these cereals need to be eliminated from the diet of a child with coeliac disease. Some children may need to avoid oats as well as they may be sensitive to a similar protein, avenin, in oats. Sometimes oats are contaminated with traces of wheat, rye or barley.

Children with undiagnosed coeliac disease or who are not following their diet may have any of the following symptoms:

- weight loss;
- poor growth;
- diarrhoea;
- nausea;
- wind;
- tiredness;
- constipation;
- anaemia;
- mouth ulcers;
- headaches;
- hair loss;
- skin problems.

Foods that should be included or eliminated in a gluten-free diet are listed in Table 19.2.

Parents and children need to check the labels on food packaging of all commercial foods for

Table 19.2 Foods to include or eliminate in a gluten-free diet

Food groups	Foods to include	Foods to eliminate	Special gluten-free foods available
1. Starchy foods: bread, rice, potatoes, pasta and other starchy foods	Rice, potatoes, yam, millet, sago, tapioca, quinoa, teff Flours made from arrowroot, buckwheat, chickpeas (gram flour), corn, lentil, maize and rice. Some brands of corn flakes and rice krispies	Any foods made from wheat, rye, barley, spelt or oats. This includes a large range of commercial bread, pasta, couscous, semolina, crackers, breakfast cereals, pizza bases, buns and pancakes	Gluten-free flours, cereals, breads, crackers and crispbreads. Some are prescribable.
2. Fruit and vegetables	Fresh, frozen, tinned and dried fruits and vegetables	Vegetable soups thickened with wheat flour	
3. Milk, cheese and yogurt	Breast milk, formula milks, cow's milk, goat's milk, yogurts, cheese and milk puddings	Milk puddings that are thickened with wheat flour	
4. Meat, fish, eggs, nuts and pulses	Meat, fish, eggs, nuts and pulses (lentils, dhal, chickpeas, hummus, kidney beans and other similar starchy beans)	Any foods coated in flour, batter or breadcrumbs	Chickpea, lentil and gram flour
5. Oils, butter and fat spreads	Cream, butter, margarines, cooking and salad oils		
6. Cakes, biscuits and puddings		Biscuits, cakes, foods with pastry	Gluten-free biscuits, cakes and pastry
7. Sauces and sweet and savoury spreads	Jam, honey and syrup,	Most commercial sauces are thickened with wheat flour Ready meals will often contain flour	
8. Sweet drinks confectionery and high fat packet snacks	Most soft drinks, smoothies and fruit juices Crisps and corn chips Water	Some drinks contain barley Some packet snacks contain wheat flour	

their suitability. Although foods are often marked as 'gluten free' on the label, the ingredients list needs to be checked for any of the following ingredients, which contain gluten or avenin: wheat, farina, flour, rusk, semolina, starch, vegetable protein, wheatgerm and wheatgerm oil, rye, barley, barley malt, oats and spelt.

Food Labelling Regulations on gluten free and low gluten foods

EU Guideline Regulation (EU) No 828/2014 requires that foods can only be labelled:

- **gluten free** if the food contains no more than 20ppm or 20mg gluten/kg food;
- **very low gluten** if a food containing wheat, rye, barley, oats or their crossbred varieties has been specially processed to reduce the gluten content, and contains no more than 100 ppm or 100 mg gluten/kg food.

Oats contained in a food presented as gluten-free or very low gluten must have been specially produced, prepared and/or processed in a way to avoid contamination by wheat, rye, barley or their crossbred varieties and the gluten content of such oats cannot exceed 20 mg/kg.

Coeliac UK (www.coeliac.org.uk) is the charity that offers support and advice to both

- families with coeliac disease and;
- food businesses with advice on food labelling of gluten content.

Their online Food and Drink Directory, which lists all the gluten-free commercial foods available in the UK is updated as recipes change. Food companies can be licensed to use their crossed grained symbol, Figure 19.1, guaranteeing that their food products contain no more than 20 ppm gluten.

Prescribable gluten-free foods

There are many specialist food companies that make gluten-free food products, and in some NHS Trusts children with coeliac disease are entitled to some gluten free bread and/or flour on prescription from their GP. However this varies over time and depends on the policy of each NHS Trust.

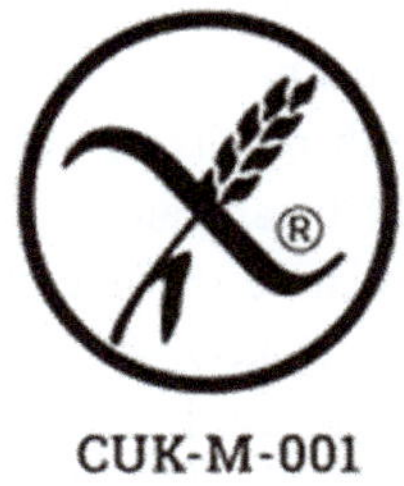

Figure 19.1 Crossed grain symbol

Cystic fibrosis

Cystic fibrosis is a genetic disorder which is inherited from both parents. It is relatively common in white populations and less so in Asian, African and Middle Eastern families. Several of the glands in the body do not function well and this causes lung disease, malabsorption of food and very salty sweat. Cystic fibrosis is usually diagnosed by measuring the amount of salt in a child's sweat.

Symptoms of the disease vary considerably between children and some may have more respiratory problems while others have more problems with malabsorption of food, particularly the fat in food.

The problems of malabsorption are due to a poor production of enzymes from the pancreas which are needed to digest foods in the small intestine so that they can be absorbed into the body. To improve the absorption of their food, about 90 per cent of children with cystic fibrosis are prescribed pancreatic enzyme supplements to be swallowed along with meals and snacks. The amount recommended varies from child to child depending on their symptoms. A vitamin and mineral supplement is also prescribed as the fat-soluble vitamins A, D, E and K are usually poorly absorbed.

Infants and children with cystic fibrosis generally need a higher energy intake than normal healthy children. To achieve this, children with cystic fibrosis need to eat more food with a higher energy content. They are encouraged to eat foods containing high amounts of fat and sugar in addition to a balanced diet based on the food groups described in Chapter 2.

Unfortunately cystic fibrosis infants and children often have a poor appetite, especially if they are often ill with respiratory illnesses. Some may have reflux which can cause pain on eating. Poor appetites often cause considerable stress for parents, who are very keen for their children to eat well to prevent more illness. Parents of toddlers with cystic fibrosis report more feeding problems than do parents of healthy toddlers.

Parents and older children usually plan the child's diet with a dietitian and he or she will advise on how many capsules of pancreatic enzymes to take with each meal and snack.

Children whose growth is inadequate may be prescribed high-calorie drinks as supplements. From time to time their calorie intake may be supplemented by tube feeding. Overnight tube feeding is commonly used, particularly in teenagers.

Diabetes

There are 2 types of diabetes:

- *Type 1 diabetes* is an autoimmune disease in which the cells in the pancreas that produce the hormone insulin are destroyed. It affects about 25,000 children in the UK and can be diagnosed at any age. It is treated with insulin.
- *Type 2 diabetes* develops when the cells in the body become resistant to insulin. It affects around 400 children in the UK, usually arising in obese teenage children. It may be controlled initially just by diet or hyperglycaemic agents but insulin treatment may be instigated as the disease progresses.

Without enough insulin or with insulin resistance, glucose in the blood will not pass into the body's cells to provide a source of energy. The glucose remains in the blood, resulting in hyperglycaemia. When this occurs before children are diagnosed they may lose weight and complain of excessive thirst. Ketones may be smelt in the breath as they are released when cells break down fat as a source of energy in the absence of glucose.

Type 1 diabetes

There are several options for giving the insulin and the medical team will discuss and agree what is the best regimen for each child. Insulin may be given via:

- 1, 2 or 3 insulin injections per day: these are usually injections of short-acting insulin or rapid-acting insulin analogue mixed with intermediate-acting insulin.
- multiple daily injection basal–bolus insulin regimens: injections of short-acting insulin or rapid-acting insulin analogue before meals, together with 1 or more separate daily injections of intermediate-acting insulin or long-acting insulin analogue.
- a small programable insulin pump which delivers fast-acting insulin either continuously or in precise amounts at pre-programmed times. It is about the size of a mobile phone and worn outside the body, often on a belt or in a pocket. It delivers the insulin into the body via an infusion set — a thin plastic tube ending in a small, flexible plastic cannula or a very thin needle. The cannula is inserted beneath the skin at the infusion site, usually in the abdomen or upper buttocks. The infusion set is kept in place for 2 to 3 days (sometimes more) and is then moved to a new location. All insulin is delivered through the infusion set.

A balanced, nutritious diet based on the food groups described in Chapter 2 is the basis of a diet for diabetic children. The diet and eating routine for each individual child is planned in consultation with a dietitian around the energy and carbohydrate needed by that child depending on:

- their age and appetite;
- activity levels;
- growth rate.

Carbohydrate is digested in the small intestine into sugars that are absorbed into the blood and transported as glucose. The amounts and timing of the carbohydrate eaten should balance the effects of the insulin administered or vice versa so that blood glucose levels remain relatively close to the normal range.

When physically active for any length of time without extra carbohydrate, blood glucose levels can fall as exercise increases the non-insulin-dependent uptake of glucose by cells as well as insulin sensitivity. Hence before extra physical activity children should eat some extra carbohydrate as rapidly absorbable sugary food (e.g. confectionery or chocolate snack bars). With experience, children and parents learn to estimate how much should be eaten to avoid hypoglycaemia during sustained physical activity.

When receiving advice on a diabetic diet, parents and older children need to understand or be taught:

- how much carbohydrate is to be consumed;
- how to distribute it through the day and load it at times just before the child is going to be particularly physically active;
- how to calculate how much carbohydrate has been ingested when the whole meal or snack is not consumed.

Often, a list of foods each containing 10 g carbohydrate is used to help work out how much food will provide the appropriate amount of carbohydrate. These food portions are called '10 g carbohydrate exchanges' and examples are listed in Table 19.3. The range is from about 13–18 exchanges of 10 g carbohydrate each day for a toddler, to 35–40 exchanges for a very active teenager going through their adolescent growth spurt.

Commercial foods state the amount of carbohydrate on the label and this can be used to work out how much carbohydrate is in a portion of food that the child eats.

Sweet puddings, confectionery and other sugary foods do not have to be cut out altogether. The overall free sugars intake can be about 5–10 per cent of total energy as for normal healthy eating. Foods with free sugars are better given at the end of meals rather than as snacks as at the end of a meal the sugar will be absorbed more slowly and therefore less likely to make the blood glucose levels rise quickly.

Special diabetic foods are not necessary and are better avoided. Sorbitol, which is a sweetener, is often used in special diabetic foods and can cause diarrhoea.

A routine of meals and snacks is recommended for those on insulin injections so that similar amounts of carbohydrate are offered at each meal and snack. A young child having 15 carbohydrate exchanges each day may have them distributed through the day like this:

Breakfast	3
Mid-morning snack	2
Midday meal	3
Mid-afternoon snack	2
Evening meal	3
Snack before bed	2
Total for the day	15

An example one-day menu for such a child is shown in Table 19.4.

Glycaemic index

The glycaemic index of the meals and snacks eaten is a measure of how quickly blood glucose levels rise after eating that meal or snack. Sugary foods, such as sweets and confectionery, have a very high glycaemic index as the blood sugar rises high very quickly when these are eaten on their own. To keep the glycaemic index of a meal or snack low so that the blood sugar rises slowly, a balanced diet as described in Chapter 2 should be offered, including foods with fibre at each meal:

- Include fruit with breakfast and at least 1 fruit and 1 vegetable with the other 2 meals.
- Encourage wholemeal varieties of bread and cereals (e.g. wholemeal bread and porridge, a mixture of brown and white rice).

Hypoglycaemia

Hypoglycaemia (low blood glucose levels) may occur when:

Table 19.3 Ten-gram carbohydrate exchanges

Food items		Quantity providing 10 g carbohydrate
Bread	Wholemeal or white slices	½ large slice or 1 small slice
	Rolls or baps	½ roll
Breakfast cereals	Porridge	7 tbsp
	Weetabix	1 biscuit
	Corn flakes/Cheerios	5 tbsp
Rice and pasta	Cooked brown or white rice	3 tbsp
	Cooked pasta shapes	3 tbsp
	Spaghetti	10 long strands
	Tinned spaghetti	⅓ small tin
Potatoes	Boiled potatoes	1 small
	Baked potatoes	1 medium
	Chips	5 thick cut
Beans	Baked beans in tomato sauce	5 tbsp
	Dried uncooked beans	2 tbsp
Fruit	Apple	1 medium
	Pear	1 medium
	Banana	1 medium
	Grapes	10
	Orange	1 medium
	Satsumas/clementines	2 small
	Dried fruit	1 tbsp
Yogurt and ice cream	Natural yogurt	1 carton
	Fruit sweetened yogurt	½ carton
	Ice cream	1 scoop
Biscuits	Oatcakes	1 large
	Crackers	2
	Crispbreads – wholewheat or rye	2
	Digestive	1
Drinks	Milk	2 glasses of 100 ml
	Unsweetened pure fruit juice	2 glasses of 50 ml pure juice diluted with 50 ml water

1 tbsp = one 15 ml tablespoon.

- a child has not had enough carbohydrate to eat – he or she may be late for a meal or a snack or may have refused to eat;
- a child has had extra exercise without eating extra carbohydrate or reducing the insulin dose;
- too much insulin has been given or it may have been given at the wrong time;

Table 19.4 Sample 1-day menu for a young child with diabetes allowed 15 carbohydrate exchanges

Meal or snack		Number of carbohydrate exchanges	Total number of carbohydrate exchanges for each meal or snack
Breakfast	2 Weetabix	2	3
	100 ml milk	½	
	½ banana sliced	½	
Mid-morning snack	½ apple sliced	½	2
	1 digestive biscuit	1	
	100 ml milk to drink	½	
Midday meal	1 large slice toast with butter	2	3
	tbsp baked beans	½	
	Cucumber and carrot sticks		
	5 grapes	½	
Mid-afternoon snack	digestive biscuits		2
	1 satsuma	½	
	Water to drink		
Evening meal	3 tbsp cooked pasta	1	3
	Bolognaise sauce		
	Broccoli florets		
	1 carton fruit yogurt	1	
	5 strawberries	½	
	50 ml fruit juice diluted with water	½	
Snack before bed	1 large slice toast with butter	2	2

- food may not have been absorbed because the child has diarrhoea or has vomited;
- alcohol has been consumed – one effect of alcohol consumption is to lower blood glucose levels.

During hypoglycaemia blood glucose levels become too low for the brain to function properly and a child will not always be able to indicate that they need more glucose to correct the hypoglycaemia.

General symptoms of hypoglycaemia are:

- pallor;
- mood swings;
- irritability;
- headache;
- hunger;
- fatigue;
- becoming uncooperative;
- becoming confused;
- finally losing consciousness and fitting.

Young children may not be able to describe any of these early symptoms but parents, teachers or carers might notice a child becoming confused or uncooperative. A young child might say he feels funny or has shaky or wobbly legs. Older children may be able to clearly recognise their early signs of hypoglycaemia.

To treat hypoglycaemia a child needs to be given some carbohydrate that will be rapidly absorbed to restore the blood glucose levels to within the normal range. Carbohydrate that is rapidly absorbed will be glucose or sugar or a sugary food or drink.

Examples are:

- glucose tablets or sweets to suck;
- about 50 ml of a glucose drink or non-diet squash or;
- 2–3 teaspoons of jam or honey or syrup.

If a child becomes confused or uncooperative it may be preferable to squeeze a glucose gel into the mouth or rub it on the gums. The glucose will be absorbed rapidly to raise blood glucose levels out of the danger zone. Glucose gels are available over the counter from pharmacies and can be prescribed. A store can be kept handy for hypoglycaemic emergencies.

If hypoglycaemia happens frequently then it is time to reassess the child's insulin regimen and carbohydrate intake. The solution may be either to increase the daily carbohydrate intake or reduce the insulin regimen.

Coping with food refusal in children with diabetes

As discussed in Chapter 12, toddlers and young children may at times refuse to eat or they may eat much less of a food than expected, particularly if they are going through a phase of food refusal. Food refusal can cause more anxiety for parents of diabetic toddlers who are concerned about hypoglycaemia. If parents begin to offer alternative foods, a child soon learns to manipulate the parent through food refusal. Force feeding should never be used and parents can try to minimise their anxiety, relying on the child becoming hungry as their blood glucose level falls. One solution is to inject insulin after meals and snacks, rather than before, calculated on how much carbohydrate has been consumed.

Adolescents may also refuse to follow their usual routine, refusing both insulin treatment and/or dietary routines for a period – just to test out the necessity of it. Some may reduce insulin intake as a means of losing weight, a condition referred to as 'Diabluminia'.

Type 2 diabetes

Dietary treatment in children with type 2 diabetes is also a nutritious, balanced, low glycaemic index diet with carbohydrate spread out evenly throughout the day. Obese children should also aim for a negative energy balance so that they lose weight because the progression of their disease will be slower in the absence of obesity.

Inflammatory bowel diseases – Crohn's disease

The intestinal inflammation in Crohn's disease is believed to be caused by an immune reaction against certain bacterial colonisation of the bowel. The inflammation can occur anywhere from the mouth to the anus although most commonly in the terminal ileum or colon. The normal food residues passing through the gastrointestinal tract are thought to be the energy source for these bacteria. To induce remission from the inflammation exclusive enteral nutrition (EEN) using a synthetic liquid diet free of all food residues for 6–12 weeks is used in preference to treatment by corticosteroids. The advantages of EEN are:

- growth support;
- avoidance of corticosteroid-associated adverse effects;
- more effective healing of the mucosa.

However strict adherence to EEN can be difficult as it requires some children to place a nasogastric tube each evening, or keep it in all day, for nocturnal continuous feeding. Some success has been seen with partial enteral nutrition regimens as maintenance therapy, such as overnight feedings with a normal daytime diet or nasogastric feeding for 1 of every 4 months (Rosen et al. 2015).

The synthetic liquid diet has one of the following as a protein source:

- single amino acids – an elemental feed;
- short chains of amino acids – an oligopeptide or hydrolysed protein feed;
- whole protein from a single source (e.g. casein).

A paediatric dietitian must ensure that the quantity of whichever feed is consumed will provide adequate energy and nutrients for the child. With the onset of the disease, often these children have a reduced appetite and may have already lost weight. Growth faltering may also be present.

The feeds are usually drunk orally but can be taken via a tube if children do not like the taste or cannot manage the required volume orally. Once the inflammation has resolved – usually after about 6–12 weeks – normal foods are introduced one by one. Any food that causes symptoms is stopped and introduction of other foods continues. The final diet is then made up of foods that do not cause symptoms. If there are any nutritional deficits, a dietitian can advise on a suitable supplement to correct the deficiency.

Neurological disabilities – cerebral palsy, Down's syndrome, muscular dystrophy and degenerative disorders

When motor function is affected in children with a neurological disability poor nutritional intake can result. The more severe the disability, the more limited the oral intake and the more likely malnutrition will arise.

Impairment of oral motor function can limit the ability to suck, drink, bite, chew, seal the lips, use the tongue effectively and swallow. Symptoms include:

- weak sucking in infants;
- poor progression through food textures during complementary feeding;
- coughing, choking and gagging on foods;
- vomiting;
- frequent respiratory infections from aspiration of food into the lungs.

Gastrointestinal muscle tone may also be impaired, resulting in limited absorption of nutrients and/or gastro-oesophageal reflux.

Feeding takes longer and usually requires a parent or carer's dedicated time as well. A multidisciplinary assessment is important:

- *Speech and language therapist* can assess biting and chewing skills and safety of swallow. Video-fluoroscopy of swallowed liquid and solids may be used to ascertain whether food/drink is spilling into the air passages and lungs causing coughing, wheezing and chest infections.
- *Occupational therapist* can advise on the most appropriate seating for mealtimes and on any eating aids that will help.
- *Physiotherapist* can advise on an ideal position for oral feeding.
- *Dietitian* can assess their nutritional intake with the current regimen and suggest improvements.
- *Paediatrician* can treat any gastro-oesophageal reflux, oesophagitis, slow gastric emptying or constipation.

Thickening liquids may help with control of swallowing liquids. However, if oral feeding is not considered safe then tube feeding directly into the stomach must be commenced. Most children will require nutritional support and tube feeding to provide partial or total nutritional intake.

Ideally, all children with neurological disabilities should have regular assessments of their:

- energy and nutrient requirements – both increase as children grow and care needs to be taken during the adolescent growth spurt when nutritional needs increase markedly to support this rapid growth rate. Overall energy requirements may be lower than the norm in children with limited mobility or higher than the norm in children who make frequent involuntary movements;
- actual nutritional intake and challenges to achieving their nutritional needs – this may change with time;
- weight and growth – this may require the use of specialist anthropological measuring equipment depending on the child's posture and muscle tone. It may be necessary to track growth through limb measurements or sitting height rather than standing height.

Down's syndrome

Children with Down's syndrome often have:

- reduced muscle tone leading to minor feeding difficulties;
- congenital heart defects which may increase their energy requirement;
- gastrointestinal problems such as constipation and gastro-oesophageal reflux.

When assessing their needs, growth must be plotted on specialist Down's syndrome charts because short stature is a component of the syndrome.

Activity 1

Plan a 1-day menu for a diabetic diet for a 12-year-old girl, with 50 per cent of her energy requirements as carbohydrate spread evenly over 3 meals and 2 snacks. Add in an extra 20 g of rapidly absorbed carbohydrate for volleyball practice after school.

Activity 2

Write a letter to a school outlining the needs and menu suggestions for a newly diagnosed 7-year-old boy with coeliac disease who wishes to continue eating school meals with his friends rather than take in a packed lunch and have to sit in another room.

Activity 3

Design a feeding regimen using a feed that provides 1 kcal/ml for a 5-year-old girl with cancer. She has lost weight and now weighs 14 kg and needs 40 per cent of her energy and nutrient requirements as an overnight feed. She is in bed from 7 pm to 6.30 am. Her parents go to bed at 11 pm.

Acknowledgements

With thanks to Vanessa Shaw, previously Head of Dietetics, Great Ormond Street Hospital for Children NHS Trust, London.

References and further reading

British Society of Paediatric Gastroenterology Hepatology and Nutrition (BSPGHAN) and Coeliac UK (2013) Guidelines for the diagnosis and management of coeliac disease in children.

Brown AC, Rampertab SD and Mullin GE (2011) Existing dietary guidelines for Crohn's disease and ulcerative colitis. *Expert Review of Gastro enterology and Hepatology* **5**(3): 411–425.

Coad J, Toft A, Lapwood S, et al. (2017) Blended foods for tube-fed children: a safe and realistic option? A rapid review of the evidence. *Archives of Diseases in Childhood* **102**(3): 274–278. doi:10.1136/archdischild-2016-311030

Eilander A, Hundscheid DC, Osendarp SJ, Transler C and Zock PL (2007) Effects of n-3 long chain polyunsaturated fatty acid supplementation on visual and cognitive development throughout childhood: a review of human studies. *Prostaglandins, Leukotrienes and Essential Fatty Acids* **76**(4): 189–203.

ESPGHAN Committee on Nutrition, Agostoni C, Braegger C, Decsi T, et al. (2011) Supplementation of N-3 LCPUFA to the diet of children older than 2 years: a commentary by the ESPGHAN Committee on Nutrition. *Journal of Pediatric Gastroenterology and Nutrition* **53**(1): 2–10.

Martínez-Costa C, Calderón C, Gómez-López L, Borraz S, Crehuá-Gaudiza E, Pedrón-Giner C (2019) Nutritional Outcome in Home Gastrostomy-Fed Children with Chronic Diseases. *Nutrients* **11**(5): 956. Published 2019 Apr 26. doi:10.3390/nu11050956

Narula N, Dhillon A, Zhang D, Sherlock ME, Tondeur M, Zachos M (2018) Enteral nutritional therapy for induction of remission in Crohn's disease. *Cochrane Database of Systematic Reviews* **4**(4): CD000542. Published 2018 Apr 1. doi:10.1002/14651858.CD000542.pub3

National Institute for Health and Care Excellence (2015) *Nice Guideline NG 20. Recognition, Assessment and Management of Coeliac Disease.* https://www.nice.org.uk/guidance/ng20 (Accessed June 2020).

National Institute for Health and Care Excellence (2016) *NICE Guideline 18.* Diabetes (type 1 and type 2) in children and young people: diagnosis and management. London: NICE. (Accessed June 2020).

Rosen MJ, Dhawan A, Saeed SA (2015) Inflammatory Bowel Disease in Children and Adolescents. *Journal of the American Medical Association Pediatrics* **169**(11): 1053–1060. doi:10.1001/jamapediatrics.2015.1982

Shaw V (2020) *Clinical Paediatric Dietetics*, 5th edn. Oxford: Wiley Blackwell

Wędrychowicz A, Zając A, Tomasik P (2016) Advances in nutritional therapy in inflammatory bowel diseases: Review. *World Journal of Gastroenterology* **22**(3): 1045–1066. doi:10.3748/wjg.v22.i3.1045

Resources

Cerebral palsy support charity (https://www.cerebralpalsy.org.uk/)

Children with Diabetes (www.childrenwithdiabetesuk.org)

Children's HIV Association (www.chiva.org.uk)

Coeliac UK (www.coeliac.org.uk)

Crohn's disease (www.crohns.org.uk)

Down's Syndrome Association (www.downs-syndrome.org.uk)

Juvenile Diabetes Research Foundation (www.jdrf.org.uk)

Answers to activities

Chapter 3

Activity 3

Your answer may include:

- lack of understanding why change is needed
- lack of confidence in the advice given by health professionals compared to their cultural traditions
- communication difficulties with language barriers and sometimes issues with literacy
- senior members of the family being held in great respect and their views on diet having considerable influence, which negatively affects compliance with guidance given by health professionals
- prior experience of receiving inappropriate and insensitive guidance ignoring cultural and religious beliefs.

Activity 4

Your answer may include:

- access to food and shops
- prices of food in accessible shops and markets
- budgeting strategies
- patterns of food choice
- social and cultural acceptability
- other pressures for allocation of limited income (e.g. rent, heating, lighting, clothes/shoes for the children)
- food preferences within the household
- concerns for food waste
- lack of education on benefits of healthy diet
- social support available for families (e.g. Healthy Start Scheme).

Activity 5

Your answer may include these items:

Nutritious choices	Lower nutrient foods that should be limited to small amounts
Bread	Fortified sugar-coated breakfast cereals
Breakfast cereals – fortified but not sugar coated	Fizzy drinks
Cheese	Fruit juices
Yogurt	Fruit smoothies
Fromage frais	Chocolate
Fish fingers	Sweets and confectionery
Frozen vegetables	Biscuits
	Cakes
	Fast food sold with little or no vegetables
	Ice cream
	Crisps and other packet snacks
	Cereal bars

Activity 6

Your answer may include:

- reduced energy expenditure as it displaces more active pastimes
- exposure to food advertising that negatively affects nutritious food choices
- misleading food advertising confuses the understanding of healthy eating.

Activity 7

Your answer could include:

- what parents/carers already 'know' about food (carers are more likely to accept, integrate and act on nutrition information that corresponds with their existing knowledge)

- established food patterns and customs and the extent to which they are followed in the household
- hierarchy within the family
- social pressures and socio-economic factors
- multicultural competencies of health professionals giving the advice, such as using the correct terminology
- access to appropriate foods in the local area
- availability of different foods.

Activity 8

Your answer may include:

- eat with their children as often as possible
- being a role model by eating the foods parents would like their children to eat
- make positive comments about the foods they want their children to eat
- plan a daily routine of 3 meals and 2–3 nutritious snacks
- always offer nutritious foods at meals and snacks
- set boundaries around food, drinks, meals and snacks and stick to them.

Activity 9

Your answer should include ideas involving:

- parental time and attention
- activities involving their parents such as playing games together, sport, visits to a park or outdoor entertainment area
- books and toys
- non-food-related activities.

Activity 10

Your answer may include:

- no strong role models for children to copy positive eating behaviours
- children adopt antisocial mealtime behaviours
- children do not learn to like the food their parents eat.

Chapter 6

Activity 1

a. An underweight woman: balanced eating plan with increased energy intake with the aim of weight gain and increased nutritional stores, exercise levels, alcohol intake, caffeine intake.
b. An overweight couple: balanced eating plan with decreased energy to reduce weight to a healthy BMI for both man and woman, exercise levels, alcohol intake, caffeine intake.
c. A couple both of normal weight: balanced eating plan to improve nutritional status, alcohol intake, exercise levels, caffeine intake, zinc supplements, hazards in the working environment.

Activity 2

Answer to include:

- reduce weight to BMI 18.5–25 kg/m^{2}at least 3–4 months prior to conception
- reduce HbAlc to below 6.1 per cent, and avoid conception if HbAlc is above 10 per cent
- follow a nutritious balanced diet with a daily supplement of 5 mg folic acid and 10 μg vitamin D.

Chapter 7

Activity 1

Answer should include:

- nutritious balanced diet
- vitamin supplementation of folic acid and vitamin D
- 3 servings of milk, cheese and yogurt per day
- encourage high-iron foods
- register for the benefits of the Healthy Start scheme.

Activity 2

Your menu should include:

- food group 1: bread, rice, potatoes, pasta and

other starchy foods – the base for each meal and some snacks using mainly wholegrain varieties
- food group 2: fruit and vegetables – 1 or more of these at each meal and some snacks
- food group 3: milk and dairy foods – 2–3 servings of milk, cheese, yogurt using low-fat varieties
- food group 4: meat, fish, eggs, beans and nuts – 2 or 3 servings
- food group 5: oils butter and fat spreads – used in food preparation
- fluid intake: 6–8 drinks.

Activity 3

Answer should include:

- reheat all food thoroughly so it is piping hot right through
- cook thoroughly all meat and eggs, and foods containing them
- avoid unpasteurised milk and milk products
- avoid pâté and mould-ripened soft cheese
- wear gloves when gardening, dealing with soil or cat litter trays
- wash fruit and vegetables thoroughly to remove any soil
- wash hands after contact with pets
- limit foods containing vitamin A
- limit oily fish to 2 servings per week.

Chapter 11

Activity 1

Preterm infants born at 30 weeks gestation will not have built up the stores of nutrients that term infants will have done. Check that the infant has been prescribed a vitamin supplement and an iron supplement. Complementary feeding can begin as early as 4 months post term age and should include high iron foods from the beginning. If the infant does not have good head control a rolled towel or muslin can be put around the back of the neck to give support.

Chapter 12

Activity

High-iron foods:

	Day 1	Day 2	Day 3
Breakfast	Egg	Baked beans	Muesli with added ground almonds
Midday meal	Chickpea	Dhal	Lentils
Evening meal	Tofu	Egg	Hummus

High-vitamin C foods:

	Day 1	Day 2	Day 3
Breakfast	Orange segments	Tomato sauce on the baked beans	Strawberries
Midday meal	Strawberries	Mango slices	Tomato in bolognaise sauce
Evening meal	Cherry tomatoes	Pepper slices	Kiwi fruit

Chapter 15

Activity 2

Your answer may include:

- developing familiarity with foods by holding cooking sessions, tasting sessions involving teachers making positive comments about the food, and classroom activities such as counting, colouring in, drawing, painting, stories, word searches, quizzes, weighing out foods as part of maths lessons and games
- involving the pupils, parents and staff in planning menus and foods available in other catering outlets

- getting the teachers to eat with the children, eat the same food and make positive comments about the foods
- amending the taught curriculum to contain the concepts of nutrients and components in food in relation to health
- introducing a garden club for pupils to set up a garden where fruits, vegetables and herbs can be grown.

Chapter 18

Activity 1

Your answer may include a range of components, including demonstrations, videos and group discussions rather than focusing on parental education alone. For example:

- planning more nutritious meals and snacks that can be substituted for the high-fat and high-sugar foods that they may normally offer
- interactive cookery demonstrations
- cook-and-eat sessions for parents to improve their cooking skills and their knowledge of healthy eating, and to empower parents to provide healthier family meals
- exploring children's activities that can be substituted for watching TV or DVDs
- increasing daily family physical activity by encouraging more walking instead of always using the car or pushing preschool children around in a buggy
- engaging in local facilities with opportunities for active play and sports.

Appendix 1: Function and Food Sources of Nutrients

Nutrient	Function in the body	Food sources
Protein – usually provides about 15 per cent of energy (kcal)	Provides structure for all the cells in the body. Enzymes and carrier molecules are made of protein. Excess protein is broken down to provide energy.	First-class protein is in milk, yogurt, cheese, meat, fish and eggs. Second-class protein sources: nuts, pulses (such as dhal, lentils, baked beans, hummus and other starchy beans: chickpeas, butter beans and red kidney beans), cereals and foods made from their flours.
Carbohydrate – provides about 50 per cent of energy There are three types: 1. 'simple' sugars, such as lactose in milk, fructose in fruit and added sugar – sucrose and glucose 2. starch 3. fibre, including prebiotics, is made up of carbohydrate complexes that are not absorbed in the intestine	Starch and sugars provide energy. Fibre keeps the gastro-intestinal tract functioning normally. Too little will cause constipation but too much can cause diarrhoea and could slow growth. Insoluble fibre passes through the small and large intestines and is found in the faeces. Soluble fibre is fermented by colonic bacteria to short chain fatty acids required for the normal functioning of the intestines. Prebiotics encourage the growth of beneficial gut bacteria.	Potatoes, yam, breakfast cereals, couscous, rice and any foods containing flour. Wholemeal varieties provide more fibre. Fruits, vegetables, pulses and nuts. The main sugar in fruit and honey is fructose. The main sugar in milk is lactose. The sugar maltose is found in starchy foods. Sweetened foods contain the sugars sucrose and glucose. Prebiotics are a type of fibre found in onions, leeks, garlic and bananas.
Fat – provides about 35 per cent of energy. It is made up of: 1. fatty acids that are: saturated, monounsaturated or polyunsaturated, including omega 3 and omega 6. 2. complex fats (e.g. cholesterol and phospholipids)	Provides energy and carries some vitamins around the body. All cells have fats in their structure.	Oils and animal fats such as lard and suet. Butter and other processed fat spreads. Fried food, cream, cheese, pastry, cakes, biscuits and ice cream. Small amounts in whole milk and yogurt, egg yolks and lean meat.

(*Continued*)

Nutrient	Function in the body	Food sources
	All the fatty acids needed can be synthesised by the human body except the omega 3 and omega 6 fatty acids. Brain, nerves and skin contain very high amounts of omega 3 and omega 6 fats.	Children need a good balance of omega 3 and omega 6 fats. Omega 6 fats are plentiful in food. Oily fish are good sources of omega 3 long-chain fats, DHA (docosahexaenoic acid) and EPA (eicosapentaenoic acid). Rapeseed oil, walnuts and walnut oil are good sources of omega 3 ALA (alpha-linolenic acid). Most pure vegetable oil in the UK is made from rapeseed. Olive and soya oils have a good balance of omega 3 and omega 6 fats.
Water	Maintaining normal hydration, blood pressure and fluid balance.	Most water comes from drinks. Milk, fruit juices and diluted squashes are all about 90 per cent water. Soups, sauces, fruit and vegetables have high water contents.
Vitamins.		
Vitamin A (retinol and carotene)	Ensures normal growth and development, strengthens the immune system, important for healthy intestines, skin and good vision.	Full fat cow's milk, egg yolks, butter and other fats spreads. Orange, red and dark green fruit and vegetables such as carrots, red peppers, tomatoes, sweet potato, pumpkin, apricots, mangoes, cantaloupe melons and broccoli. Oily fish. Liver and liver pâté have very high levels so only one portion per week is recommended.
B vitamins: thiamine, folate, niacin, riboflavin, pyridoxine, biotin, pantothenic acid, vitamin B12	Growth and development of healthy nervous system.	Liver pâté and yeast extracts such as Marmite are the only foods that contain all the B vitamins.

(*Continued*)

Nutrient	Function in the body	Food sources
	Necessary for the processes that convert food into energy.	Meat, milk, yogurt, cheese, fish, eggs, seeds, bread and vegetables. Most children's breakfast cereals are fortified with extra B vitamins.
Vitamin C (ascorbic acid)	Absorption of iron from non-meat sources. Is part of the immune system and protects cells from damage. Maintains blood vessels, cartilage, muscle and bone.	Most fruit and vegetables contain some. The richest sources are blackcurrants, kiwi fruit, citrus fruits, tomatoes, peppers and strawberries. Potato, sweet potatoes and mangoes are also good sources. Certain fruit juices such as blackcurrant and orange have higher levels than other fruit juices.
Vitamin D	Absorption of calcium into the body and regulation of blood calcium levels. Bone health and a component of the immune system.	Most vitamin D is made in exposed skin when outside during the summer months, i.e. April–September in the UK. The few food sources are oily fish and foods fortified with vitamin D, which include some yogurts and fromage frais, some breakfast cereals and formula milks.
Vitamin E	Antioxidant that protects cell structures throughout the body.	In a wide variety of foods. Rich sources are vegetable oils and margarine, avocados, almonds, meat, fish and eggs.
Vitamin K	Blood clotting and bone health.	Mainly produced by bacteria in the large bowel. Food sources are green leafy vegetables and broccoli.
Minerals.		
Calcium	Bone structure and density, teeth, muscle contractions, the structure and functioning of all cells and the working of nerves.	Richest sources are milk, cheese, yogurt and fortified drinks, which are milk substitutes.

(Continued)

Nutrient	Function in the body	Food sources
		White bread is fortified with calcium. Ground almonds. Canned fish with bones such as sardines.
Copper	Energy and protein production.	In small amounts in most foods.
Fluoride	Strengthens tooth enamel making it resistant to attack by the bacteria that cause tooth decay.	Fluoride toothpaste on toothbrush when cleaning teeth twice a day provides enough. It is in tap water in some areas of the UK where tap water is fluoridated, or the water naturally contains adequate levels of fluoride. However, large areas of the UK have water that contains very, very little fluoride.
Iodine	Part of the hormone thyroxine, which is involved in energy production from food and is needed for mental and physical development.	Fish, milk, yogurt, cheese and eggs.
Iron	Necessary for carrying oxygen around the body in the blood and needed for muscle development, energy metabolism and the immune system.	Best sources are red meat (beef, lamb and pork) and dark poultry meat (e.g. chicken legs and thighs). White meat such as chicken breast has less. Other sources are fortified breakfast cereals, nuts, dhal, lentils, hummus, poppadums made with lentil flour, bhajis and Bombay mix made with chickpea flour. Smaller amounts are in fruit and vegetables.
Magnesium	Bone development, making protein and converting food into energy.	Best sources are wholegrain breakfast cereals, milk and yogurt. Also in meat, egg, dhal, lentils, hummus, potatoes and some vegetables.
Phosphorus	Bone and teeth formation, protein and energy production.	Richest source is milk and it is present in most other foods.

(*Continued*)

Nutrient	Function in the body	Food sources
Potassium	Fluid balance, muscle contraction and nerve conduction.	Milk, vegetables and potatoes. Bananas, dried apricots, prunes, dates and kiwi fruit are also good sources.
Selenium	Antioxidant and necessary for production of the thyroid hormone thyroxine.	Bread, meat, fish, nuts, eggs and foods made from flour.
Sodium	Regulation of fluid balance and blood pressure.	Salt is the main source of sodium and salt is used in preserving bacon, ham, cheese and bread. Salt is added to bread, most ready meals, sauces, soups, snacks and other processed foods. Sodium is also found naturally in small quantities in most fresh foods particularly meat, fish, eggs, milk and yogurt. Foods with added salt such as crisps and processed foods should be kept to a minimum.
Zinc	Wound healing and the functioning of many enzymes and hormones.	Best sources are meat, fish, shellfish and eggs. Other good sources are milk, wholegrain breakfast cereals, porridge and bread. Some in potatoes, dhal, lentils, hummus and leafy vegetables.
Other bioactive substances.		
Phytochemicals in plants provide long-term protection against cancer and heart disease. Also called flavonoids, flavanols and isoflavones (e.g. lycopene, lutein and quercetin).	Among other things, they act as antioxidants protecting all cells from damage and they are a key part of the immune system.	Fruits, vegetables, spices, herbs, nuts and foods made from cereals – particularly those that are brightly coloured. Cocoa and chocolate.
Probiotics are bacteria that colonise the intestine and provide health benefits	Increase the number of beneficial bacteria in the intestine and consequently reduce the effects of harmful bacteria that may cause infection.	Fermented foods such as live yogurt, kefir, cheese, kimchi, natto, sauerkraut and sour dough bread.

Appendix 2: Growth Charts

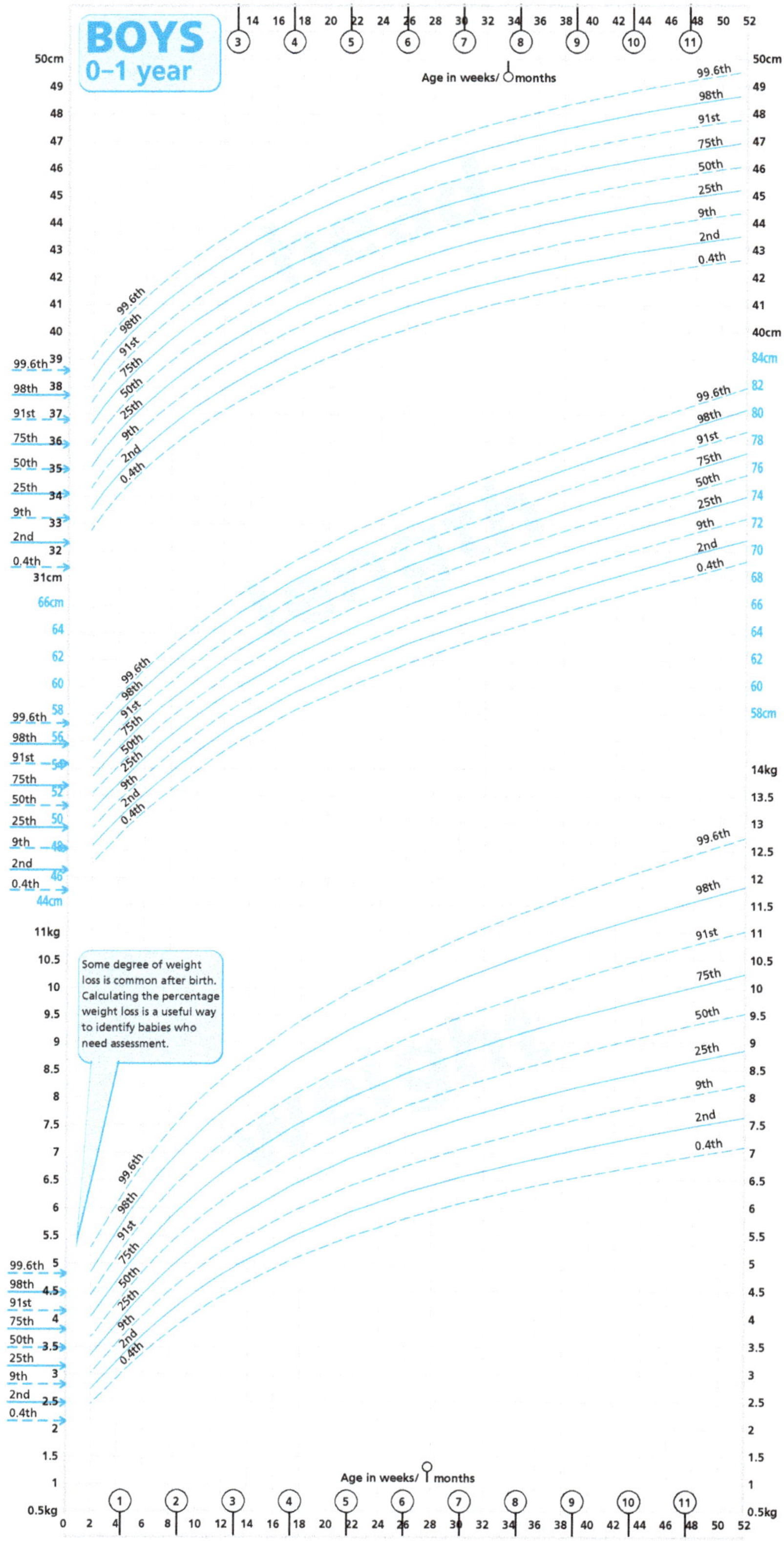
BOYS
0–1 year
Age in weeks/ months
50cm
40cm
31cm
84cm
58cm
66cm
44cm
14kg
11kg
0.5kg
99.6th
98th
91st
75th
50th
25th
9th
2nd
0.4th
Some degree of weight loss is common after birth. Calculating the percentage weight loss is a useful way to identify babies who need assessment.
Age in weeks/ months

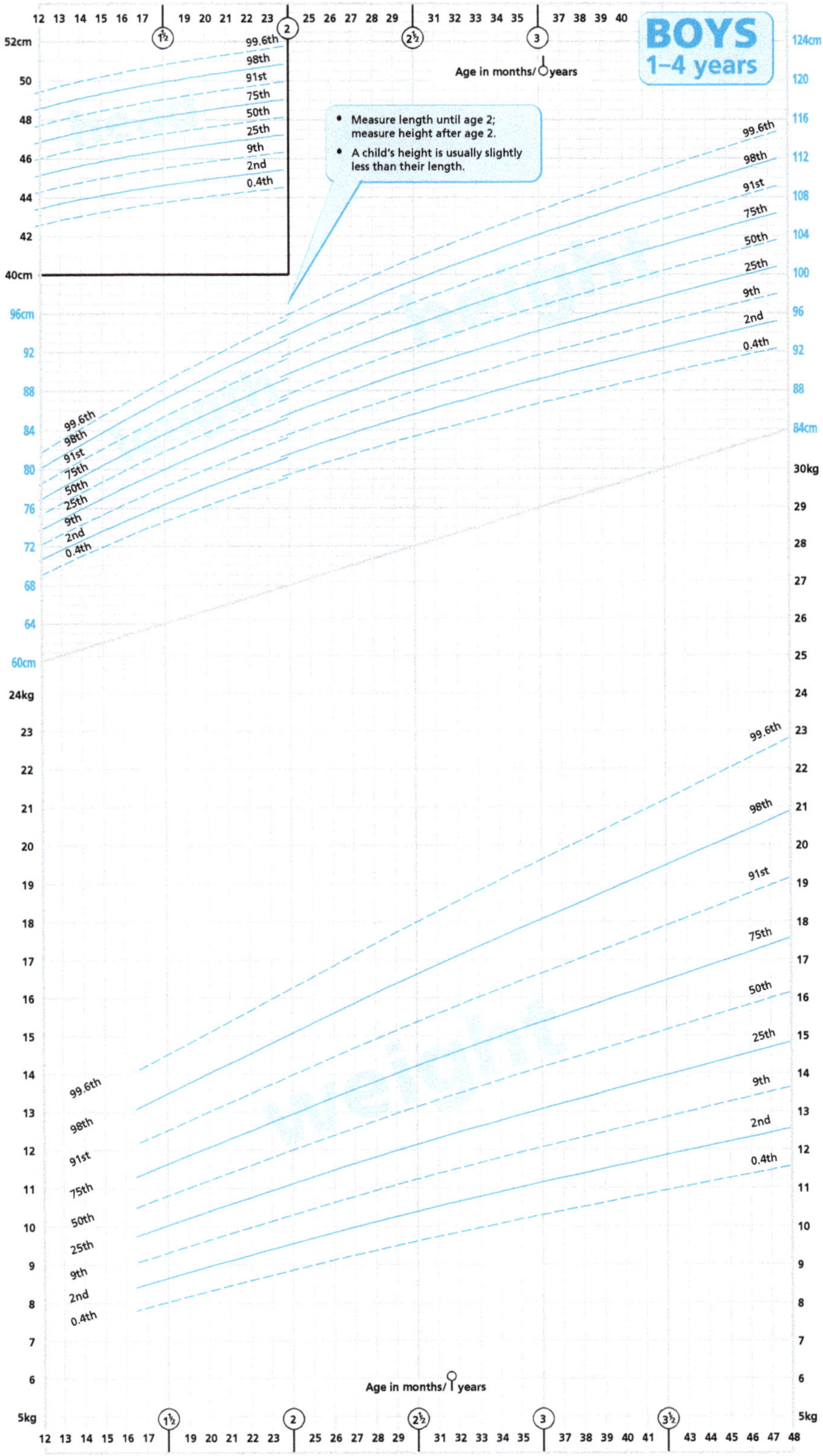
BOYS
1–4 years
Age in months/ years
Measure length until age 2; measure height after age 2.
A child's height is usually slightly less than their length.
length
height
weight
99.6th
98th
91st
75th
50th
25th
9th
2nd
0.4th
52cm
40cm
124cm
96cm
84cm
60cm
24kg
30kg
5kg

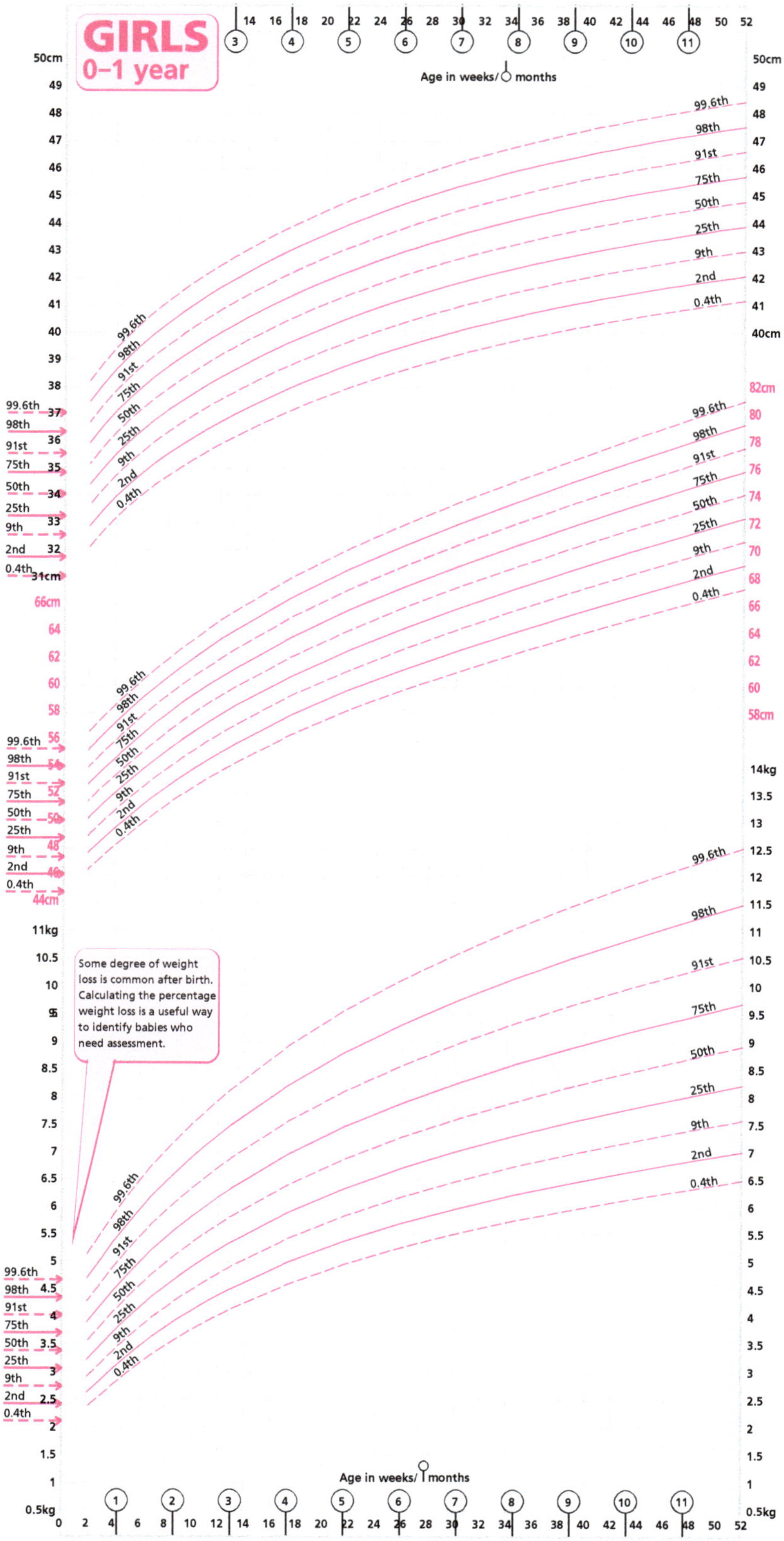
GIRLS
0–1 year
Age in weeks/months
50cm
40cm
82cm
58cm
66cm
44cm
31cm
14kg
11kg
0.5kg
99.6th
98th
91st
75th
50th
25th
9th
2nd
0.4th
Some degree of weight loss is common after birth. Calculating the percentage weight loss is a useful way to identify babies who need assessment.

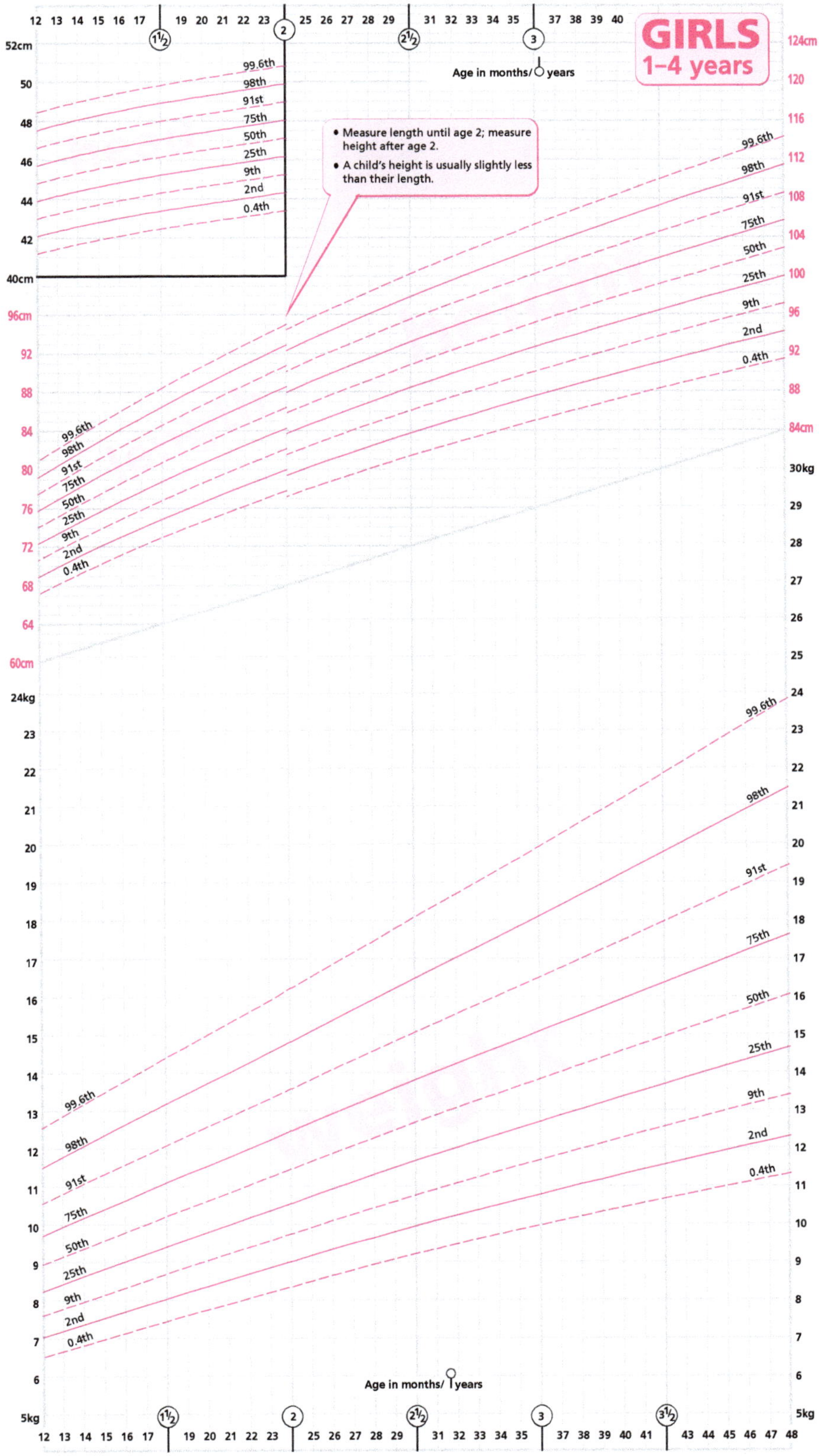
GIRLS
1–4 years
Age in months/ years
• Measure length until age 2; measure height after age 2.
• A child's height is usually slightly less than their length.
99.6th
98th
91st
75th
50th
25th
9th
2nd
0.4th
52cm
40cm
96cm
60cm
124cm
84cm
30kg
24kg
5kg
Age in months/ years
12 13 14 15 16 17 19 20 21 22 23 25 26 27 28 29 31 32 33 34 35 37 38 39 40 41 43 44 45 46 47 48
1½
2
2½
3
3½

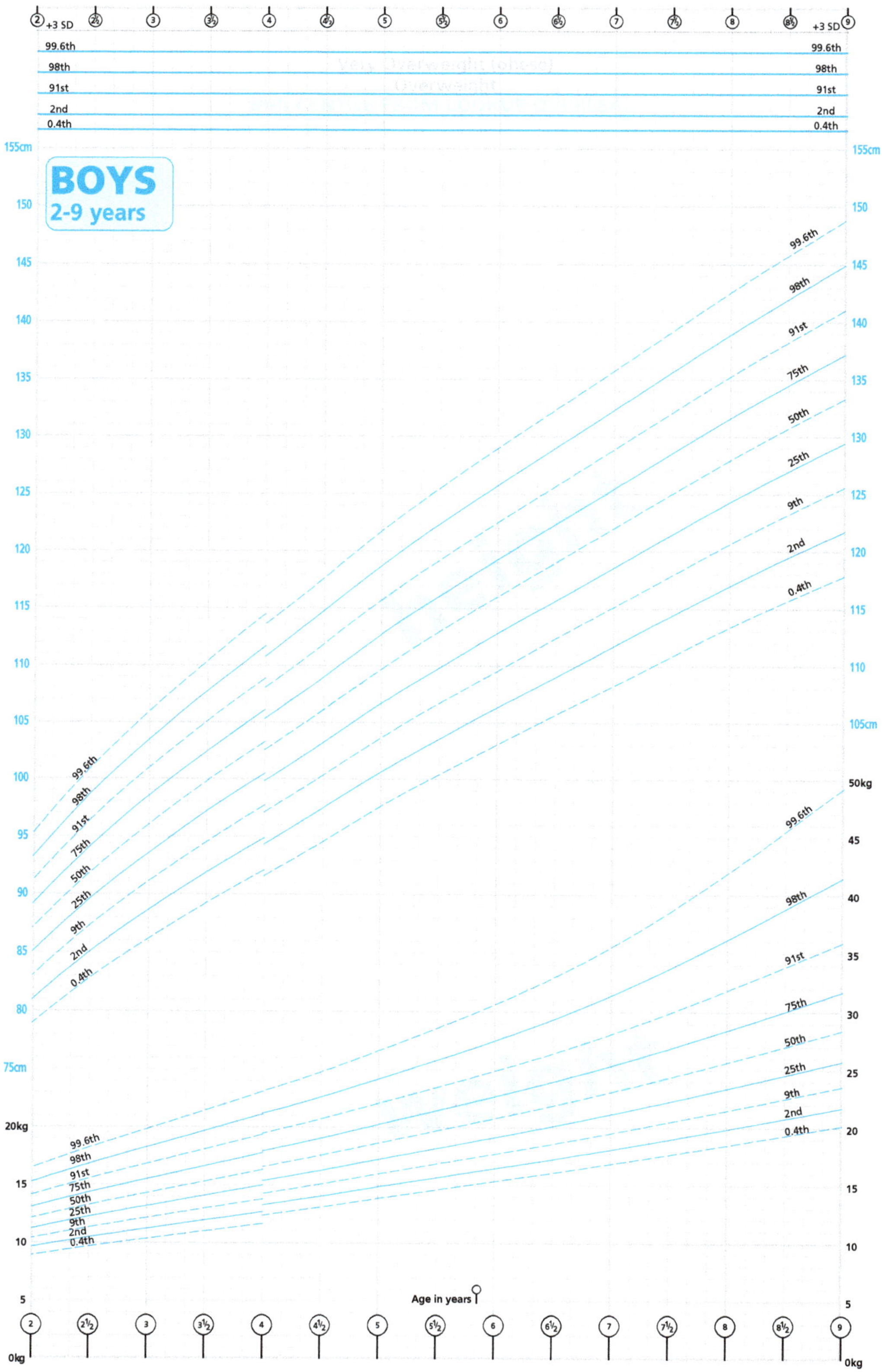
BOYS
2-9 years
+3 SD
99.6th
98th
91st
2nd
0.4th
155cm
150
145
140
135
130
125
120
115
110
105
105cm
100
95
90
85
80
75cm
50kg
45
40
35
30
25
20kg
20
15
10
5
0kg
99.6th
98th
91st
75th
50th
25th
9th
2nd
0.4th
Age in years
2
2½
3
3½
4
4½
5
5½
6
6½
7
7½
8
8½
9

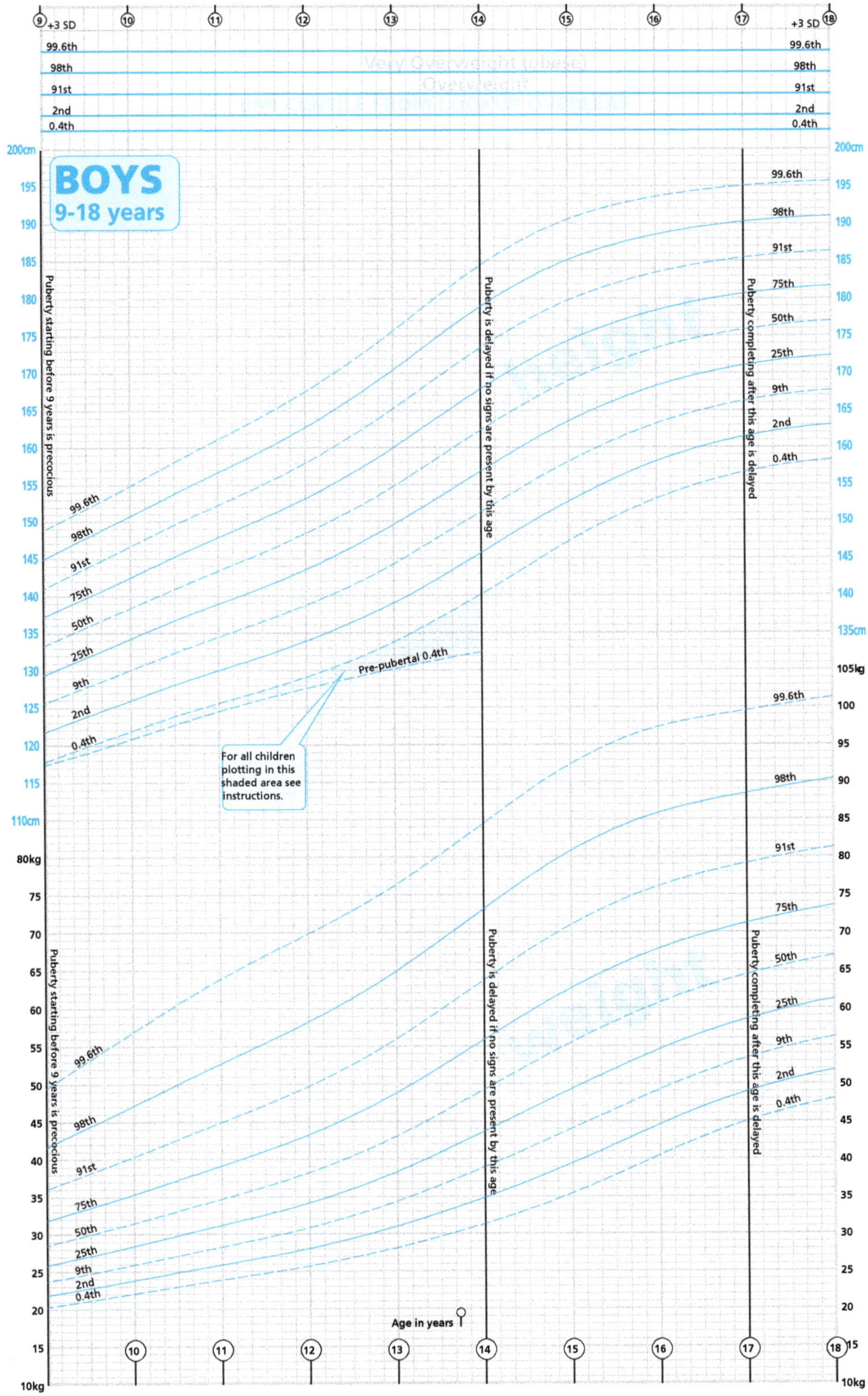
BOYS
9-18 years
+3 SD
99.6th
98th
91st
75th
50th
25th
9th
2nd
0.4th
200cm
195
190
185
180
175
170
165
160
155
150
145
140
135cm
130
125
120
115
110cm
105kg
100
95
90
85
80kg
75
70
65
60
55
50
45
40
35
30
25
20
15
10kg
Puberty starting before 9 years is precocious
Puberty is delayed if no signs are present by this age
Puberty completing after this age is delayed
Pre-pubertal 0.4th
For all children plotting in this shaded area see instructions.
Age in years
9
10
11
12
13
14
15
16
17
18

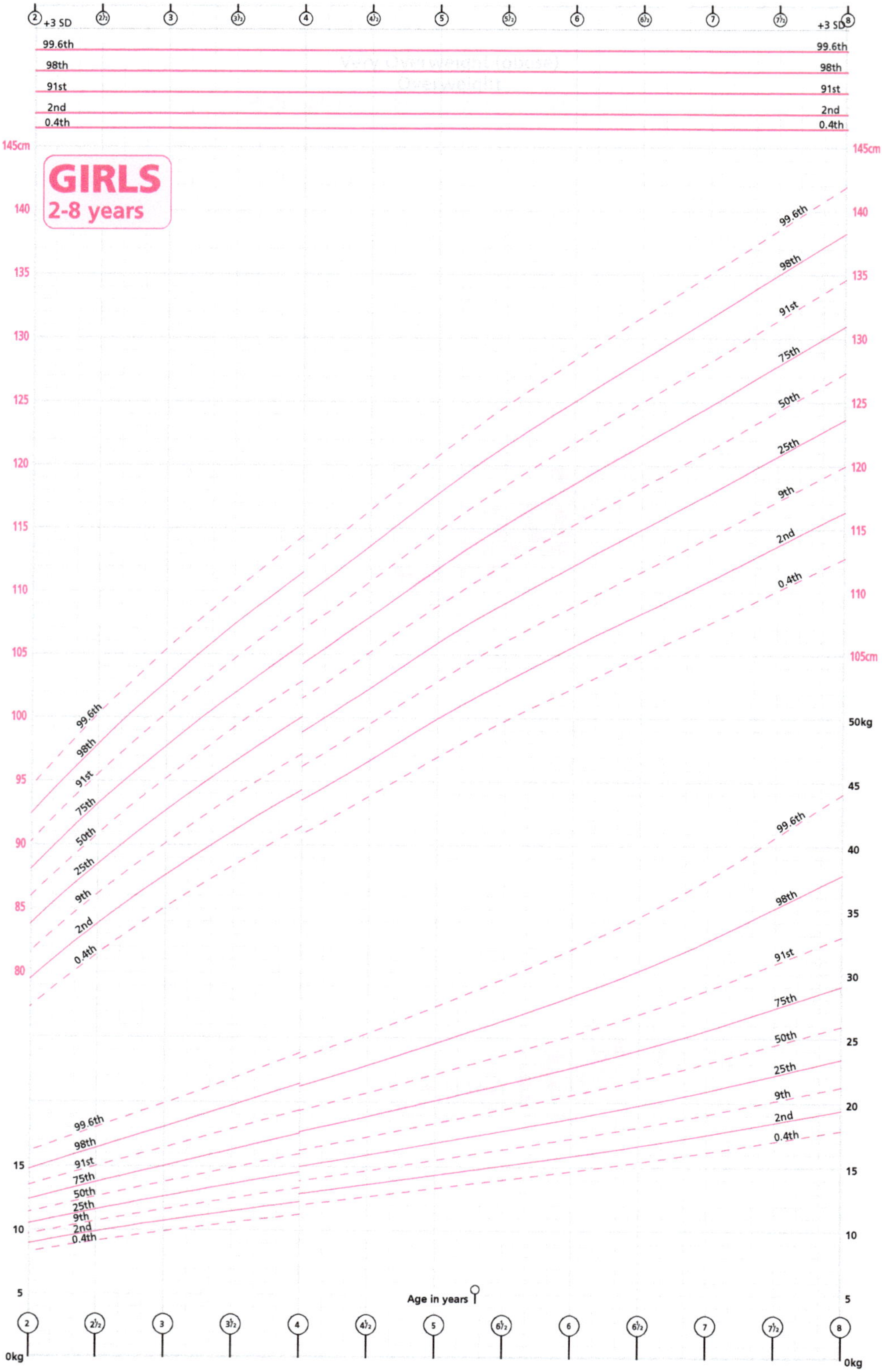
GIRLS
2-8 years
+3 SD
99.6th
98th
91st
2nd
0.4th
145cm
140
135
130
125
120
115
110
105
100
95
90
85
80
105cm
50kg
45
40
35
30
25
20
15
10
5
0kg
99.6th
98th
91st
75th
50th
25th
9th
2nd
0.4th
Age in years
2
2½
3
3½
4
4½
5
5½
6
6½
7
7½
8

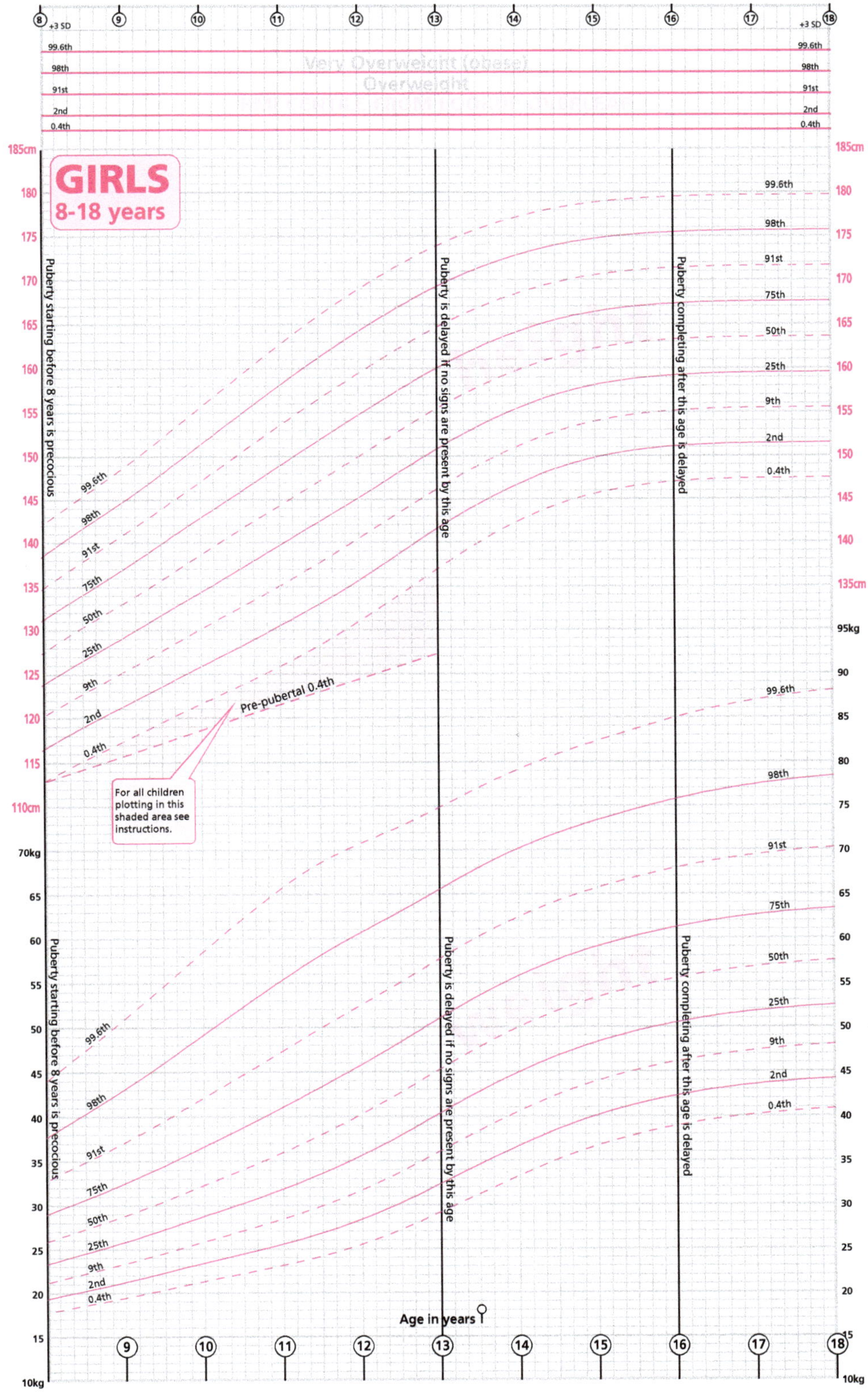
GIRLS
8-18 years
Very Overweight (obese)
Overweight
+3 SD
99.6th
98th
91st
2nd
0.4th
185cm
180
175
170
165
160
155
150
145
140
135cm
110cm
70kg
95kg
Puberty starting before 8 years is precocious
Puberty is delayed if no signs are present by this age
Puberty completing after this age is delayed
99.6th
98th
91st
75th
50th
25th
9th
2nd
0.4th
Pre-pubertal 0.4th
For all children plotting in this shaded area see instructions.
Age in years
10kg

Appendix 3: BMI and Waist Circumference Charts

BOYS BMI CHART

Birth - 20 yrs UK cross-sectional body mass index reference chart. 2008/1

BMI equation: weight [kg] ÷ height [m²]

IDENTIFICATION

Name...

D.O.B. [DDMMYY] ☐☐ / ☐☐ / ☐☐☐☐

NHS No. ☐☐☐ ☐☐☐ ☐☐☐☐

Mother
Weight [kg] ☐ Height [m] ☐ BMI ☐

Father
Weight [kg] ☐ Height [m] ☐ BMI ☐

Body Mass Index (BMI)

Although highly correlated with weight, body mass index [BMI] is not a direct measure of body fat and rapid changes in BMI can occur in normal childhood growth. By itself it should therefore be interpreted with caution. Waist circumference and body type should be evaluated before intervention or referral is considered.

The blue shaded area indicates a healthy BMI range bordered by the international cut-offs for the degrees of overweight and thinness. The Royal College of Paediatrics & Child Health has stated that severe or progressive obesity should be referred to a paediatrician before age 2.

Referrals of infants showing signs of concerning overweight/underweight in their early months [shaded grey] should be based on the 1st year weight charts with 95%/5% thrive lines.

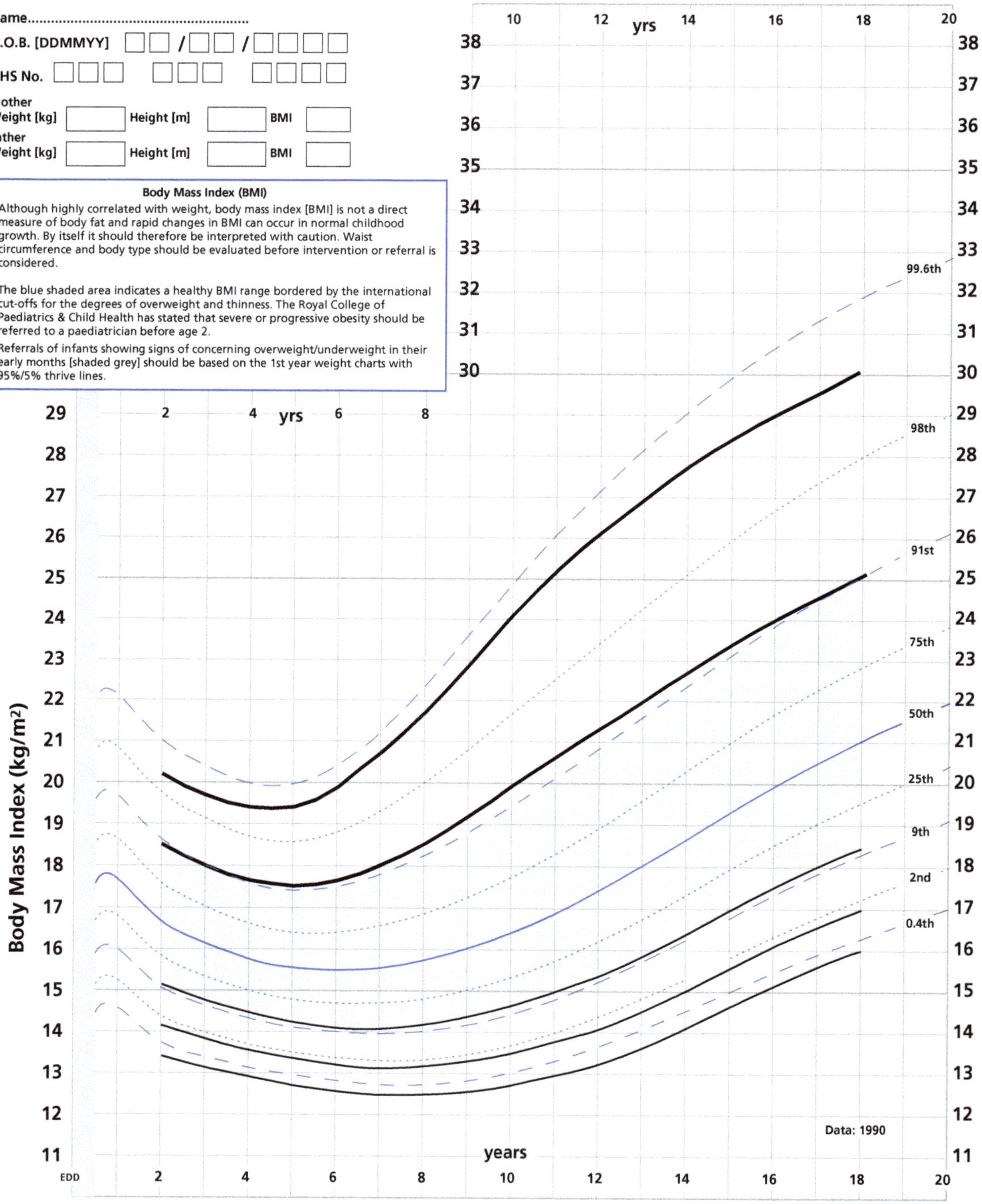

Body mass index reference curves for the UK, 1990 (Cole TJ, Freeman JV, Preece MA) *Arch Dis Child* 1995; **73:** 25-9
Establishing a standard definition for child overweight and obesity: international survey (Cole TJ, Bellizzi MC, Flegal KM, Dietz WH) *BMJ 2000;* **320:** 1240-3
Body mass index cut-offs to define thinness in children and adolescents: international survey (Cole TJ, Flegal KM, Nicholls D, Jackson AA) *BMJ 2007;* **335:** 194-7

BOYS WAIST CIRCUMFERENCE

D.O.B. [DDMMYY] ☐☐ /☐☐ /☐☐☐☐

Because a high BMI by itself may not be a guarantor of obesity/overweight, a high waist centile added to a high BMI centile will confirm fatness more conclusively. The shaded area represents a healthy waist range.

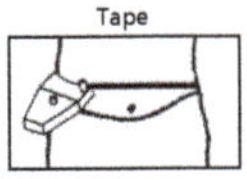

Measuring the Waist

The waist is defined as the mid-way point between the lowest rib cage and the iliac crest and should be measured, preferably, with a special tension tape [see illustrations below].

When measuring his waist, the boy should ideally be wearing only underclothes. Ask him to stand with his feet together and weight evenly distributed with his arms relaxed. Ask him to breathe normally and take the waist measurement at the end of a normal expiration.

The waist can also be identified by asking him to bend to one side. Measurement is taken at the point of flexure.

If he is wearing a shirt or vest, deduct 1cm before recording and plotting the waist measurement.

There is no consensus about how to define paediatric obesity using waist measurement. For clinical use the 99.6th or 98th centiles are suggested cut-offs for obesity and the 91st centile for overweight, like the BMI [see chart overleaf].

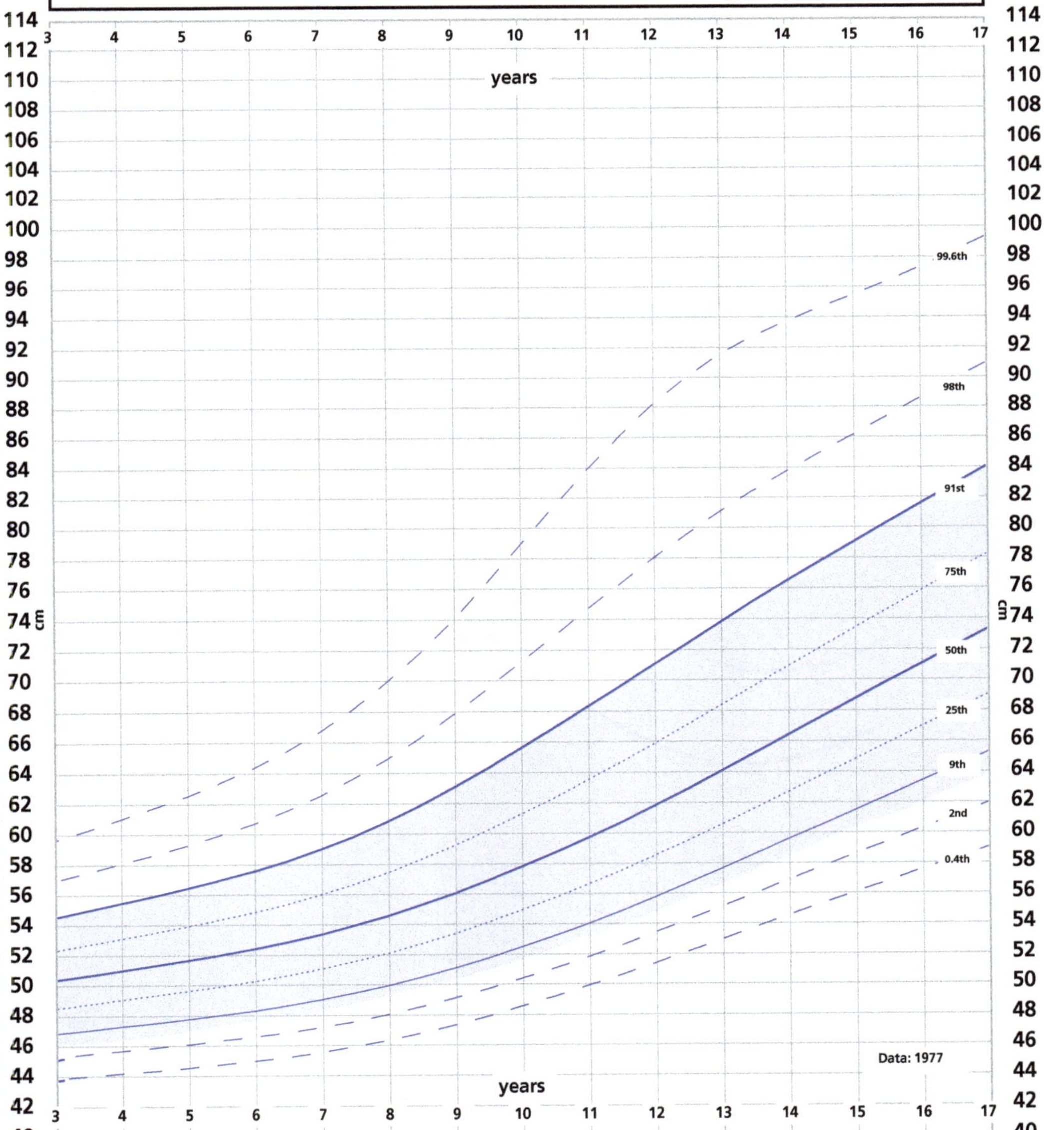

Reference
The development of waist circumference percentiles in British children aged 5-16.9 yrs: (McCarthy HD et al) *European Journal of Clinical Nutrition* (2001): **55:** 902-907.

GIRLS BMI CHART

Birth - 20 yrs UK cross-sectional body mass index reference chart. 2008/1

BMI equation: weight [kg] ÷ height [m²]

IDENTIFICATION

Name...

D.O.B. [DDMMYY] ☐☐ / ☐☐ / ☐☐☐☐

NHS No. ☐☐☐ ☐☐☐ ☐☐☐☐

Mother Weight [kg] ☐ Height [m] ☐ BMI ☐

Father Weight [kg] ☐ Height [m] ☐ BMI ☐

Body Mass Index (BMI)

Although highly correlated with weight, body mass index [BMI] is not a direct measure of body fat and rapid changes in BMI can occur in normal childhood growth. By itself it should therefore be interpreted with caution. Waist circumference and body type should be evaluated before intervention or referral is considered.

The red shaded area indicates a healthy BMI range bordered by the international cut-offs for the degrees of overweight and thinness. The Royal College of Paediatrics & Child Health has stated that severe or progressive obesity should be referred to a paediatrician before age 2.
Referrals of infants showing signs of concerning overweight/underweight in their early months [shaded grey] should be based on the 1st year weight charts with 95%/5% thrive lines.

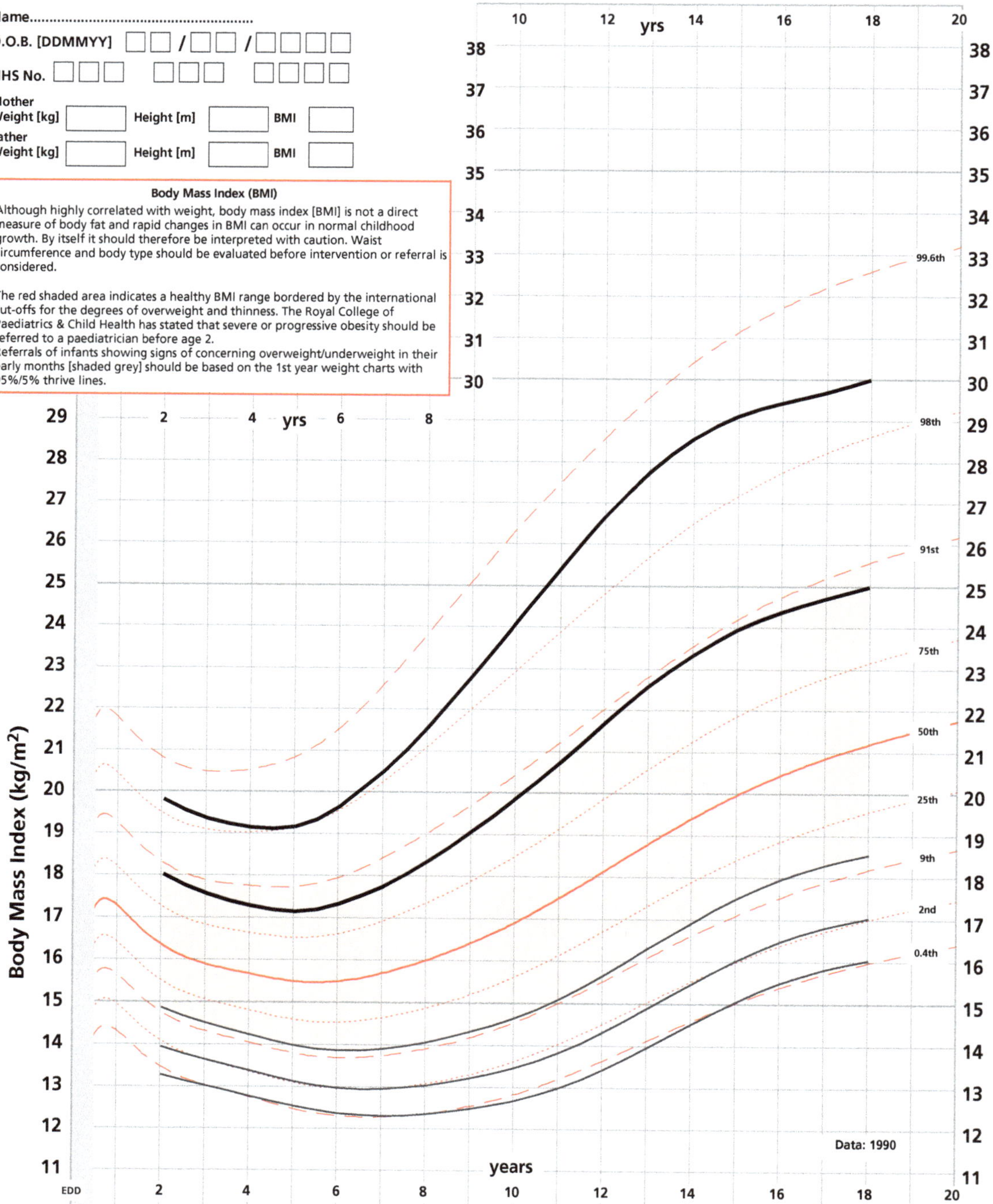

Manufacture 22 June 12 BMIBG

Body mass index reference curves for the UK, 1990 (Cole TJ, Freeman JV, Preece MA) *Arch Dis Child* 1995; **73:** 25-9
Establishing a standard definition for child overweight and obesity: international survey (Cole TJ, Bellizzi MC, Flegal KM, Dietz WH) *BMJ 2000;* **320:** 1240-3
Body mass index cut-offs to define thinness in children and adolescents: international survey (Cole TJ, Flegal KM, Nicholls D, Jackson AA) *BMJ 2007;* **335:** 194-7

GIRLS WAIST CIRCUMFERENCE

D.O.B. [DDMMYY] ☐☐/☐☐/☐☐☐☐

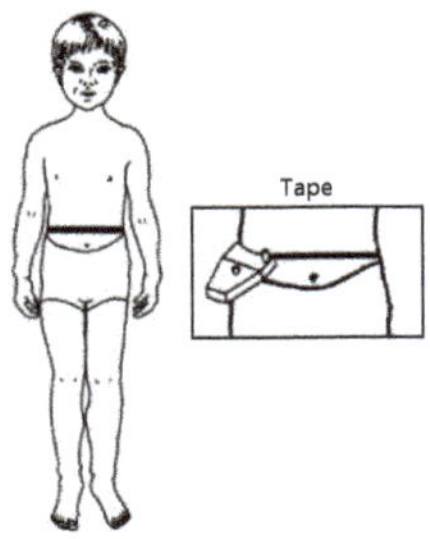

Because a high BMI by itself may not be a guarantor of obesity/overweight, a high waist centile added to a high BMI centile will confirm fatness more conclusively. The shaded area represents a healthy waist range.

Measuring the Waist

The waist is defined as the mid-way point between the lowest rib cage and the iliac crest and should be measured, preferably, with a special tension tape [see illustrations below].

When measuring her waist, the girl should ideally be wearing only underclothes. Ask her to stand with her feet together and weight evenly distributed with her arms relaxed. Ask her to breathe normally and take the waist measurement at the end of a normal expiration.

The waist can also be identified by asking her to bend to one side. Measurement is taken at the point of flexure.

If she is wearing a shirt or vest, deduct 1cm before recording and plotting the waist measurement.

There is no consensus about how to define paediatric obesity using waist measurement. For clinical use the 99.6th or 98th centiles are suggested cut-offs for obesity and the 91st centile for overweight, like the BMI [see chart overleaf].

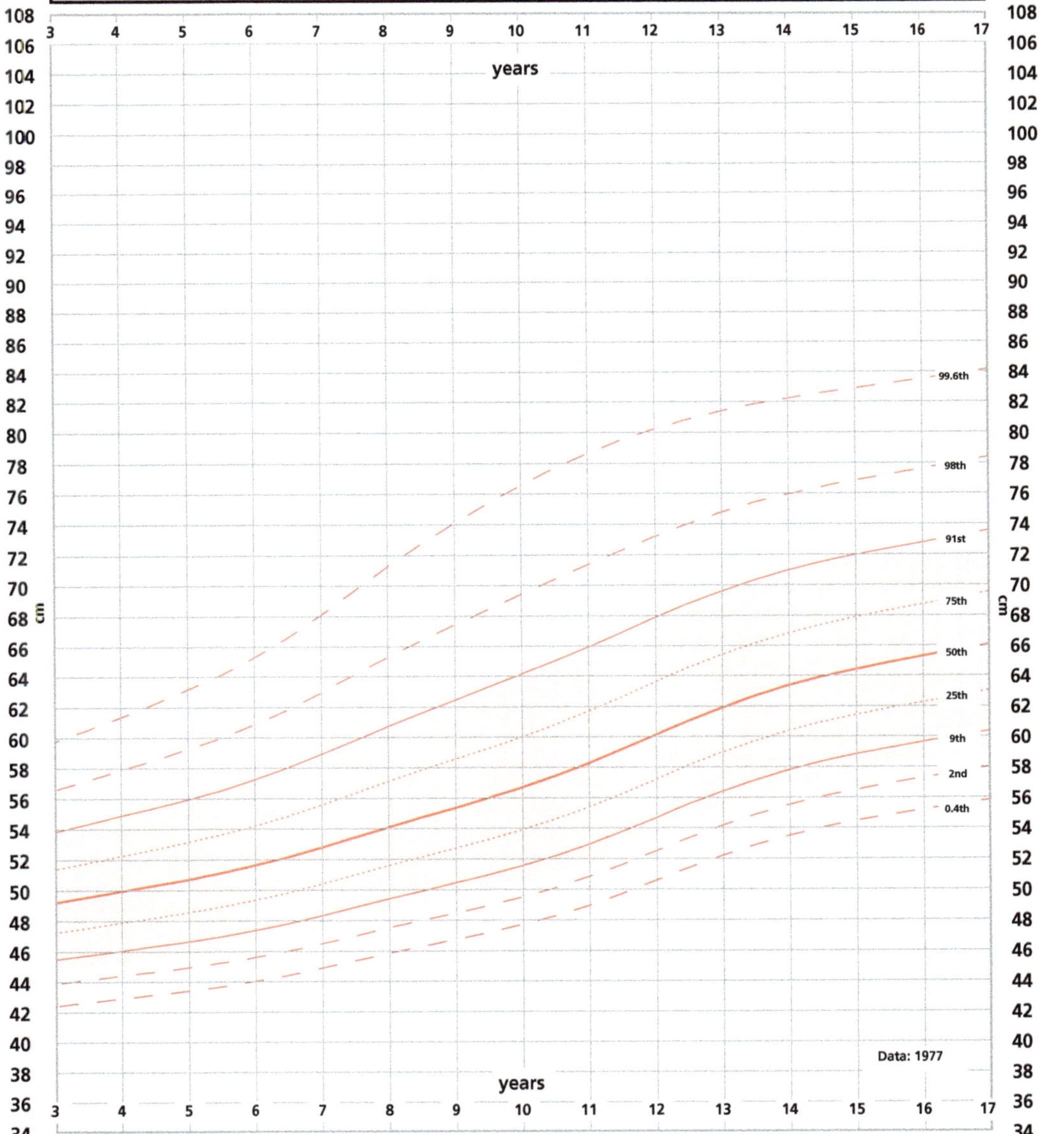

Reference
The development of waist circumference percentiles in British children aged 5-16.9 yrs: (McCarthy HD et al) *European Journal of Clinical Nutrition* (2001): **55:** 902-907.

Glossary

Allergen – A substance that causes an immune response.

Allergy – A hypersensitivity reaction initiated by specific immunological mechanisms.

Amino acids – A group of compounds that proteins are made of. Essential amino acids are those that we cannot make ourselves and therefore we must eat them in food. Non-essential amino acids are those that we can make for ourselves if our diets are adequate.

Anaphylaxis – Severe difficulty breathing and heart malfunction due to a fall in blood pressure, usually as a result of a serious allergic reaction. It can result in death, but if adrenaline is administered, the body is quickly restored to normal.

Apnoea – A transient absence of spontaneous respiration. It may occur during sleep in very obese children.

Asperger's syndrome – One of several autism spectrum disorders (ASD) characterised by difficulties in social interaction and by restricted and stereotyped interests and activities.

Atopy – A characteristic making one susceptible to develop immediate allergic reactions to substances such as pollen, food, dander and insect venoms and manifested by hay fever, asthma, food allergies, eczema or similar allergic conditions.

Autism – Autistic spectrum disorders (ASD) are a spectrum of psychological conditions characterised by widespread abnormalities of social interactions and communication, as well as severely restricted interests and highly repetitive behaviour.

Autoimmune disease – A disease in which the body produces antibodies that attack its own tissues.

Body mass index (BMI) – An index calculated by dividing body weight in kilograms by the height in metres squared.

Cardiomyopathy – Disease of the heart muscle that can lead to heart failure.

Coeliac disease – An autoimmune disease in which the protein gluten causes the production of destructive antibodies that damage the tissue of the small intestine causing malabsorption of food.

Corrected age – The age of a child born preterm minus the weeks the baby was born early.

Cushing's syndrome – Disorder caused by excessive levels of the hormone cortisol, which causes rapid weight gain, particularly of the trunk and face.

Dehydration – Condition that results from excessive loss of body water. This may occur due to a high temperature and excessive sweating or it may be due to normal water losses through skin, breathing, passing water and stools coupled with an inadequate intake of water.

Dyslipidaemia – An excess of lipids in the blood, usually the lipids cholesterol and triglycerides.

Estimated date of delivery (EDD) – For a premature baby, this is the date they were expected to be born if they had remained in the womb for a normal-length pregnancy of 40-weeks gestation.

Encopresis – Involuntary faecal soiling of underwear in children who are already toilet trained.

Endocrine disorders – Abnormalities of hormone secretion or action.

Eosinophilic esophagitis – An allergic inflammatory reaction in the eosinophils (a type of white blood cell) in the esophagus. It is a cause of feeding difficulties and poor weight gain in children as it causes decreased appetite due to difficulty in swallowing, food impaction, stomach pains, regurgitation or vomiting.

Epigenetics – Heritable changes in which genes are turned on and off without actually changing an individual's DNA.

Free sugars-All monosaccharides and disaccharides added to foods by the manufacturer, cook, or consumer, plus sugars naturally present in honey, syrups, and fruit juices and smoothies

Food allergy – An abnormal or exaggerated immunological response to specific food proteins.

Gag on food – Food is not successfully swallowed and comes back into the mouth.

Gastro-oesophageal reflux – The contents of the stomach flow backwards: back up out of the stomach into the oesophagus.

Glucose – A form of sugar. Sugar in the blood is always in the form of glucose.

Gluten – A protein found in wheat, rye and barley. Oats contain a very similar protein.

Growth hormone – A hormone secreted by the pituitary gland, which stimulates growth and cell reproduction.

Halal – Means 'lawful' and relates to meat that is acceptable to Muslims. Animals must be ritually slaughtered to provide meat that is Halal.

Hypoglycaemia – Blood sugar levels are lower than the normal range for blood sugar.

Hypothyroidism – Insufficient production of thyroid hormone by the thyroid gland.

Hyperglycaemia – Blood sugar levels are higher than the normal range for blood sugar.

Hypersensitivity – Objectively reproducible symptoms or signs initiated by exposure to a defined stimulus at a dose tolerated by normal persons.

Hypertension – Raised blood pressure.

Infant – A child under 12 months of age.

Kangaroo care – The practice of securing a very young or preterm infant against the mother's skin, usually on her chest between her breasts to maximise body contact. The benefits include reduced morbidity and mortality.

Kosher – This means that animals and birds have been slaughtered by the Jewish method, carried out by a trained and authorised person.

Leptin – A hormone secreted by adipose tissue that plays a key role in regulating energy intake and energy expenditure, including the regulation of appetite and metabolism.

Oesophagus – The part of the digestive canal that food and drinks pass through between the mouthdown to the stomach.

Palmar grasp – Grasping with the thumb opposite the fingers and holding an object in the palm of the hand.

Personal Child Health Record (PCHR) – A record of a child's growth, development and uptake of preventive health services (e.g. immunisations), designed to enhance communication between parents and health professionals.

Pesticide – Chemicals including herbicides, insecticides and fungicides used to kill pests.

Phytochemicals – Compounds that occur naturally in plants (phyto means 'plant' in Greek), which may have biological significance but are not established as essential nutrients. They are responsible for some colour and smell, such as the deep purple of blueberries and smell of garlic. In the diet, they play a role in the immune system and provide long-term protection against cancer and heart disease. They include the brightly coloured pigments in fruits and vegetables and are also called flavanoids, flavanols or isoflavones.

Phyto-oestrogens – Plant chemicals that behave the same way in the body as the hormone oestrogen.

Pincer grasp – Picking up objects with the thumb and forefinger.

Prader-Willi syndrome – A condition caused by a chromosomal abnormality. Babies are floppy at birth and go on to develop obesity due to an excessive appetite and overeating. Other characteristics are small hands and feet, mental retardation, poor emotional and social development and immature development of sexual organs and other sexual characteristics.

Prebiotics – Fibre that encourages the growth of good bacteria in the intestine.

Preterm babies – Babies born before 37-weeks gestation.

Probiotics – Bacteria present in fermented food that colonise the intestinal tract and improve the intestinal microbial balance. Examples are bifidobacteria and lactobacilli.

Protein – A complex molecule consisting of a particular sequence of chains of amino acids. Proteins are essential constituents of all living things.

Pulses – A group of foods that includes lentils, peas and starchy beans but excludes green beans. Examples of starchy beans are chick peas, black eye beans, baked beans, white and red kidney beans and flageolet beans.

Reflux – See gastro-oesophageal reflux.

Retch – Make an involuntary effort to vomit.

Stool – Evacuated faecal matter passed through the anus.

Supine – Lying on the back.

Teratogenesis – The development of physical defects in the embryo or fetus.

Term babies – Babies born after 37-weeks gestation.

Index

A
abscess, breast 106–107
acidic drinks and caries 177, 198
additives 110, 223
ADHD *see* deficit hyperactivity disorder
adiposity rebound 56, 233, 236
adolescence
cooking skills 214
crossing centiles during 56
diabetic, food refusal 258
eating disorders 212–213
emotional changes and food choices 205–207
food portion sizes 208–209
factors contributing to nutritional imbalances 209–213
alcohol consumption 213
consumption of sugar-containing foods and soft drinks 209
dieting/slimming 209, 211–212
eating disorders 212–213
inadequate intake of fruits, vegetables and milk-based foods 209
insufficient nutrient intakes 209
snacking or 'grazing' 209
vegetarianism and veganism 209, 211
food portion sizes and number 208–209
guidelines on healthy eating 207
healthier snack foods and take-away meals 210
SACN recommendations for macronutrient intakes 210
health risks with obesity 236
healthy eating for 207
high energy requiring conditions
pregnancy 214
sports training 213–214
nutritional requirements in 206
calcium and phosphorus 206
iron 207
macronutrient intakes 207
minerals 206–207
during pregnancies 206
vitamins 206–207
physical development 205
pubertal progress 205
nutritional status and early date of menarche 77
overweight or obese during 234
adrenaline auto-injector pens 221, *222*
advertising, food 39
age
centile chart 198
growth data for different ages 50
growth rates changing with 50–51
preterm baby age correction 55
alcohol
adolescents and teenagers 213
breastfeeding mothers and 110
preconception 75–76, 77
during pregnancy 77, 90
allergy, food *see* food allergy
ALSPAC *see* Avon Longitudinal Study of Parents and Children
amenorrhoea 77, 212
amino acids
essential 5, 24
non-essential 5
amines, biogenic 222
amino acid formulas 144
anaemia 199
iron-deficiency 10
dietary risk factors 178
in preschool children 178
anaphylaxis 221
anorexia nervosa 77, 212
fertility and 77
primary school children 198
anovulation 77
anthropometric measurement 51
antioxidants 11
anti-reflux fundoplication surgery 180
anti-reflux medications 180
appetite, poor/inadequate 10, 254
in cystic fibrosis 254
iron deficiency and 178
nutritional support for children with 247–248
primary school children 198
ARFID *see* avoidant restrictive food intake disorder
ascorbic acid *see* vitamin C
Asperger's syndrome, diet for 251
attention deficit hyperactivity disorder (ADHD) 246, 251
authoritarian parenting style 41
authoritative parenting style 41
autistic spectrum disorders, diet for 251
avoidant restrictive food intake disorder (ARFID)
and faltering growth 184
in preschool children 183
autumn-time meals plan, for preschoolchildren 169
Avon Longitudinal Study of Parents and Children (ALSPAC) 68, 141

B
baby foods, commercial 133
balanced/healthy diet
Brazilian 10 steps to 23–24
principles of 30
promotion in childcare setting 191
basal metabolic rate 4
BDD *see* body dysmorphic disorder
benzoic acid intolerance 222
bigorexia 212
binge drinking 90, 110
binge eating disorders 212
biogenic amine intolerance 222
biological drivers of growth 49–50
biotin, safe intakes 15
birth weight 55
BMI-for-age centile charts, gender-specific 55–56
body dysmorphic disorder (BDD) 212
body mass index (BMI) 51, 55–56, 233–234
assessment 51–52
body fat and 55–56
charts 54
girls *vs.* boys 55–56
body weight
and fertility 76–77
preconception 76
bottle caries 124
bottle (formula)-feeding
choice of formula types 107
components 111
constipation and 139–140
food hypersensitivity and 141–145
growth faltering in formula-fed babies 141–145
preterms 154
and discharge home from neonatal unit 155
feeding routes 150
bran, unprocessed 179
bread, sandwich fillings for preschool children 190
breadsticks and dips, for packed lunches for preschool children 191
breakfast 67
adolescents not having 209
plans 28, 29
diabetic child 255, 256, 257
preschool children 167, 168, 169, 170

vegetarian 30
recording intake 65
example case 65
breast (mother's)
abscess 106–107
blocked ducts 106
engorgement 106
breastfeeding 42, 99–100, 99–100
attachment for 103–104
good attachment 104
poor attachment 104
benefits of 101
and bottle feeding 107
contraindications to 99
duration of 43
expressing breast milk 107–108
breast pump, use of 108
hand expression 108
for new-born infants 108–109
storage of milk 109
food hypersensitivity 108
frequency and length of breastfeeds 103
good attachment 104
kangaroo care 153
mature milk 102
mothers returning to work and 109
nutrients in breast milk 111–113
and nutritional needs for mothers 110
poor attachment 104
positioning for 103
preterms 153–154
discharge home from neonatal unit 155
feeding routes 150
problems and difficulties 105
assessment of 105
blocked ducts 106
breast abscess 106–107
engorgement 106
inadequate milk supply 107
mastitis 106
sore or cracked nipples 105–106
tongue-tie 107
problems and solutions
constipation 139–140
food hypersensitivity 141–145
progression of breastfeed 104–105
supporting mothers to breastfeed 103, 105
transitional milk 102
twins and multiples 105
vitamin D supplement with 102
vs. formula feeding 42–43, 101
breast milk
adequate supply 107
benefits of 101, 151
composition/components 101
preterms 152
expressing 107–108
new-born infants 108–109
preterms 151–152
inadequate milk supply 107
nutritional components in 111–113
for preterms 151–152
fortification 152
trophic feeding of 149–150
stages of 101
colostrum 101–102
mature milk 102
transitional milk 102
supplements for 152–153
breast pump 108
British Lion Mark 134
Buddhist 37
bulimia nervosa 77, 212
fertility and 77

C

caffeine 26, 90
fertility and 90
calcium 10
in breast milk with preterms 152
in formula feeds
constipation related to 139–140
very low 144
reference nutrient intakes 14
calcium carbonate 10
carbohydrate 5–6
dietary requirements 15
as energy source 5
exchanges
sample 1-day menu 257
ten-gram 255, 256
intakes
school-age children 196
carbonated (fizzy) drinks 115
adolescents 206, 210
preschool children 165
cardiomyopathy 9, 83
caries (dental decay)
fluoride and 10
free sugars and 25
in preschool children 177–178
school-age children 198–199
carotene 8
centile charts 51 *see also* growth charts
central obesity, preconception 77
childcare setting, feeding preschool children in
food and drinks offered in, nutritional standards for 188–189
food for celebrations 189
healthy lifestyle/eating promotion 191
opportunities and challenges 188–189
packed meals/lunches 189–191
selective eaters, feeding to 187–188
choking
infants 133–134
preschool children 172–173
cholecalciferol *see* vitamin D
cholesterol 6
chondrogenesis 49
Christian traditions 37
chromium, safe intakes 15
Clinical Paediatric Dietetics 245
clothing, weight and length measurement without 53
coeliac disease 29
diet for 251–253
colic 137–138
colostrum 43, 101–102
colours and preservatives, in food and drinks 26
COMA *see* Committee on Medical Aspects of Food Policy
commercial baby foods 133
gluten-free 253
for infants and young children 133
labelling on, checking 252–253, 255
saturated fat in 4
Committee on Medical Aspects of Food Policy (COMA) 13
complementary feeding
see also complementary foods (CFs)
age to begin 121–122
breast milk with 121, 124
drinking cup, use of 124
hunger cues 126
learning to like new tastes 126
learning to manage new textures 126–127
milk feeds with 124
purpose of 121
recommendations from various agencies 123
responsive feeding environment 125
safe positioning for 156
satiety cues 126
spoon feeding and finger foods 126
complementary foods (CFs) 121
commercial baby foods 133
dental care 133
foods to avoid until 12 months 125
items from food groups 125
menu planner
for 6–7 months 130
for 7–9 months 130
for 9–12 months 132
nutrient and energy density of 123–124
progressing through feeding stages 127
stage 1 (4–6 months) 127–128
stage 2 (6–9 months) 129–130
stage 3 (9–12 months) 131–132
safety concerns
choking prevention 133

foods to limit and avoid 134
hygiene 133–134
vegetarian foods 133
vitamin D supplement 125
constipation
exacerbating factors 179
infants 139–140
preschool children 179
symptoms 141
treatment 179
copper 14
reference nutrient intakes 14
cravings in pregnancy 93
Crohn's disease, diet for 258–259
cutlery 38
cystic fibrosis, diet for 253–254

D
daily nutritional requirements of preterms in parenteral or enteral nutrition 148–149
dehydration 92, 93, 214
diarrhoea and gastroenteritis 139
dental disease, fluoride tablets for prevention of 10
dental health
brushing teeth 25
fluoride and 10
free sugars and 25–26
regular dental checkups 25
see also caries (dental decay)
diabetes
coping with food refusal in 258
insulin injections for 254–255
nutritional support 254–258
type 1 254–255
type 2 254, 258
see also hypoglycaemia
diabetic diet 254–255
diabluminia 258
diarrhoea 225
infants 139
preschool children 180
dietary analysis software 68
dietary diary 62
dietary folates 82–83
dietary guidelines for St. Lucia 22
dietary history, taking of 61
dietary intake, assessment of 61
assessing nutritional adequacy of food diaries 62–68
biomarkers for 71
for epidemiological data 68
food and drink diary 61, 62
food frequency questionnaire 61, 62
dietary modifications
for chronic medical conditions 245–247
effect of non-compliance with dietary treatment 247
feed and feeding regimen, selection 250
high-energy drinks, prescribable 248
individualised advice 245, 247
medical conditions requiring
Asperger's syndrome 251
attention deficit hyperactivity disorder (ADHD) 251
autistic spectrum disorders 251
cancer 251
coeliac disease 251–253
Crohn's disease 258–259
cystic fibrosis 253–254
diabetes 254–258
Down's syndrome 259–260
neurological disabilities 259–260
parenteral feeding for children with poor gut function 250
sip feeds 248
tube feeding 248–249, 248–250
dietary treatments
of constipation 179
of gastro-oesophageal reflux disease 180
diet(s)
balanced 17–18
omega 3 and omega 6 fats in 7
vegan 24–25
vegetarian *see* vegetarian diet
Down's syndrome, diet for 259–260
drinks/beverages 18
with meals or snacks 27
'no added sugar' 165
offered in childcare settings 188–189
recommended daily servings 20
as rewards, treats or for comfort 41
drug(s)
in gastro-oesophageal reflux disease 180
sugar-containing medicines 26

E
eating disorders 198
during adolescence 212–213
anorexia nervosa 198, 212
bigorexia 212
binge eating disorders 212
body dysmorphic disorder (BDD) 212
bulimia nervosa 212
female athlete triad 77, 213
fertility and 75–76, 77
muscle dysmorphia 212
during pregnancy 89
eating environment 38
Eatwell Guide 21
EBM *see* expressed breast milk
EEN *see* exclusive enteral nutrition
energy (and calories) 4–5
adequate intake 15
estimated average requirement 4
requirements for preschool children 161–163
energy intake 15
school-age children 196
enteral nutrition, preterms 150
ESPGHAN *see* European Society for Paediatric Gastroenterology, Hepatology and Nutrition
essential amino acids 5
essential fats 7
estimated average requirement (EAR) 13
for energy 4–5
European Food Safety Authority 84, 102
European Society for Paediatric Gastroenterology, Hepatology and Nutrition (ESPGHAN) 148–149, 150
evening meal 67
plans 28, 29
diabetic child 255, 256, 257
preschool children 167, 168, 169, 170
vegetarian 30
recording intake 65
example case 65
exclusion diets 226
exclusive enteral nutrition (EEN) 258
expressed breast milk (EBM) 109
extremely low birthweight babies 148

F
family meals 40–41
fasting tradition 35, 37
fat (body)
girls vs boys 56
preconception, excessive or low 75
fat (dietary lipid) 6–7
dietary requirements 15
as energy source 5
fat-soluble vitamins 8
feeding
assessments, in specialist clinics 184–185
breastfeeding *see* breastfeeding
formula *see* bottle (formula)-feeding
gastrostomy 249
infants 99–156
routes for preterms 149–51
self-feeding 38
sociocultural influences 42
feeding clinics, specialist 184–185
female athlete triad 77, 213
fertility 75–78
improving 76
and iron status 77
nutritional influences decreasing 76–77, 78
alcohol, smoking and drug misuse 77
body weight 76–77
eating disorders 77

extreme levels of exercise 77
poor iron stores 77
weight loss and undernutrition 77
nutritional status and 75
festivals
nursery celebrations 189
religious 35, 38
fibre 6
preschool children 162
primary school children 196
flour, folate fortification 82
fluid
constipation and intake of 140
requirements 116 *see also* water
fluoride 10
safe intakes 15
in toothpaste 25
folate/folic acid
children 13
preconception 76
pregnancy 81–82
supplementation 85
food allergy
additives 223
adrenaline auto-injectors for 221, *222*
appearance of symptoms 223
coeliac disease and 223
common allergenic foods in UK 220–221
diagnosis of 223–225
clinical tests 224
gold standard test 224
NICE guidelines 223–224
severity of symptoms 225
egg allergy 219–220
immunoglobulin E (IgE)-mediated 221
non IgE-mediated 222
peanut allergy 219–220
risk factors 221
food challenges 224–225
food choice/traditions 33
cultural food traditions 33–35
cultural variations in 38
feeding practices
cultural variations in 38
family, influence of 40–41, 42
festivals and 35, 38
food fashions and 39–40
infant feeding choices, socio-cultural influences on 42–43
in low-income families 36
marketing and media influences on 38–39
neophobia, preschool children 173–174
parenting skills, influence of 41–42
religion and 35, 37, 38
socio-economic factors, influence of 36–37
food fashions 39–40
negative impact on children 39–40
positive 39
food frequency questionnaires (FFQ) 62
food groups 17–18
daily meal plans 27–29
drinks 18, 20, 27
for lunchbox 190
nutritional adequacy, assessment of 29, 30, 62–68
pictorial guides for 18–24
in pregnancy, recommended daily intake 82
and recommended number of daily portions 19–21
food hypersensitivity 220–225
classification of 220
eating outside home, challenges 231
environmental factors 219
ezcema and 220
in infants 220
management of 225–228
adapting family foods 230–231
clinical 225–226
exclusion diets 226
foods to avoid 226–228
oral immunotherapy (OIT) 226
prevention strategies 220
food intolerance 220, 222–223
coeliac disease and 223
diagnosis of 223–225
food labels 228–230
'free-from' lists 230
food neophobia, in preschool children 173–174
food policy 189
food portion sizes
for children 4-10 years 197
for children 11-18 years 208
for preschool children 164
food(s)
to avoid during hypersensitivity/allergy 226–228
eggs 226
milk 226–228
peanuts 226
rice milk 228
sesame 226
soya and soya formula milk 227–228
tree nuts 226
wheat 228
beneficial components other than classical nutrients 11–13
phytochemicals 11–12
probiotics 12–13
for celebrations at nurseries 189
choice/selection/preferences/tastes
adolescents
sociocultural influences 33–43
colours and preservatives in 26
'free-from' 230
with high fibre content 179
offered in childcare settings 188–189
as rewards, treats or for comfort 41
food safety and hygiene
infants 133–134
pregnant women 89–90
preschool children 172–173
formula foods
role in early weight gain 235
formula milks, for preterm infants 154–155
hydrolysed preterm formula 154
nutrient-enriched post-discharge formula 154, 155
preterm formulas 154
'free-from' foods 230
free sugar(s) 6
and dental health 25
fizzy drinks and squashes with 165
intake
school-age children 196
fructose 5
fruits
preschool children 162
and diarrhoea 180
portion sizes 164

G

gastroenteritis, infants 139
gastro-oesophageal reflux disease (GORD) 139
in infants 138–139
in preschool children 180
thickening feeds for 143
gastrostomy feeding 249
blended diets for 249–250
gluten-free foods 251–253
food labelling regulations on 253
prescribable 253
glycaemic index 255
GORD *see* gastro-oesophageal reflux disease
growth
abnormal 56–58
assessment/measurement 49–58
anthropometric measurement 51
equipment for 53
growth charts 53–55
biological drivers of 49–50
energy requirements 4
faltering 198, 259
ARFID and 184
in infancy 56–57
in preschool children 57, 183–184
normal 55–56
prenatal 50
pubertal spurt 50, 51, 56

rates throughout childhood 50
growth (centile) charts 53–55
plotting on 54–55
preterm infants, classification and assessment 147–148
growth faltering in formula-fed babies 140

H
haem iron 10
healthy eating
pregnancy 81–82
Healthy Start scheme 37, 88, 118, 214
heartburn in pregnancy 93
height
abnormal 58
drivers of 50
following centiles in first 2 years 55
measurement 51, 52
infants, difficulties 52
without clothing 53
high-carbohydrate diet 214
Hindu traditions 37
histamine intolerance 222
hunger cues 126
hungry infant milk 113 *see also* infant formula
hyperemesis gravidarum 92
hypoglycaemia 255–258, 256–258
blood glucose levels 257
causes of 255–257
symptoms of 257
treatment 257–258

I
iMap Milk Ladder 228, 229
immunoglobulin E (IgE)-mediated food allergy 221
indulgent parenting style 41
infant(s)
faltering growth in 56–57
feeding 99–156
complementary *see* complementary feeding
milk *see* bottle (formula)-feeding, breastfeeding
routes for preterms 149–51
self-feeding 38
sociocultural influences 42
growth
charts 53
measurement recommendations 51–52
measuring weight of 51–52
nutritional requirements of 3
preterm *see* preterm infants
small-for-gestational-age, classification of 147–148
weight gain in 55
weight loss after birth 55
infertility
male 77–78
nutritional influences 78
ovulatory 76–77
insoluble fiber 6
intrauterine growth restriction babies 148
iodine 10
during pregnancy 84
reference nutrient intakes 14
iron
in breast milk
with preterms 152
deficiency
in preschool children 178
fertility and iron status 77
reference nutrient intakes 14
requirement during adolescence 207
iron-deficiency anemia 199
iron-rich foods, in pregnancy 83

J
jejunostomy feeding 249
Jewish traditions 37

K
kangaroo care 153
ketogenic diet 251

L
lactation
maintenance through expression of milk (for preterms) 152
lacto-ovo vegetarian 24
lactose 6
lactose-free formula 139
lactose intolerance 222
lacto-vegetarian 24
late and moderately preterm (LMPT) 147, 148 *see also* preterm infant
LBW *see* low birthweight
LMPT *see* late and moderately preterm
low birthweight (LBW) 147
lower reference nutrient intakes (LRNIs) 13
adolescents 207, 211
lunchbox *see* packed meals/lunches

M
macronutrients 5–7
carbohydrate 5–6
dietary requirements 13–15
fat 6–7
intakes
adolescents and teenagers 207, 210
school-age children 196
protein 5
magnesium 10–11
reference nutrient intakes 14
malabsorption of food 199, 248–249, 251, 253
male infertility 77–78
see also boys
malnutrition 247–248
in adolescents and teenagers 209–213
in school-age children 196–198
maltose 6
mastitis 106
meal and snack routine 27, 165–166
advantages of 42
meal plans
breakfast 28, 29
evening 28, 29
food groups 27–29
midday meal 28, 29
vegetarian diet 29, 30
mealtime routines 38
advantages of 42
for preschool children 165–166
men, infertility 77–78
menarche and nutritional status 77
micronutrients 7–11
dietary requirements 15
minerals 10–11
safe intakes for 15
vitamins 7–9 *see also* minerals; vitamin(s)
midday meal
plans 28, 29
diabetic child 255, 256, 257
preschool children 167, 168, 169, 170
vegetarian 30
recording intake 65
example case 65
mid upper arm circumference (MUAC) 51
milk feeding 3, 99 *see also* breastfeeding; infant formula
choice of 99–100
breastfeeding 99–100
infant formula 99–100
HIV-positive mothers and 100
Milk Subsidy Scheme 201
minerals 10–11
for preschool children 163
see also specific minerals
minimal enteral feeding 149–150
molybdenum, safe intakes 15
monosodium glutamate (MSG) 251

intolerance 223
monounsaturated fats 7
muscle dysmorphia 212
Muslim traditions 37
My Healthy Plate 22
MyPlate 22

N

nasogastric tube feeding 249
National Diet and Nutrition Survey (NDNS) 68, 196
National Institute for Health and Clinical Excellence recommendations
constipation 179
obesity
in pregnancy 87
parenteral nutrition 149
preconception body weight 76
pregnancy
alcohol 90
diabetes 87
obesity 86
vitamin D 83
National School Breakfast Programme 201
nausea in pregnancy 91–92
neglectful parenting style 41
Neonatal and Infant Close Monitoring Chart 147
neonatal unit, preterms in
discharge home 155
feeding routes 149–150
neonates/newborns
bottle-feeding 116
neural tube defects (NTDs)
and folate 82
in pregnancy, recommended daily intake 82
niacin 13
nipples, sore/cracked 105–106
non-haem iron 10
non IgE-mediated food allergy 222
nurseries
food for celebrations at 189
menu planning for 188
nutritional guidance for 189
see also childcare setting, feeding preschool children in
nutrient/nutritional intake
adolescents and teenagers 206–207
for chronic medical conditions 245, 246–247
options for improving 248
preconception stage 75–76
school-age children 196
support for children with inadequate appetite 247–248
nutrient(s) 5–11
adequate intake of 15
classification 5
macronutrients 5–7
micronutrients 7–11
in pregnancy, key 82–85
requirements for preschool children 161–163
nutritional intake and adequacy, assessment of 61–71
biochemical measures used for 71
computer software programmes 68
dietary history 61
for epidemiological data 68–71
by food groups 62–68
individual child's diet knowledge 61
nutritional problems, in preschool children
anaemia, iron-deficiency 178
avoidant restrictive food intake disorder 183
caries 177–178
constipation 179
diarrhoea 180
faltering growth 183–184
gastro-oesophageal reflux disease 180
obesity 179
selective eating behaviour 180–183
management of 182–183
specialist feeding clinics 184–185
vitamin D deficiency or rickets 185
nutritious puddings 27

O

obesity and overweight 76
child
preschool 179
rapid weight gain 58
as a form of malnutrition 196
portion sizes, effect of 196
preconception 76
pregnancy 76
obesity in children 234
assessment 234
definition 233–234
factors associated with 234–236
adiposity rebound 236
early infancy weight gain 235–236
genetic and epigenetic differences 235
medical causes 235
parental obesity 235
risk 235
health risks associated with 236
percentage classified as obese 234–235
prevention of
in children under 5 years 238–239
in children 5–18 years 239
good sleep 239
limiting sedentary behaviour 239
nurseries and childcare facilities, role of 239
nutrition education 237
physical activities 237–238
portion sizes 237
postnatal 236
prenatal 236
in preschool and primary school children 237
in secondary school children 237
treatment 239–242
change in dietary habits 240
drug therapy and bariatric surgery 242
lifestyle changes 242
parental intervention 240–242
reward system 242
self-monitoring 241–242
SMART goal setting 241
stimulus control foods and triggers 241
in UK 234
oily fish, in pregnancy 90
OIT *see* oral immunotherapy
omega 3 fats 7
in breast milk 7
importance of 7
in oily fish 84
from plant sources 24
during pregnancy 84, 89
supplements 84
vegetarian and vegan diets 88–89
omega 6 fats 7
oral feeding 153–154
bottle feeding 154
breastfeeding 153–154
oral immunotherapy (OIT) 226
orogastric tube feeding 149, 249
overweight in children
assessment 234
definition 233–234

P

packed lunches/meals 189–191
dips for breadsticks or vegetable sticks 191
ideas for 190
items include in 190
pudding or second course in 191
salads 191
sandwich fillings in 190
pantothenic acid, safe intakes 15
parenteral nutrition
preterms 149, 150
parenting styles 41
partial vegetarian 24
pescatarian 24
phosphorus 11
in breast milk with preterms 152
reference nutrient intakes 14
physical activity

energy requirement for 4
during pregnancy 86
phytochemicals 11–12
in cancer prevention 12
in cardiovascular disease prevention 12
phytoestrogen 113
polyunsaturated fats 7
portion sizes 21–22
adolescents and teenagers 208–209
obesity and 196
in obesity prevention 237
school-age children 196, 197–198
see also food portion sizes
posseting 138–139
potassium 11
reference nutrient intakes 14
preconception 75–78
body weight, optimal 76
diabetes control in diabetic women 76
nutritional advice 75–76
nutritional status and fetal growth 75
pre-existing medical conditions in pregnancy 87–89
pregnancy 81–93, 203, 214
allergy prevention during 91
common dietary problems 91–93
food safety 89–90
healthy eating 81–82
key nutrients 82–85
low vitamin D levels during, effects of 83
nutritional status of woman during, influence of 81
overweight/obese women and 86
poor nutrition during 81
promoting breastfeeding during 93
recommended daily intake during 82
supplements during 85
underweight women and 86
vitamin D *see also* vitamin D
weight gain during 86
preschool children
dental health 172
drinks 163, 165 *see also* drinks/beverages
faddy eating 173
feeding in childcare settings 160–191, 187–191
food groups with
combining 162–163
in packed lunches 189–191
food neophobia in 173–174
food refusal 173
reasons for 180–181
food safety 172–173
meal plans 166–170
for autumn 169
for spring 167
for summer 168
vegetarian diet 172
for winter 170
meal routines 165–166
mineral supplements 163
nutrient and calorie requirements, achieving 161–163
nutrients at risk 171
nutritional problems in 177–185
portion sizes 163
recommendations 164
selective eating 173
self-feeding 38
snacks
nutritious 170
routine for 165–166
specialist feeding clinics 184–185
vegetarian diet for 171–172
meal plans 172
vitamin supplements 163
preterm infants 147–155
age correction for measurements 55
benefits for 151
breastfeeding progression 153
breast milk for 151–153
classification of 147–148
complementary feeding 155
enteral nutrition 150
formula milks for 154–155
hydrolysed preterm formula 154
nutrient-enriched post-discharge formula 154, 155
preterm formulas 154
nasogastric tube 151
with nasogastric tube 151
nutritional requirements 148–149
oral feeding 153–154
parenteral nutrition 149
trophic feeds 149
principles of healthy eating 30
probiotics 12–13
proteins 5
in breast milk
with preterms 152
as energy source 5
essential amino acids in 5
function of 5
intakes
school-age children 196
UK Reference Nutrient Intakes for 12, 13
puberty, physiological changes during 50, 51

R

rapid growth 58
Rastafarian food traditions 37
raw shellfish, and food poisoning 91
Red Book (Personal Child Health Record) 54
reference nutrient intake (RNI) 13, 17
for minerals 14
sodium/salt 11
for protein 12, 13
for vitamins 13
vitamin D 9
Reference Nutrient Intakes (RNIs), adolescence
folate intakes 207
for iron 207
for vitamins 206
refrigerated or frozen breast milk
warming or thawing 116
re-introduction of food 228, 229–230
restricted diet 25
retinol *see* vitamin A
Reynaud's syndrome 106
riboflavin 13
rickets 9, 83, 118, 185
RNIs *see* Reference Nutrient Intakes (RNIs)

S

SACN *see* Scientific Advisory Committee on Nutrition
salicylate intolerance 222
saliva, and dental decay 178
salt 11, 26
excess use of 11
recommendations on intake of 11
saturated fat 6, 15, 26
saturated fat intake
school-age children 196
school-age children
average dietary intakes 196
dental caries in 198–199
energy and nutrient intakes 196
food tastes and preferences 195–196
parental influence 195
inappropriate dieting among 198
malnutrition 196–198
portion sizes 196, 197–198
risk of anemia in 199
underweight 198
vitamin D deficiency among 199
school food and drinks
breakfasts 201
fruits and vegetables 201
government funded schemes 201
milk and milk products 201–202
packed lunches 200–201
popular meals 200
nutritional improvements 200
standards and guidance 199–200
in England 199, 202
in Northern Ireland 200, 202
in Scotland 200, 202
in Wales 200, 202
Scientific Advisory Committee on Nutrition (SACN) 5, 13
recommendations RNIs of macronutrients 15
on salt/sodium intake 11

scurvy 8
selective eating behaviour, in preschool children 180–183
growth and dietary intake, assessment of 182
management of 182–183
mismanaging mealtimes and 181–182
parental anxiety and 181
selenium 11
reference nutrient intakes 14
self-feeding, by infants and toddlers 38
Sikh traditions 37
Singapore My Healthy Plate 18, 22
skin, vitamin D synthesis in 83
factors affecting 8–9
small for gestational age babies 148
snacks 27
daily eating plans 28, 29
routines
advantages of 42
for preschool children 165–166
for toddlers at nursery 188
sociocultural influences on food choice 33–43
sodium 11
reference nutrient intakes 14
soluble fibre 6
sorbitol 255
sore nipples 105–106
soya-based infant formula 113–115
specialist feeding clinics 184–185
spina bifida and folate 82
sports beverages 214
sports training, high energy requirements in 213–214
spring-time meals plan, for preschool children 167
standards, nutritional
pre-school childcare settings 188
primary school 199
starch 5
stimulus control, in obesity treatment 241
storage
breast milk 109
formula milk 115–116
sucrose 6
sugars 5–6
disaccharides 6
free sugars 6
monosaccharides 5
naturally occurring 6
in non-processed fruits/vegetables 6
summer-time meals plan, for preschool children 168
sunlight (UV) and vitamin D synthesis 83
sunscreens 9
sunshine vitamin *see* vitamin D
surgery
bariatric 240
gastro-oesophageal reflux disease 180
synthetic liquid diet 258

T
take-away meals, adolescents 207, 210
tap water, fluoride in 10
teenage pregnancy 87–88
ten-gram carbohydrate exchanges 255, 256
teratogenesis, retinol foods and 90
texture of complementary foods 126–127
4-6 months 127
6-9 months 127, 129
9-12 months 127, 131
Thailand, Nutrition Flag 22
thiamin 13
toddlers *see* preschool children
tooth brushing, in infancy 133
toothpaste, fluoride-containing 10
trace minerals, safe intakes 15
trans fats 6–7
trophic feeds, preterms 149–150
tube feeding 248–249
considerations when initiating 250
feeds available for 249
gastrostomy feeding 249
nasogastric 249
orogastric 249
support for home 250
24-hour recall 61
twins, breastfeeding 105

U
UK 90 reference data 53
UK-WHO growth charts 54
ultraviolet (UV) and sunlight and vitamin D synthesis 83
undernutrition
adolescents 206
preconception 77
pregnancy 81–82
underweight
preconception 77
pregnancy 86
primary school children 198
unsaturated fats 6, 7
urine collection, 24-hour 71

V
vegan diets 24–25
for preschool children 172
vegetarian diet 24–25
meals plans 29, 30
for preschool children 171–172
very low birthweight babies 148
vitamin A 8
children 13
vitamin and mineral intakes 253
school-age children 196
vitamin B 8
safe intakes 15
vitamin C 8, 199
children 13
vitamin D 8–9
children 13
deficiency
among school-age children 199
in preschool children 185
in pregnancy 83
vitamin E 9
vitamin K 9
vitamin(s) 7–9
in breast milk with preterms 152
fat-soluble 8
for preschool children 163
water-soluble 8

W
waist circumference centile charts 234
water 3–4
in infant milk feeds 3
with meals or snacks 27
see also dehydration; fluid
water-soluble vitamins 8
weight (woman)
preconception 75–77
loss 77
optimization 76
weight gain, in infancy 55
see also growth
weight loss, after birth 55
weight monitoring 57–58
winter-time meals plan, for preschool children 170
whey-dominant infant formula 110, 114
see also infant formula
women with diabetes, preconception guidelines for 76
World Health Organization (WHO)
Child Growth Standards 53
on iron-deficiency anaemia 178
Ten Steps to Successful Breastfeeding 100
on weaning 121

Z
zinc 11
reference nutrient intakes 14

For Product Safety Concerns and Information please contact our EU
representative GPSR@taylorandfrancis.com
Taylor & Francis Verlag GmbH, Kaufingerstraße 24, 80331 München, Germany

www.ingramcontent.com/pod-product-compliance
Ingram Content Group UK Ltd.
Pitfield, Milton Keynes, MK11 3LW, UK
UKHW052048230926
475702UK00025B/955

* 9 7 8 0 3 6 7 5 5 4 5 6 9 *